Stroke: Evidence-Based Management

Stroke: Evidence-Based Management

Editor: Vin Lopez

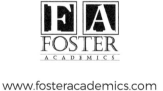

www.fosteracademics.com

www.fosteracademics.com

Cataloging-in-Publication Data

Stroke : evidence-based management / edited by Vin Lopez.
    p. cm.
Includes bibliographical references and index.
ISBN 978-1-63242-496-9
1. Cerebrovascular disease. 2. Ischemia. 3. Reperfusion injury. 4. Brain--Hemorrhage. I. Lopez, Vin.
RC388.5 .S77 2017
616.81--dc23

Foster Academics,
118-35 Queens Blvd., Suite 400,
Forest Hills, NY 11375, USA

ISBN 978-1-63242-496-9 (Hardback)

Printed and bound in the United States of America.

Contents

Preface

Strokes are a medical condition that can be characterized by the disruption of blood flow to the brain causing interference in brain function and mental capability. This book outlines the various risk factors of strokes which include, high blood pressure, diabetes mellitus, etc. It elaborately compiles the different diagnostic techniques that are used around the globe like CT scan, MRI, etc. This book contains some path-breaking studies in the field of stroke diagnosis and management. With state-of-the-art inputs by acclaimed experts of this field, this text targets students, professionals and medical professions working in this field. The extensive content of this book provides the readers with a thorough understanding of the subject.

After months of intensive research and writing, this book is the end result of all who devoted their time and efforts in the initiation and progress of this book. It will surely be a source of reference in enhancing the required knowledge of the new developments in the area. During the course of developing this book, certain measures such as accuracy, authenticity and research focused analytical studies were given preference in order to produce a comprehensive book in the area of study.

This book would not have been possible without the efforts of the authors and the publisher. I extend my sincere thanks to them. Secondly, I express my gratitude to my family and well-wishers. And most importantly, I thank my students for constantly expressing their willingness and curiosity in enhancing their knowledge in the field, which encourages me to take up further research projects for the advancement of the area.

Editor

Long-Term Survival of Human Neural Stem Cells in the Ischemic Rat Brain upon Transient Immunosuppression

Laura Rota Nodari[1], Daniela Ferrari[1], Fabrizio Giani[1], Mario Bossi[2], Virginia Rodriguez-Menendez[2], Giovanni Tredici[2], Domenico Delia[3], Angelo Luigi Vescovi[1,4]*, Lidia De Filippis[1]*

1 Department of Biotechnologies and Biosciences, University Milano Bicocca, Milan, Italy, **2** Department of Neurosciences and Biomedical Technologies, University Milano Bicocca, Milan, Italy, **3** Department of Experimental Oncology, Fondazione IRCSS Istituto Nazionale Tumori, Milan, Italy, **4** IRCCS Casa Sollievo della Sofferenza, Opera di San Pio da Pietralcina, San Giovanni Rotondo, Italy

Abstract

Understanding the physiology of human neural stem cells (hNSCs) in the context of cell therapy for neurodegenerative disorders is of paramount importance, yet large-scale studies are hampered by the slow-expansion rate of these cells. To overcome this issue, we previously established immortal, non-transformed, telencephalic-diencephalic hNSCs (IhNSCs) from the fetal brain. Here, we investigated the fate of these IhNSC's immediate progeny (i.e. neural progenitors; IhNSC-Ps) upon unilateral implantation into the corpus callosum or the hippocampal fissure of adult rat brain, 3 days after global ischemic injury. One month after grafting, approximately one fifth of the IhNSC-Ps had survived and migrated through the corpus callosum, into the cortex or throughout the dentate gyrus of the hippocampus. By the fourth month, they had reached the ipsilateral subventricular zone, CA1-3 hippocampal layers and the controlateral hemisphere. Notably, these results could be accomplished using transient immunosuppression, i.e administering cyclosporine for 15 days following the ischemic event. Furthermore, a concomitant reduction of reactive microglia (Iba1+ cells) and of glial, GFAP+ cells was also observed in the ipsilateral hemisphere as compared to the controlateral one. IhNSC-Ps were not tumorigenic and, upon in vivo engraftment, underwent differentiation into GFAP+ astrocytes, and β-tubulinIII+ or MAP2+ neurons, which displayed GABAergic and GLUTAmatergic markers. Electron microscopy analysis pointed to the formation of mature synaptic contacts between host and donor-derived neurons, showing the full maturation of the IhNSC-P-derived neurons and their likely functional integration into the host tissue. Thus, IhNSC-Ps possess long-term survival and engraftment capacity upon transplantation into the globally injured ischemic brain, into which they can integrate and mature into neurons, even under mild, transient immunosuppressive conditions. Most notably, transplanted IhNSC-P can significantly dampen the inflammatory response in the lesioned host brain. This work further supports hNSCs as a reliable and safe source of cells for transplantation therapy in neurodegenerative disorders.

Editor: Colin Combs, University of North Dakota, United States of America

Funding: This work was supported by CARIPLO Foundation; Neurothon ONLUS Foundation; Italian Association for Cancer Research (AIRC); Italian Ministry of Health Ricerca Finalizzata. The funders had no role in study design, data collection and analysis, decision to publish, or preparation of the manuscript.

Competing Interests: The authors have declared that no competing interests exist.

* E-mail: lidia.defilippis@unimib.it (LDF); angelo.vescovi@unimib.it (ALV)

Introduction

The isolation of multipotent neural stem cells (NSCs) from the human central nervous system (CNS) has spurred the investigation of new cell-therapy approaches for brain injuries and neurodegenerative diseases. NSCs, which reside in specialized regions of the adult CNS, in particular in the subventricular zone (SVZ) [1–3] and the dentate gyrus of the hippocampus (DG), possess life-long self-renewal and the ability to generate neurons, astrocytes and oligodendrocytes. Although NSCs play a central role in CNS development and cellular homeostasis throughout adulthood [2,4,5], limited spontaneous recovery is known to occur following brain damage [6,7]. Nonetheless, the integration of functional new neurons following injury can be achieved by the mobilization of endogenous stem cells [8,9] or by transplanting new cells from different sources, as shown in experimental models of ischemia [10–12].

Also owing to the resilience of hNSCs (human neural stem cells) to expansion ex vivo, a relatively limited number of studies has investigated the use of hNSCs for the experimental treatment of cerebral ischemia [13]. An initial solution to this issue has come from the establishment of non-transformed, v-myc immortalized hNSCs, to give rise to stable cell lines (IhNSCs) [14], that can be rapidly expanded in vitro and retains the features of parental NSCs, such as proliferation, self-renewal, functional stability and multipotency.

In this paper, we demonstrate that the IhNSC's immediate progeny, represented by neural progenitors undergoing early differentiation phases (IhNSC-Ps) exhibit widespread integration ability and long-term survival when transplanted into the brain of adult rats lesioned by transient global ischemia. IhNSC-Ps generated both glial cells and mature neurons, both in the cortex and the corpus callosum. We also found that IhNSC-P-derived neuronal cells were able to establish heterotypic synaptic junctions with the host tissue after 4 months from transplantation.

Although several studies have reported a weak host' immunogenic response against transplanted hNSCs and their progeny in the brain, this issue has never been unraveled [15–18]. Thus, we investigated the immunogenic response of our immortal hNSCs' progeny and were able to show that grafted IhNSC-Ps have the ability to integrate in the post-ischemic, inflammatory environment that develops in the brain after injury, also dampening the local inflammatory reaction at the integration sites. All of the above was accomplished even using transient immunosuppression.

Materials and Methods

Transient Global Ischemia

All animal experimental protocols were approved by the Ethics Review Committee for Animal Experimentation of the Italian Ministry of Health (protocol number 37/2007-B). Adult male Sprague-Dawley rats (350–400 gr) were anesthetized with ketamine (60 mg/Kg) and Xylazine (10 mg/Kg). The common carotid arteries were exposed bilaterally by means of a ventral midline incision and occluded with microvascular clips for 10 minutes. The body temperature of the rats was mantained at $37°\pm0.5°C$ by a heating pad provided with a rectal probe. All physiological parameters were monitored and recorded throughout the surgery with BIOPAC Data Acquisition System. During the 10 minutes of carotid occlusion, mean blood pressure was maintained at 50 mmHg by withdrawal of blood from the femoral artery previously exsposed and incannulated with PE50 tubing connected to a BIOPAC system and to a collector. After the removal of the clips from the carotid arteries, the blood was reinjected into the femoral artery. After the surgery, the rats were daily treated with subcutaneous injections of antibiotics (Enrofloxacin 10–15 mg/Kg) and painkillers (Carprofen 5 mg/Kg) for one week.

Cell Preparation

To generate IhNSC-Ps for transplantation, IhNSC neurospheres, cultured as described in De Filippis et al. 2007, were mechanically dissociated and transferred onto laminin (Roche, Base, Switzerland, http://www.roche-applied-science.com)- coated tissue culture flasks (or glass coverslips for immunostaining assays) at a density of 1×10^4 cells per cm^2 in the presence of FGF2 (20 ng/ml) for 3 days. The day of transplant IhNSC-Ps were collected with VERSENE (Gibco, Aukland, NZ) and transferred into control medium ad the density of 1×10^5 cells/µL.

Characterization was performed by immunostaining assays with primary antibodies β-TubulinIII (β-Tub, TUJ-1, 1:400, Covance), Galactocerebroside C (GalC, 1:100, Chemicon), Glial fibrillary acidic protein (GFAP, 1:500, Chemicon), Green Fluorescent Protein (GFP, 1:500, Sigma), Microtubule-associated protein 2 (MAP2, 1:200, Sigma), Doublecortin (DCX, 1:200, Santa Cruz) and Neural Cell Adhesion Molecule (NCAM, 1:100, Santa Cruz).

Transduction of IhNSC with lenti-gfp

Transduction of IhNSC with a lentiviral vector carrying the gfp gene was carried as described in [19,20] and the percentage of GFP+ IhNSC reached 95%. After 4 passages they were used for transplantation.

Cell Transplantation

Experimental design (Figure S3) included the following animal groups: healthy control animals (n = 4), healthy control animals transplanted with IhNSC-Ps in the corpus callosum (n = 2/each time point), healthy control animals transplanted with IhNSC-Ps in the hippocampal fissure (n = 2/each time point) and lesioned animals transplanted with IhNSC-Ps (n = 2/each time point) and GFP+ IhNSC-Ps cells (n = 3/each time point) [19] in the corpus callosum (n = 5 tot/each time point) or in the hippocampal fissure

(n = 5 tot/each time point). The four groups of transplanted animals were transiently immunosuppressed with cyclosporine (see below) and sacrificed at 7 days, 2 weeks, 1 month, 3 and 4 months from transplantation and analyzed in parallel with healthy controls.

In the paralel a set of lesioned animals was transplanted with GFP+ IhNSC-Ps in the periventricular region next to cc (n = 3 each time point) or in the hippocampal fissure (n = 3 each time point), constitutively immunosuppressed and sacrificed 1, 3 and 4 months later.

Rats were anesthetized with an intraperitoneal injection of ketamine (60 mg/Kg) and Xylazine (10 mg/Kg), placed in a sterotactic frame (David Kopf Instruments, Tujunga, CA) and injected with 2 µL of cell suspension (1×10^5 cells/µL control medium) using a Hamilton syringe to the hippocampal fissure (anteroposterior: −5.3; lateral: +3.0; dorsoventral: −3.0) or to the posterior periventricular region in the cc (anteroposterior: −5.3; lateral, +3; dorsoventral: −2). All animals were immunosoppressed with Cyclosporine A (15 mg/Kg; Sandimmun, Novartis) administered subcutaneously starting 2 days before transplantation and for the duration of the study or for 14 days for transient immunosuppression experiments.

Tissue Processing and Immunohistochemistry

Rats were anesethized with an intraperitoneal injection of Avertin (300 mg/Kg) and transcardially perfused-fixed with 4% paraformaldehyde. Brains were fixed overnight in 4% paraformaldeyde at 4°C, then sequentially transferred in 10%, 20% and 30% sucrose solutions. Brains were then cryopreserved (Killik, Bio-Optica, Italy), frozen and stored at −80°C. Coronal sections (18 µm thick) were obtained using a cryostat, transferred onto Super Frost/Plus object glasses (Menzel-Glaser, Braunschweig, Germany) and stored at −20°C. Sections were let dry at room temperature for 1 hour, rehydrated in phosfate-buffered saline and blocked with phosphate-buffered saline containing 10% Normal Goat Serum and 0,3% Triton X-100 for 90 minutes at room temperature. The following primary antibodies and dilutions were used: Human Specific Nuclei (HuN, 1:100, Chemicon), β-TubulinIII (TUJ-1, 1:400, Covance), Gamma-aminobutyric acid (GABA, 1:500, Sigma), Glial fibrillary acidic protein (GFAP, 1:500, Chemicon), Green Fluorescent Protein (GFP, 1:500, Sigma), Glutamate (GLUTA, 1:500, Sigma), Microtubule-associated protein 2 (MAP2, 1:200, Sigma), Doublecortin (DCX, 1:200, Santa Cruz), Neural Cell Adhesion Molecule (NCAM, 1:100, Santa Cruz), human specific Ki67 (Ki67, 1:200, Novocastra), Iba1 (1:100, Wako). The fluorescent secondary antibodies used were labelled with Cy3 (1:800, Jackson), Cy2 (1:200, Jackson), Alexa Fluor 546 and 488 (1:800, Molecular Probes). DAPI (ROCHE) was used as nuclear marker. Immunofluorescence-labeled sections were viewed under a fluorescence microscope (Zeiss Axioplan 2 imaging) and a confocal microscope (Leica Dmire2).

Quantification of cell death in the CA1 layer, survival of transplanted cells and micro/astroglial cells

The percentage of dying cells was assessed by counting the pyknotic nuclei over total nuclei into the CA1 layer of lesioned and healthy control animals in serial brain sections (each 200 µm) as described below (n = 3 rats/time point).

At different time points, the rate of survival of IhNSC-Ps was evaluated by counting GFP+ or HuN+ cells in serial brain sections (each 200 µm apart) spanning the graft area of n = 3 rats per time point. The total number of surviving transplanted cells was calculated for the whole graft using Abercrombie formula [21]. Data is presented as the percentage of surviving cells over total transplanted cells (200.000), calculated as the mean average among the animals of each experimental group.

The percentage of Iba1+ or GFAP+ cells was counted by sampling three field in the hippocampal region of healthy or lesioned rats at 3, 7, 14 and 30DAI.

For all the quantifications an average number of 3 sections was counted per rat spanning about 500 μm along the antero-posterior axis.

Statistical analysis was performed by one-way ANOVA. Data is reported as means±SEM. (*P<0.05. **P<0.01, ***P<0.001).

GFP immunolabeling and electron microscopy

Animals were perfused with 4% paraformaldehyde in phosphate buffer (0.12 M, pH 7.4). Brain samples were then cut using a vibratome (section thickness 30–40 μm). Free-floating brain slices were washed in Tris-buffered saline (TBS) and pre-incubated in 3% goat normal serum (NGS) in TBS for 30 min. Cells were also fixed with 4% formaldehyde and rinsed in TBS. Sections and cells were subsequently incubated with a rabbit anti-GFP antibody (1:250 for brain slices, 1:650 for cell cultures; Chemicon International) overnight at 4°C in 1% NGS/TBS. A secondary antibody (goat anti-rabbit HRP-labeled, 1:250 dilution; PerkinElmer, Boston, MA) was used for 1 h at room temperature before developing the immunoreactive signal determined by the reaction of 3,3'-diaminobenzidine tetrahydrochloride (DAB; Sigma, St. Louis, MO) with H_2O_2.

Immunolabeled samples were post-fixed in 1% OsO_4 in cacodylate buffer (0.12 M, pH 7.4) for 45 60 min, dehydrated and embedded in Epoxy resin. Ultramicrotome (Ultracut E, Reichert-Jung) 60 nm sections (both rat hippocampus and cultured cells) were then examined by a Philips CM 10 transmission electron microscope. Images were taken with a Mega View II digital camera (Soft Imaging System).

Results

We have previously shown that IhNSC transplantated into the immunodficient SCID mice brain can survive for as long as 6 months [14]. Nonetheless, pre-clinical and, most important, clinical neural transplantation are based on the concept that continuous immunosuppressive treatments are to be used to avoid donor cell rejection [18]. In addition, the possibility that the stroke heavy inflammatory environment (see Fig. 1) might enhance cell rejection compounds the problem further. In this view, we performed experiments in which animals transplanted with GFP-expressing IhNSC-Ps were treated with cyclosporine, either continuously (starting on the first day after ischemia (DAI 1) till the end of the experiment) or only transiently, i.e. for only two weeks, starting on DAI 1 and finishing on DAI 14. Tissues were analyzed 1, 3 and 4 months after implantation. Much to our surprise, no significant differences in the survival or integration were detected in transiently immunosuppressed animals (56.7%; n = 17/30) as compared to those receiving cyclosporine for the whole duration of the experiments (66.7%; n = 10/15). In considering that the two types of immunosuppressive protocols yielded overlapping results, the data presented below refer to milder one, i.e the transient administration of cyclosporine administered in the peri-transplantation period (two days before cell injection, all the way to 12 days after the latter took place).

Evaluation of the ischemic lesion

The lesion generated by transient global ischemia in the central nervous system is widespread and involves most brain districts. Notwithstanding, cortical areas and the CA1 layer of the hippocampus (Figure S1A–C) are known to be the most affected by this type of injury [22,23]. In this view, in order to assess the ability of I-hNSC-P to integrate following ischemic brain tissue damage, we focused our study on the hippocampal region and standardized our investigation by quantifying the fraction of pyknotic nuclei in the CA1 layer, as detected by hematoxilin-eosin staining (Fig. 1A and B and Figure S1C). Therein, the fraction of dead cells amounted to approximately 75% of the total CA1 cells at 3 and 14 DAI, with their number progressively decreasing to 60% at 90 DAI, as compared to the physiological 25% fraction in control animals (Fig. 1C and Figure S1F). Given the inflammatory nature of this kind of ischemic injury, we also investigated the activation of microglia and astroglia during the subacute phase of the lesion, that is at 3 days (Figure S1D–F) and 1 week from ischemia: no significative changes in the inflammatory environment were detected between these two time points. In the lesioned brain, Iba1+ cells presenting an ameboid morphology, typical of reactive, macrophagic microglia (Fig. 1D and E) – in sharp contrast with the star-shaped resting microglia found in the non-lesioned brain (Fig. 1F) – were dramatically increased both in the CA1 layer and in the hilus of the dentate gyrus (Fig. 1G) as compared to control animals (Fig. 1H). This was consistent with the data concerning the analysis of reactive gliosis by GFAP immunostaining, showing a striking alteration of astrocyte morphology (Fig. 1I) characterized by thicker and shorter processes in the lesioned brain as compared the healthy controls (Fig. 1L).

IhNSC-Ps efficiently survive after transplantation into the ischemic rat brain

In order to contribute to the neural regeneration in the early phases following tissue damage, IhNSC-Ps cells were transplanted nearby the CA1 layer soon after lesioning. Previous results with various transplantation paradigms in several animal models have shown that transplantation of undifferentiated NSCs cells from neurospheres generate mainly glial progenitors upon engraftment [20,24] or remain undifferentiated in vivo [25,26]. Hence, we decided to commit the IhNSCs' progeny in vitro, prior to implantation. To do this, we pre-differentiated IhNSCs for 3 days in the presence of FGF2 in order to induce early neuronal progenitors' proliferation and to favour their fate choice towards the neuronal lineage [27,28]. By this, the IhNSC-Ps used for transplantation contained cells of the neuronal lineage, that expressed both the early markers Dcx and NCAM (21.97±4.21% and 21.11±4.5%, of the total differentiated cells, respectively; Figure S2A, B and F), and the late markers β-Tub (13.37±2.71%, Figure S2C and F) and MAP2 (6.12±4.1%, Figure S2D and F), as well as astroglial GFAP+ (15.91±3.91% Figure S2C and F) and oligodendroglial GalC+ (8.6±2.65%, Figure S2E and F) cells. This was quite different from IhNSC cultured in the presence of EGF and FGF2 (neurospheres) which, in turn, contained only sporadic β-Tub+ cells and low percentages of MAP2+ (3.57±1.75%) and GalC+ (5.25±0.77%) cells. As expected for a population intended to contain early transient dividing progenitors, most IhNSC-Ps were actively proliferating, with 71.1±6.6% (Figure S2F) being positive for Ki67 (Figure S2A, B and D), as compared to 46.4±3.5% in undifferentiated IhNSC.

The IhNSC-Ps were injected into the posterior periventricular region, next to the corpus callosum or in the hippocampal fissure of rats at 3 DAI (Figure S3). Integrated surviving cells were detected in approximately 60.6% (n = 37/61) of the transplanted, injured animals, as compared to 25% (n = 7/28) in the control animals (not lesioned) receiving the same cells. This is in agreement with previous findings showing that the presence of

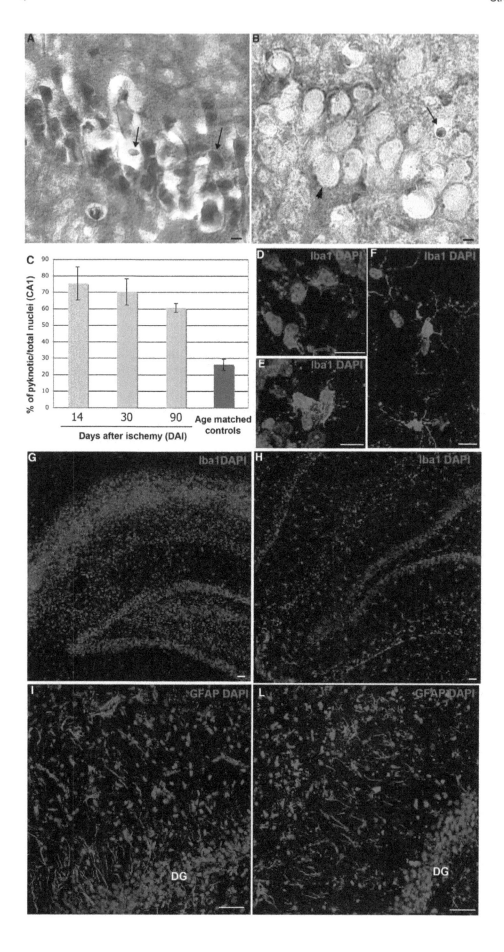

Figure 1. Neuronal loss and inflammation in the ischemic hippocampus. (A–B) Damaged cells at 14DAI (pyknotic nuclei, arrows) versus normal CA1 cells (B arrowhead). (C) Quantification of damaged cells in control and lesioned animals. (D–F) Iba1+ microglial cells with ameboid (lesioned hippocampus D–E) or stellate (control F) morphology. (G–H) Increase of microglia (Iba1+ cells) in the lesioned hippocampus (G, 7DAI) with respect to control (H). (I–L) Morphology of astroglial cells in the lesioned hippocampus (I, 7DAI) and control (L). Scale bars: A, B: 5 μm, D, E and F: 10 μm, G, H, I and L: 50 μm.

CNS injury is required to favor engraftment of exogenous cells in the adult brain tissue [29]. In the injured animals where engraftment was successful, the average survival rate of IhNSC-Ps was 19.5±1,4% of the total transplanted cells and remained unchanged for over 4 months. Fourteen days after transplantation into the posterior periventricular region, donor cells were found to be located close to the injection site (n = 4), (Fig. 2A). By 30 DAI, IhNSC-Ps migrated medially and laterally, along the myelin fibers of the corpus callosum and clusters of donor cells displayed long neuronal-like processes, which were directed towards the corpus callosum, with some of the cells migrating to the upper cortical layer (n = 3) (Fig. 2B and C', C").

At 14 DAI, IhNSC-Ps injected into the hippocampus were found to integrate into the DG (n = 3) (Fig. 2D) and in the subgranular zone (SGZ) (n = 3) (Fig. 2E and F), crossing the hilus and reaching the lower SGZ by 30 DAI. A subset of IhNSC-Ps presented a stem cell-like morphology [30,31], with the cell body nested in the SGZ and tangential processes extending along the border of the granule cell layer and hilus (Fig. 2F, arrow). No IhNSC-P cells were detected in the contralateral hemisphere at 2 and 4 weeks after transplantation. In control (unlesioned) animals, IhNSC-Ps were confined to the injection site (data not shown). The colocalization of GFP with the human specific antigen HuN (Fig. 2F inset) confirmed the identity of these cells as donor cells.

This analysis demonstrates that IhNSCs efficiently survive in vivo and that their engraftment and migration capacities are improved in a lesioned brain, which is consistent with previous results showing that injury generates a local environment permissive for the integration of xenotransplanted cells [17,29,32].

IhNSC-Ps give rise to neuronal cells in vivo

Next, we evaluated the differentiation of IhNSC-Ps into specific neuronal and glial phenotypes following transplantation into the ischemic environment by analyzing the colocalization of selective markers for neurons, astroglial and oligodendroglial cells with the anti-human specific antibody anti-huN. This was carried out on IhNSC-Ps that were not tagged with GFP, in order to rule out possible effects on their differentiation properties, as consequence of viral transduction with the GFP expression construct.

At one and three months post transplantation, IhNSC-Ps migrating through the corpus callosum and localizing into the DG were found to be relatively immature neuronal cells, expressing NCAM protein (corpus callosum, Fig. 3A) or Dcx (dentate gyrus, Fig. 3B). A subset of HuN+ cells had further matured into neuronal cells expressing β-Tub+ ($11.3 \pm 0.8\%$ over total HuN+ cells) (Fig. 3C) and MAP2+ (marker of dendritic neuronal processes), found in sporadic cell clusters or as isolated elements (Fig. 3D) within the corpus callosum and cortex. Such clusters seemed to have arisen through the in vivo, transient proliferation of single donor cells, as supported by the sporadic expression of Ki67 observed in HuN+ cells (Fig. 3E and inset). This would be in agreement with recent data reporting that ischemic injury

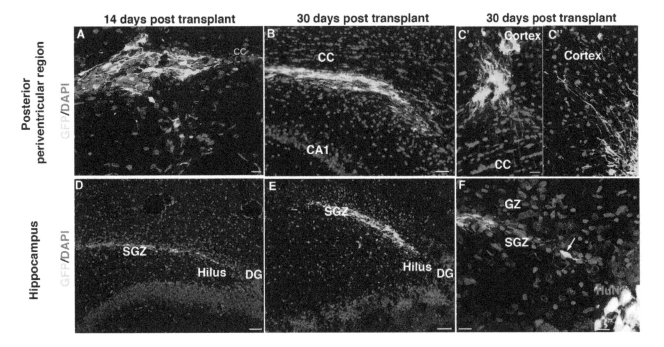

Figure 2. GFP-IhNSC-Ps survive in the ischemic brain. (A–C") IhNSC-Ps into the cc at 14 (A) and 30 (B) days post transplant. Long processes from donor cells directed toward the cc (C') and the upper cortical layer (C"). (D–F) Distribution of IhNSC-Ps along the SGZ at 14 days (D) and migrating to the lower SGZ at 30 days (E). Single GFP-IhNSC-Ps with tipical stem cell phenotype in the SGZ (F, arrow). Confocal analysis of colocalization of HuN with GFP (inset in F). cc: corpus callosum, GZ: granular zone, SGZ: subgranular zone, DG: dentate gyrus. Scale bars: A, F, F inset: 10 μm, C' and C": 20 μm, B, D, E: 50 μm.

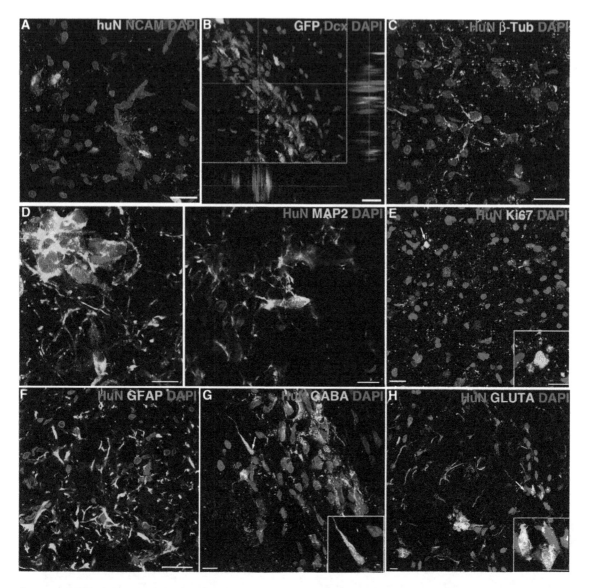

Figure 3. Differentiation of transplanted IhNSC-Ps in vivo. (A–F) IhNSC-Ps at 3 months post transplantation differentiate into both NCAM+HuN+ (A, cc) and Dcx+/GFP+ (B, dentate gyrus) neuronal progenitors and β-Tub+HuN+ (C) and MAP2+HuN+ (D) mature neurons in the cortex. (E) Sporadic proliferating cells (Ki67+HuN+, arrow and inset magnification). (F) GFAP+HuN+ astroglial cells in the cortex. (G–H) IhNSC-Ps at 1 month from transplantation generate GABAergic (GABA+HuN+, arrow in G and inset magnification) and Glutamatergic neurons (GLUTA+HuN+, arrow in H and magnification). Scale bars: A, B, C, E, F: 20 μm, D, inset in E, G, H, inset in H: 10 μm, inset in G: 5 μm.

generates in the cortex an environment favoring the proliferation of local precursors [33]. We also observed IhNSC-P-derived, stellate GFAP+/HuN+ astrocytes (29.7±3.03% over total HuN+ cells) amongst the engrafted, surviving cells (Fig. 3F), but failed in detecting oligodendroglial cells.

Altogether, the results above show that IhNSC-Ps can differentiate towards the neuronal and astroglial lineages in the ischemic brain. Both immature migratory neuroblasts and more mature β-Tub+ and MAP2+ neuronal cells are produced throughout this process.

Neuronal subtypes derived from grafted IhNSC-Ps

We have previously shown that IhNSCs [14] can differentiate in vitro into GABAergic and Glutamatergic neurons, similar to their wild-type counterpart [34]. Therefore, we analyzed the expression of such neurotransmitters among the IhNSC-Ps' progeny that successfully engrafted in our model. We found both cells exhibiting

the GABAergic (Fig. 3G and inset) and glutamatergic (Fig. 3H and inset) phenotypes in the corpus callosum and cortex, as early as 1 month after transplantation, which were still detectable 4 months from transplantation. These findings show, for the first time, that IhNSCs progeny can engraft in the adult brain as mature neuronal cells expressing the GABAergic or the glutamatergic phenotypes.

Long-term survival of IhNSC-Ps

At the later time tested, i.e. 4 months (Fig. 4A, n = 3) the presence of IhNSC-P-derived cells was obvious in the corpus callosum, wherein they migrated tangentially (4.3±0.6 mm medially and 4.5±0.45 mm laterally, n = 3, Fig. 4B and C), also spreading into the controlateral hemisphere (Fig. 4B). GFP+ cells were also detected along the injection tract in the hippocampal fissure, along the SGZ of the dentate gyrus (n = 4) (average distance of migration 400 μm medially and 380 μm laterally to the injection site up to the

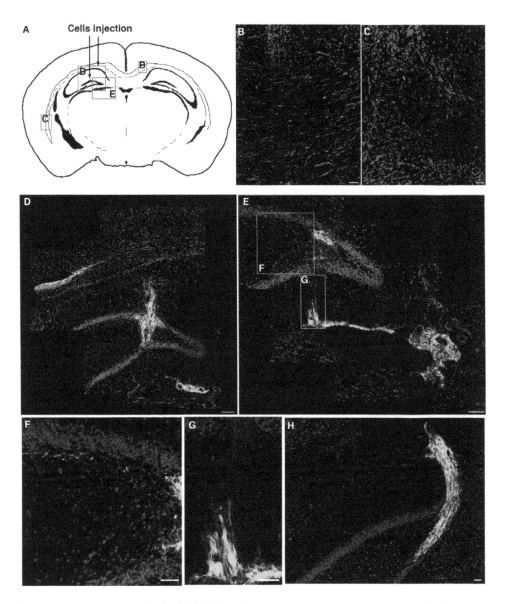

Figure 4. Long-term survival of IhNSC-Ps after transient immunosuppression. (A) Map of the brain areas colonized by IhNSC-Ps in transiently immunosuppressed ischemic rats 4 months following transplantation. Letters in boxed area refer to the figures B–E. IhNSC-Ps migrate extensively through the cc (B–C) and along the dentate gyrus (D, E and H) to the underling SVZ (D, E). F and G magnifications of boxed areas in E. Scale bars: B,C,E,F,G and H: 50 μm; D: 100 μm.

SVZ, wherein they migrated 1.2±0.53 mm (n = 3) medially along the ventricles (Fig. 4D–H). These results support the concept that, immunologically, transplanted human cells are well tolerated by the adult brain and that even a quite mild immunosuppression, like the transient one used here, may be sufficient to accomplish their efficient integration in the lesioned CNS tissue.

Migration of IhNSC-Ps' progeny and long-term integration into the CA1 layer

The CA1 layer of the hippocampus is one of the areas most prominently damaged in transient global ischemia. In addition, neurons newly generated by adult neurogenesis in the CA1 pyramidal layer also die, due to the persistence of inflammatory conditions [35]. Consistently with these findings, we were unable to detect IhNSC-Ps in the CA1 pyramidal layer at 1, 2 or 3 months after transplantation. At 4 months after ischemia, we found that some IhNSC-Ps did integrate along the CA3 layer (n = 2), sending processes toward the CA1 layer (Fig. 5A–D) and migrating to the underlying SVZ (Fig. 5C). Unexpectedly, IhNSC-Ps were also found as irregular clusters, distributed along the CA1 layer (n = 4), with their nuclei organized according to the classic multilayer pattern of the CA1 layer (Fig. 5E). These observations show that, despite the persistence of inflammation in this region [35], IhNSC-Ps retain the ability to interact with the to host endogenous neurogenic pathways, suggesting that they can undertake appropriate differentiation and contribute to the local regeneration of the damaged hippocampal tissue.

IhNSC-P derived neurons establish synaptic junctions in vivo

Since neither electrophysiological recordings on adult rat brain slices nor high resolution immunofluorescence analysis

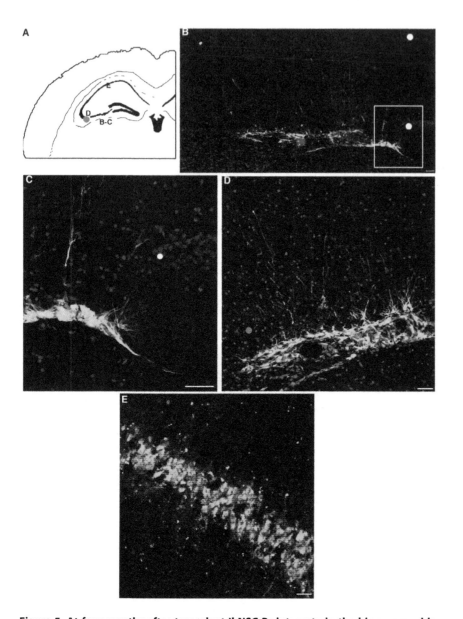

Figure 5. At four months after transplant IhNSC-Ps integrate in the hippocampal layers under transient immunosuppression. (A) Schematic map of the hyppocampal layers colonized by IhNSC-Ps in transiently immunosuppressed ischemic rats. The letters are positioned next to the regions referred to the figures B–E. (B–D) At 4 months following transplantation IhNSC-Ps were found integrated into the CA3 layer and in the underling SVZ (B), emitting long processes toward the dentate gyrus (boxed area in B, shown at higher magnification in (C) and CA1 layer (B–D). (E) At this time IhNSC-Ps were also found distributed along the CA1 layer. Scale bars: in B–D: 50 μm, in E: 30 μm.

could be performed because of the ischemia-induced decay of tissue cytoarchitecture, we assessed the ultrastuctural features of GFP-expressing IhNSC-Ps progeny located in the CA1 layer, 4 months after transplantation (Fig. 5E). In the hippocampus, GFP immunoreactivity was present within IhNSC-P-derived cell processes, mainly distributed along the cytoskeleton. Despite the disorganization of the ischemic tissue, we observed reci-pient axons (GFP-negative, a in Fig. 6A-C), possibly pyramidal neurons in the CA1 layer of the hippocampus, making synaptic contacts with the GFP-labeled processes (d in Fig. 6A-C). GFP-labeled myelinated axons were also detected (Fig. 6D and E). This was similar to the GFP-labeling pattern observed in cultured IhNSC-Ps, which was associated with microtubular structures (Fig. 6G) and could not be oserved in the non-transduced control cells (Fig. 6F).

This supports the notion that surviving IhNSC-Ps progeny have the ability to integrate into the lesioned CA1 area, therein establishing heterotypic synaptic junctions with host cells.

IhNSC-Ps can modulate the inflammatory response in the post-ischemic hippocampus

NSCs can act as immunomodulators in pathological, inflam-matory brain environments [20,26,36–38]. We have analyzed both the quantitative reduction and morphological changes in reactive microglial Iba1+ cells and GFAP+ astrocytes, in post-ischemic hippocampal area after IhNSC-Ps transplantation. As shown in Fig. 7A, B, 1 week after transplantation, the inflammatory reaction was significantly reduced in the transplant-ed hemisphere as compared to the controlateral one (Fig. 7C, D), which displayed an inflammation pattern comparable to that

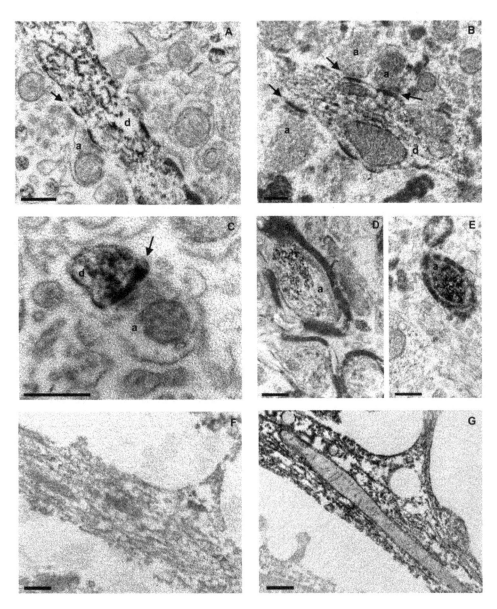

Figure 6. IhNSC-Ps form synapses into the rat hippocampus. Representative electron micrographs of rat hippocampus (A–E) and IhNSC-Ps differentiated *in vitro* (F–G), immunostained for GFP. (A–C) GFP immunopositive dendrites (d) on which unstained axons (a) project, making synaptic contacts (arrows). (D, E) GFP immunopositive myelinated axons (a). (F) Sham transfected IhNSC-Ps in culture. (G) GFP expressing IhNSC-Ps in culture. To note, GFP is mainly associated to microtubular structures. Scale bars: 500 nm.

observed earlier on, i.e. at 3DAI (Figure S1D–F). Indeed the fraction of Iba1+ cells in the ipsilateral emisphere amounted to 9.45±3.06% of total cells in the area as compared to 14,71±3.23% in the controlateral one (n = 3). Similarly GFAP+ cells in the ipsilateral side were 8.63±1.07% of the total cells, much less than the 13.13±2.69% detected controlaterally. This difference was even more striking at a later time, i.e. at 14 DAI (Fig. 7E and F), when the inflammatory reaction induced by the lesion is known to reach its peak: the fractions of Iba1+ cells were 10.57±2.64% and 29.36±7.8% and those of GFAP+ cells 6.9±2% and 31.65±3.11% in the transplanted and control hemispheres, respectively (n = 3 each). Moreover, the morphology of both Iba1+ and GFAP+ cells appeared to shift from ameboid and globular, typical of a reactive phenotype, to branching and star-shaped, like in resident cells. At 1 month after lesion inflammation had subsided in both sides and, no significant

differences were detectable between the two hemispheres (Fig. 7A and B, G and H).

It is worth noting that immunosuppression by cyclosporine, be it administered transiently or even continuously, did not affect inflammatory response in lesioned animals, as assessed by immunofluorescence using anti-Iba1 antibody (not shown).

Discussion

Cell survival and migration

In the adult brain, ischemia and brain trauma increase neurogenesis in the SVZ and migration of newly generated NSC-derived progenitors to the sites of injury [39,40]; however this self-repair process is limited [7], so that cell therapy through transplantation of exogenous neural cells has been envisioned as a candidate therapeutic approach [13,41–43]. The present study

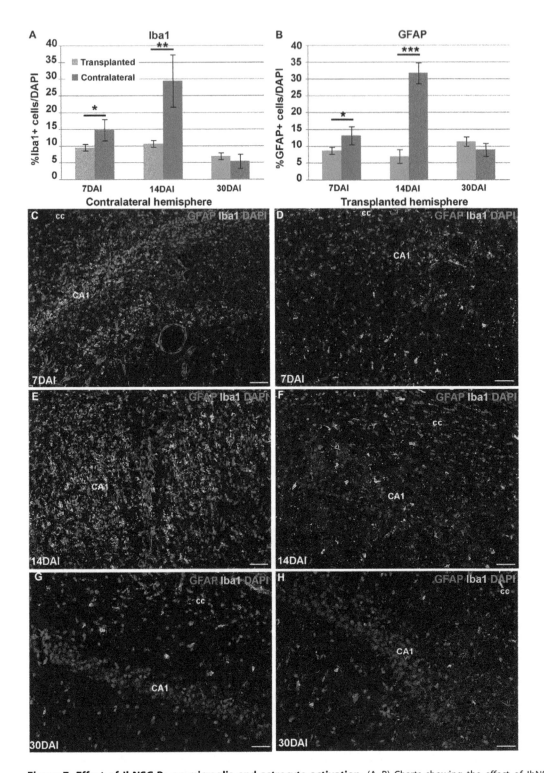

Figure 7. Effect of IhNSC-Ps on microglia and astrocyte activation. (A–B) Charts showing the effect of IhNSC-Ps transplantation on the number of microglia (Iba1+, A) and astroglial cells (GFAP+, B) in the hippocampal region at 7, 14 and 30 DAI. (C–H) Representative images of the hippocampal regions, showing the morphology and density of Iba1+ cells (green) and GFAP+ cells (red) in not transplanted (C, E, and G) and transplanted (D, F and H) brain hemispheres at 7, 14 and 30 DAI. Abbreviations: cc = corpus callosum. Scale bars: 50 μm.

aimed at defining the capacity of IhNSCs for engraftment, migration and differentiation in the adult brain following and ischemic lesion, in view of their perspective use in modeling neural transplantation of human neural cells in ischemia and as a source of cells for cell replacement therapy.

IhNSCs can generate significant percentages of mature neurons and oligodendrocytes *in vitro* [14]. Thus, we investigated their ability to do the same *in vivo*, in the brain of adult rats which suffered transient global ischemia, causing a widely distributed brain injury that primarily affects the neocortical and the hippocampal CA1 layers [22,23]. As the survival of fetal neural tissue is markedly impaired when grafted within the severely lesioned area in ischemic lesion, but not in the surrounding area [44], the latter was chosen as elective site of injection of the cells. More specifically, IhNSC-Ps were transplanted in the posterior periventricular region, below the neocortical layers and in the hippocampal fissure below the damaged CA1 region. The first evidence to emerge was that the survival rate of the grafts was higher when cells were injected into the posterior periventricular region next to the cc (81.2% of cc transplanted animals, n = 13/16) than in hf (53.3% of hf transplanted animals, n = 8/15). Also, quite remarkably, IhNSC-Ps which were transplanted in the cc showed a preferential tropism for the lesioned cortex, while IhNSC-Ps injected into the hf migrated primarily to colonize the NSC niche in the DG (SGZ). This seems to suggest the existence of differential, locoregional instructive cues in these brain regions, although this phenomenon shall require a specific investigation to be fully unraveled, also considering the proximity of the two injection sites.

We found that, even upon the transient immunosuppression conditions used here, IhNSC-Ps integrated into the cortex, corpus callosum and DG of the hippocampus as early as 14 DAI, also migrating along preferential neurogenic pathways [31], acquiring a typical neuronal morphology. By 30 DAI, IhNSC-Ps injected in the periventricular region were migrating tangentially along the cc, as shown by previous studies [45]. Consistent with this pattern, IhNSCP-derived cells were found in the controlateral hemisphere, diffusely spreading through the white matter, 4 months post implantation. When injected in the proximity of the DG, IhNSC-Ps migrated along the SGZ (30 DAI), possibly attracted by endogenous environmental cues secreted by the activated stem cell niche layer [32]; in accordance with these observations, at the endpoint of the analysis, we detected IhNSCP-derived cells being distributed all along the medial dorsal wall of the SVZ in the 3rd–4th ventricle. The evidence above seems to suggest the existence of differential, locoregional instructive cues in the cc and DG, although this phenomenon shall require a full blown study to be fully unraveled.

At least 19% of the grafted human cells survived 1 month after transplantation, a percentage similar to that observed after 4 months. This would suggest a quite stable profile of integration and survival of the transplanted cells over a quite long period. Nonetheless, it is also possible that this apparent stability in the overall number of grafted cells may be the consequence of a dynamic balance between two competing processes, the death of engrafted cells and the birth of new ones through cell proliferation. In fact, it is well known that stroke-associated hypoxia enhances the proliferation of neuronal precursors [40,46,47] and, in agreement with this, we documented the sporadic presence of Ki67+ elements among our donor cells.

Only 7 out of 28 of the transplanted control (unlesioned) animals showed appreciable cell engraftment and survival with respect to 37 out of 61 in lesioned animals. Furthermore, in control animals, engrafted cells were mainly localized next to the injection site (not shown). These results are in good agreement with previous studies, showing that both IhNSC-Ps survival and migration are enhanced by the presence of a brain lesion as compared to the healthy CNS tissue [29]. Finally, the transplanted IhNSC-Ps were not tumorigenic, in accordance with our earlier findings in SCID mice [14]. Our findings are also consistent with studies carried out with primary cultures of human progenitors [40,48,49] and provide the initial evidence that neural progenitors that are continuously produced by a renewable source of hNSCs can undergo targeted migration to different areas in the adult brain affected by a global ischemic lesion.

IhNSC-Ps proliferation and differentiation

Others and us have previously shown that NSCs undergo prevalent glia differentiation after transplantation in neurodegenerative disease animal models such as metachromatic leukodystrophy (MLD) [20], focal demyelination [24] and multiple sclerosis (MS) [38]. In order to enhance the neuronogenic potential of IhNSCs, in this study we transplanted neural progenitors derived from IhNSCs (IhNSC-Ps) which were pre-committed to differentiation in vitro and cultured at 5% oxygen, a condition approximating the physiological range of oxygen in the SVZ and DG [50]. As early as 1 month from transplantation into the brain of ischemic adult rats, clusters of HuN+ cells expressed markers of early neuronal progenitors (Dcx+ and NCAM+), and we also identified HuN+/β-Tub+ and HuN+/MAP2+ neurons with ramified morphology and typically star-shaped HuN+/GFAP+ astrocytes. The expression of these markers was maintained at 4 months from transplantation when IhNSC-Ps appeared widely distributed in the corpus callosum and cortex, where we could detect HuN+ cells bearing GABAergic or Glutamatergic phenotypes, consistent with their physiological prevalence in these brain areas and with the pattern of in vitro differentiated hNSCs and IhNSCs [14,34]. To note, the synthesis of GABA by newborn neurons and active cortical neurogenesis by resident progenitors of layer 1 have been recently shown to be a fundamental requisite to restore neuronal function after stroke [33,51]. Intriguingly, we also found sporadic MAP2+/humanKi67+ cells at 3 months post ischemia, which completely disappear at 4 months, indicating that at least a fraction of IhNSC-Ps undergo transient short–term proliferation, also favoured by the local specific environmental cues [33]. Most importantly, our findings show the expression of both GABA and Glutamate neurotransmitters by a renewable source of human cells transplanted in a lesioned adult rodent brain.

IhNSC-Ps are not immunogenic under transient immunosuppression treatment

A wide array of studies have shown that NSCs are not susceptible to immunological rejection [15–18] even when transplanted in animal models like EAE, characterized by a constitutively activated immunological response [25,26]. Notably, others and us have documented the ability of NSCs to somewhat modulate or even dampen immunological response upon transplantation [26,36,38,43]. This phenomenon may, in fact, participate in the low immunogenic response that these cells seem to elicit in the CNS. Notwithstanding, it is also true that some level of immune surveillance is maintained in the adult brain upon NSCs engraftment, which explains the widespread need to use immune suppression [18] in experimental and clinical intracerebral transplantation [15,17].

The succesful use of transient immunosuppression described here, supports the twofold notion of limiting toxicity in an experimental model plagued by high animal mortality and of preventing the bias introduced by the known neuroprotective effects of cyclosporine following hypoxia-ischemia [52], and proposes a suitable milder approach to immunosuppression for the prospective use hNSCs for clinical purposes. That the discontinuous treatment with cyclosporine does not affect integration of transplanted cells in most of the brain regions, which to all effects emerge as immunopriviledged when considering hNSCs, is in good accordance with most recent findings [18]. It should also be noted that the rate of survival of our transplanted IhNSC-Ps appeared more prominent than that observed in xenografts of embryonic human neural precursor cells [53], transplants of fetal tissue into patients with Parkinson's Disease [15] or of adult human NPCs in ischemic rats [17].

Generation of mature neurons and reduction of the inflammation by IhNSC-Ps in ischemia

Our ultrastructural analysis determined the full maturation of IhNSCs progeny by detecting the presence of newly established synaptic junctions between rat axonal terminals and IhNSC-Ps progeny dendritic spines in the CA1 layer, 4 months after transplantation. This is consistent with previous observations, showing the ability of IhNSCs to generate post-synaptic structures and to fire spontaneous action potentials in culture [14] and is further supported by the detection of GFP labeled axons enveloped by a multilayered myelin structure. Given the prolonged timing required by human neural progenitors to mature in vivo, analysis at further time points could provide additional details on the functional integration of transplanted cells in the damaged neuronal circuitry. Unfortunately, the age and size of adult rats, combined with the dysplastic condition of the ischemic brain tissue allowed neither electrophysiological studies, nor an ultrastructural investigation beyond the 4 month end/point.

Besides neurodegeneration *per se*, one of the hallmarks characterizing most neurodegenerative disorders like stroke, AD, PD, ALS, MLD [37], is the development of an inflammatory environment, which can contribute to tissue damage. Recent studies have shown that NSCs may also exert their therapeutic potential through an immunomodulatory action [26,36,38]. Our study reports that transplantation of IhNSCs can effectively decrease reactive astrogliosis and dumpen microglial activation in the injuried areas. This effect occurred exclusively in the transplanted regions and was most prominent at 15 days from transplantation, when the inflammatory reaction appeared to reach its nadir. There was an obvious effect on the state of activation of microglia, whose cells shifted from the activated, macrophagic-amoeboid phenotype to the resting, stellate one, with a concomitant shift of astrocytes from fibrotic and globular to star-shaped and long-branching in the transplanted areas.

Conclusion

Transient global ischemia is a commonly accepted model of vascular dementia, since it resembles the pathological features of Alzheimer's Disease. In this view, the findings presented in this manuscript lend to the idea of using IhNSCs as a suitable tool to model transplantation of hNSCs in pre-clinical settings. This is particularly relevant in view of the fact that the first phase I clinical trial exploiting cell therapy has been authorized and is currently underway. The trial uses non-immortalized neural cells similar to those described here, which may thus be considered for a prospective use in clinical settings. This is particularly true,

considering the suitable migration and differentiation pattern of our IhNSCs in the ischemic brain, their negligible rejection, their ability to establish synaptic interaction with host cells and their capacity to generate appropriate neurotransmitter phenotypes in ischemia target areas, such as the hippocampus and cortex. The ability of transplanted IhNSC-Ps to dampen reactive astrogliosis and microglia activation provide an extra positive element when considering hNSCs for therapeutic purposes in neurodegenerative disorders.

Supporting Information

Figure S1 Analysis of the lesioned brain at 3DAI. (A–C) Hematoxylin-eosin showing the pyknotic nuclei present in the lesioned (A, arrows) respect to the control cortex (B), and in the lesioned CA1 layer (C). (D–E) Microglial (Iba1+, D) and astroglial (GFAP+, E) reaction in the hippocampal region of lesioned animals at 3DAI. (F) Quantification of pyknotic nuclei in the CA1 layer and of Iba1+ and GFAP+ cells in the hippocampal region. Scale bar: A and B: 50 µm, C: 5 µm, D and E: 75 µm.

Figure S2 *In vitro* differentiation of IhNSC. (A–E) IhNSC-P used for transplantation contained early neuronal progenitors (Dcx+, A and NCAM+, B), neurons (β-Tub+, C and MAP2+, D), astrocytes (GFAP+, C), oligodendrocytes (GalC+, E) and a percentage of residual proliferating cells (Ki67+, A, B and D). (F) Quantification of the neural cell lineages in IhNSC-P. Scale bars: A–E: 10 µm.

Figure S3 Experimental design. (A) Schematic representation showing the experimental plan with transplanted animals undergoing transient or constitutive immunosuppression. Healthy not transplanted animals (n = 4) have been excluded. (B) Table showing the numerosity of the transplanted animal groups. Abbreviations: cc: corpus callosum, hf: hippocampal fissure, AP: anteroposterior, L: lateral, DV: dorsoventral.

Acknowledgments

We thank David Della Morte, Cristina Zalfa and Elena Fusar Poli for technical support in obtaining and analyzing the global ischemia animal model. We also thank Pietro De Filippis, Patrizia Karoschtiz, Cesare Rota Nodari, Loredana Turani, Antonio Tomaino, Maurizio Gelati for precious suggestions.

Author Contributions

Conceived and designed the experiments: LDF. Performed the experiments: LRN DF FG MB VRM LDF. Analyzed the data: LRN DF FG MB VRM ALV LDF. Contributed reagents/materials/analysis tools: GT ALV. Wrote the paper: LRN DF DD LDF.

References

1. Gritti A, Parati EA, Cova L, Frolichsthal P, Galli R, et al. (1996) Multipotential stem cells from the adult mouse brain proliferate and self-renew in response to basic fibroblast growth factor. J Neurosci 16: 1091–1100.
2. Reynolds BA, Weiss S (1992) Generation of neurons and astrocytes from isolated cells of the adult mammalian central nervous system. Science 255: 1707–1710.
3. Weiss S, Reynolds BA, Vescovi AL, Morshead C, Craig CG, et al. (1996) Is there a neural stem cell in the mammalian forebrain? Trends in neurosciences 19: 387–393.
4. Temple S, Alvarez-Buylla A (1999) Stem cells in the adult mammalian central nervous system. Curr Opin Neurobiol 9: 135–141.
5. Gage FH, Kempermann G, Palmer TD, Peterson DA, Ray J (1998) Multipotent progenitor cells in the adult dentate gyrus. J Neurobiol 36: 249–266.
6. Popa-Wagner A, Buga AM, Kokaia Z (2009) Perturbed cellular response to brain injury during aging. Ageing Res Rev.

7. Romanko MJ, Rola R, Fike JR, Szele FG, Dizon ML, et al. (2004) Roles of the mammalian subventricular zone in cell replacement after brain injury. Prog Neurobiol 74: 77–99.
8. Craig CG, Tropepe V, Morshead CM, Reynolds BA, Weiss S, et al. (1996) In vivo growth factor expansion of endogenous subependymal neural precursor cell populations in the adult mouse brain. J Neurosci 16: 2649–2658.
9. Kuhn HG, Winkler J, Kempermann G, Thal LJ, Gage FH (1997) Epidermal growth factor and fibroblast growth factor-2 have different effects on neural progenitors in the adult rat brain. J Neurosci 17: 5820–5829.
10. Bang OY, Lee JS, Lee PH, Lee G (2005) Autologous mesenchymal stem cell transplantation in stroke patients. Ann Neurol 57: 874–882.
11. Kondziolka D, Wechsler L, Goldstein S, Meltzer C, Thulborn KR, et al. (2000) Transplantation of cultured human neuronal cells for patients with stroke. Neurology 55: 565–569.

12. Modo M, Rezaie P, Heuschling P, Patel S, Male DK, et al. (2002) Transplantation of neural stem cells in a rat model of stroke: assessment of short-term graft survival and acute host immunological response. Brain research 958: 70–82.

13. Daadi MM, Davis AS, Arac A, Li Z, Maag AL, et al. (2010) Human Neural Stem Cell Grafts Modify Microglial Response and Enhance Axonal Sprouting in Neonatal Hypoxic-Ischemic Brain Injury. Stroke.

14. De Filippis L, Lamorte G, Snyder EY, Malgaroli A, Vescovi AL (2007) A novel, immortal, and multipotent human neural stem cell line generating functional neurons and oligodendrocytes. Stem Cells 25: 2312–2321.

15. Bjorklund A, Dunnett SB, Brundin P, Stoessl AJ, Freed CR, et al. (2003) Neural transplantation for the treatment of Parkinson's disease. Lancet Neurol 2: 437–445.

16. Mendez I, Vinuela A, Astradsson A, Mukhida K, Hallett P, et al. (2008) Dopamine neurons implanted into people with Parkinson's disease survive without pathology for 14 years. Nature medicine 14: 507–509.

17. Olstorn H, Moe MC, Roste GK, Bueters T, Langmoen IA (2007) Transplantation of stem cells from the adult human brain to the adult rat brain. Neurosurgery 60: 1089–1098; discussion 1908-1089.

18. Wennersten A, Holmin S, Al Nimer F, Meijer X, Wahlberg LU, et al. (2006) Sustained survival of xenografted human neural stem/progenitor cells in experimental brain trauma despite discontinuation of immunosuppression. Exp Neurol 199: 339–347.

19. Amendola M, Venneri MA, Biffi A, Vigna E, Naldini L (2005) Coordinate dual-gene transgenesis by lentiviral vectors carrying synthetic bidirectional promoters. Nature biotechnology 23: 108–116.

20. Givogri MI, Bottai D, Zhu HL, Fasano S, Lamorte G, et al. (2008) Multipotential neural precursors transplanted into the metachromatic leukodystrophy brain fail to generate oligodendrocytes but contribute to limit brain dysfunction. Dev Neurosci 30: 340–357.

21. Abercrombie (1946) Estimation of nuclear population from microtome sections. Anat. Rec 94: 239–247.

22. Bendel O, Alkass K, Bueters T, von Euler M, von Euler G (2005) Reproducible loss of CA1 neurons following carotid artery occlusion combined with halothane-induced hypotension. Brain research 1033: 135–142.

23. Pulsinelli WA, Brierley JB, Plum F (1982) Temporal profile of neuronal damage in a model of transient forebrain ischemia. Ann Neurol 11: 491–498.

24. Neri M, Maderna C, Ferrari D, Cavazzin C, Vescovi AL, et al. (2010) Robust generation of oligodendrocyte progenitors from human neural stem cells and engraftment in experimental demyelination models in mice. PloS one 5: e10145.

25. Pluchino S, Quattrini A, Brambilla E, Gritti A, Salani G, et al. (2003) Injection of adult neurospheres induces recovery in a chronic model of multiple sclerosis. Nature 422: 688–694.

26. Pluchino S, Zanotti L, Rossi B, Brambilla E, Ottoboni L, et al. (2005) Neurosphere-derived multipotent precursors promote neuroprotection by an immunomodulatory mechanism. Nature 436: 266–271.

27. Gritti A, Cova L, Parati EA, Galli R, Vescovi AL (1995) Basic fibroblast growth factor supports the proliferation of epidermal growth factor-generated neuronal precursor cells of the adult mouse CNS. Neurosci Lett 185: 151–154.

28. Vescovi AL, Reynolds BA, Fraser DD, Weiss S (1993) bFGF regulates the proliferative fate of unipotent (neuronal) and bipotent (neuronal/astroglial) EGF-generated CNS progenitor cells. Neuron 11: 951–966.

29. Boockvar JA, Schouten J, Royo N, Millard M, Spangler Z, et al. (2005) Experimental traumatic brain injury modulates the survival, migration, and terminal phenotype of transplanted epidermal growth factor receptor-activated neural stem cells. Neurosurgery 56: 163–171; discussion 171.

30. Seri B, Garcia-Verdugo JM, McEwen BS, Alvarez-Buylla A (2001) Astrocytes give rise to new neurons in the adult mammalian hippocampus. J Neurosci 21: 7153–7160.

31. Ming GL, Song H (2005) Adult neurogenesis in the mammalian central nervous system. Annu Rev Neurosci 28: 223–250.

32. Park KI, Hack MA, Ourednik J, Yandava B, Flax JD, et al. (2006) Acute injury directs the migration, proliferation, and differentiation of solid organ stem cells: evidence from the effect of hypoxia-ischemia in the CNS on clonal "reporter" neural stem cells. Exp Neurol 199: 156–178.

33. Ohira K, Furuta T, Hioki H, Nakamura KC, Kuramoto E, et al. (2010) Ischemia-induced neurogenesis of neocortical layer 1 progenitor cells. Nat Neurosci 13: 173–179.

34. Vescovi AL, Parati EA, Gritti A, Poulin P, Ferrario M, et al. (1999) Isolation and cloning of multipotential stem cells from the embryonic human CNS and establishment of transplantable human neural stem cell lines by epigenetic stimulation. Exp Neurol 156: 71–83.

35. Bueters T, von Euler M, Bendel O, von Euler G (2008) Degeneration of newly formed CA1 neurons following global ischemia in the rat. Exp Neurol 209: 114–124.

36. Bacigaluppi M, Pluchino S, Peruzzotti Jametti L, Kilic E, Kilic U, et al. (2009) Delayed post-ischaemic neuroprotection following systemic neural stem cell transplantation involves multiple mechanisms. Brain 132: 2239–2251.

37. Glass CK, Saijo K, Winner B, Marchetto MC, Gage FH (2010) Mechanisms underlying inflammation in neurodegeneration. Cell 140: 918–934.

38. Pluchino S, Gritti A, Blezer E, Amadio S, Brambilla E, et al. (2009) Human neural stem cells ameliorate autoimmune encephalomyelitis in non-human primates. Ann Neurol 66: 343–354.

39. Doetsch F (2003) A niche for adult neural stem cells. Curr Opin Genet Dev 13: 543–550.

40. Arvidsson A, Collin T, Kirik D, Kokaia Z, Lindvall O (2002) Neuronal replacement from endogenous precursors in the adult brain after stroke. Nature medicine 8: 963–970.

41. Chu K, Kim M, Jeong SW, Kim SU, Yoon BW (2003) Human neural stem cells can migrate, differentiate, and integrate after intravenous transplantation in adult rats with transient forebrain ischemia. Neurosci Lett 343: 129–133.

42. Englund U, Bjorklund A, Wictorin K (2002) Migration patterns and phenotypic differentiation of long-term expanded human neural progenitor cells after transplantation into the adult rat brain. Brain Res Dev Brain Res 134: 123–141.

43. Lee ST, Chu K, Jung KH, Kim SJ, Kim DH, et al. (2008) Anti-inflammatory mechanism of intravascular neural stem cell transplantation in haemorrhagic stroke. Brain 131: 616–629.

44. Kelly S, Bliss TM, Shah AK, Sun GH, Ma M, et al. (2004) Transplanted human fetal neural stem cells survive, migrate, and differentiate in ischemic rat cerebral cortex. Proc Natl Acad Sci U S A 101: 11839–11844.

45. Wong AM, Hodges H, Horsburgh K (2005) Neural stem cell grafts reduce the extent of neuronal damage in a mouse model of global ischaemia. Brain research 1063: 140–150.

46. Fagel DM, Ganat Y, Silbereis J, Ebbitt T, Stewart W, et al. (2006) Cortical neurogenesis enhanced by chronic perinatal hypoxia. Exp Neurol 199: 77–91.

47. Parent JM, Valentin VV, Lowenstein DH (2002) Prolonged seizures increase proliferating neuroblasts in the adult rat subventricular zone-olfactory bulb pathway. J Neurosci 22: 3174–3188.

48. Aboody KS, Brown A, Rainov NG, Bower KA, Liu S, et al. (2000) Neural stem cells display extensive tropism for pathology in adult brain: evidence from intracranial gliomas. Proc Natl Acad Sci U S A 97: 12846–12851.

49. Hurelbrink CB, Armstrong RJ, Dunnett SB, Rosser AE, Barker RA (2002) Neural cells from primary human striatal xenografts migrate extensively in the adult rat CNS. Eur J Neurosci 15: 1255–1266.

50. Santilli G, Lamorte G, Carlessi L, Ferrari D, Rota Nodari L, et al. (2009) Mild hypoxia enhances proliferation and multipotency of human neural stem cells. PloS one 5: e8575.

51. Gu W, Gu C, Jiang W, Wester P (2009) Neurotransmitter synthesis in poststroke cortical neurogenesis in adult rats. Stem Cell Res.

52. Domanska-Janik K, Buzanska L, Dluzniewska J, Kozlowska H, Sarnowska A, et al. (2004) Neuroprotection by cyclosporin A following transient brain ischemia correlates with the inhibition of the early efflux of cytochrome C to cytoplasm. Brain Res Mol Brain Res 121: 50–59.

53. Le Belle JE, Caldwell MA, Svendsen CN (2004) Improving the survival of human CNS precursor-derived neurons after transplantation. J Neurosci Res 76: 174–183.

2

I_{Ks} Protects from Ventricular Arrhythmia during Cardiac Ischemia and Reperfusion in Rabbits by Preserving the Repolarization Reserve

Xiaogang Guo[1], Xiuren Gao[1]*, Yesong Wang[1], Longyun Peng[1], Yingying Zhu[2], Shenming Wang[3]*

1 Department of Cardiology, The First Affiliated Hospital of Sun Yat-sen University, Guangzhou, China, **2** Intensive Care Unit, Central Hospital, Tai'an, China, **3** Department of Vascular Surgery, The First Affiliated Hospital of Sun Yat-sen University, Guangzhou, China

Abstract

Introduction: The function of the repolarization reserve in the prevention of ventricular arrhythmias during cardiac ischemia/reperfusion and the impact of ischemia on slowly activated delayed rectifier potassium current (I_{Ks}) channel subunit expression are not well understood.

Methods and Results: The responses of monophasic action potential duration (MAPD) prolongation and triangulation were investigated following an L-768,673-induced blockade of I_{Ks} with or without ischemia/reperfusion in a rabbit model of left circumflex coronary artery occlusion/reperfusion. Ischemia/reperfusion and I_{Ks} blockade were found to significantly induce MAPD90 prolongation and increase triangulation at the epicardial zone at 45 min, 60 min, and 75 min after reperfusion, accompanied with an increase in premature ventricular beats (PVBs) during the same period. Additionally, I_{Ks} channel subunit expression was examined following transient ischemia or permanent infarction and changes in monophasic action potential (MAP) waveforms challenged by β-adrenergic stimulation were evaluated using a rabbit model of transient or chronic cardiac ischemia. The epicardial MAP in the peri-infarct zone of hearts subjected to infarction for 2 days exhibited increased triangulation under adrenergic stimulation. KCNQ1 protein, the α subunit of the I_{Ks} channel, was downregulated in the same group. Both findings were consistent with an increased incidence of PVBs.

Conclusion: Blockade of I_{Ks} caused MAP triangulation, which precipitated ventricular arrhythmias. Chronic ischemia increased the incidence of ventricular arrhythmias under adrenergic stimulation and was associated with increased MAP triangulation of the peri-infarct zone. Downregulation of KCNQ1 protein may be the underlying cause of these changes.

Editor: Bernard Attali, Tel Aviv University, Israel

Funding: This work was supported by the Guangdong Science and Technology Department of China [grant number 2008A030201011] and National Natural Science Foundation of China [grant number 81170172]. The funder had no role in study design, data collection and analysis, decision to publish or preparation of the manuscript.

Competing Interests: The authors have declared that no competing interests exist.

* E-mail: xiurengao@yahoo.com (X. Gao); shenmingwang@vip.shou.com (SW)

Introduction

Slowly activated delayed rectifier potassium (I_{Ks}) current serves as a repolarizing current in the ventricular cardiomyocytes of humans and various mammals. Together with the rapid (I_{Kr}) and inwardly rectifying potassium (I_{K1}) current, it provides multiple mechanisms for normal repolarization, which was termed "repolarization reserves" by Roden et al. [1]. Loss of function in one of these currents may not necessarily result in clinical consequences.

Functionally, I_{Ks} constitutes one of the critical repolarization reserves that compensate for reductions in other repolarizing currents, particularly I_{Kr}, that are caused by mutations in hereditary long QT syndrome (LQT2) or drugs in acquired LQT syndrome. This is supported by the observation that pharmacological I_{Ks} inhibition played a minor role in the *in vitro* lengthening of action potential duration (APD) in the absence of β-adrenergic stimulation [2,3]. In contrast, certain drugs, for example sotalol, erythromycin, chlorpromazine, and methadone,

or diseases, for example heart failure, diabetes, and cardiac hypertrophy, can trigger a life-threatening arrhythmia in the absence of the repolarization reserve provided by I_{Ks} [4].

Cardiac ischemia and reperfusion are known to change the outward currents responsible for repolarization. For example, when cardiac ischemia was induced, the contribution of adenosine triphosphate sensitive potassium current (I_{KATP}) to repolarization was increased, while those of IKr and IK1 were lessened in comparison, which led in turn to a shortening of the APD [5]. The shortening of the APD induced by ischemia is gradually restored by reperfusion, however a temporary prolongation of APD during early reperfusion was observed by Ducroq et al. and Bes et al. in an *in vitro* model of simulated ischemia and reperfusion in isolated cardiomyocytes [6,7]. This phenomenon, which directly involved repolarization ion current function, has not yet been well explained. In addition, little is currently known about the role played by the repolarization reserve in acute ischemia/reperfusion-induced ventricular arrhythmias. In canine hearts infarcted for 5 days, chronic ischemia decreased I_{Ks} current density and downregulated the

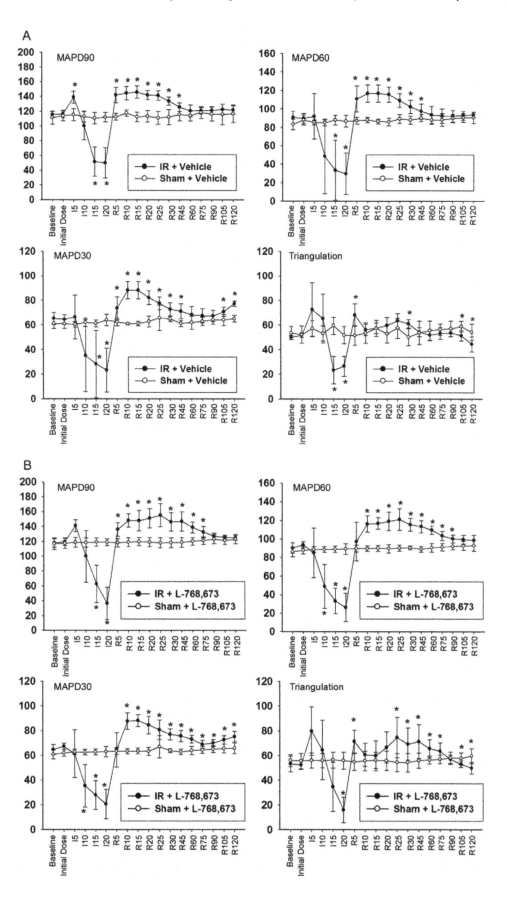

Figure 1. Comparison of epicardial monophasic action potential changes between groups. (**A**) Epicardial monophasic action potential durations (MAPDs) and triangulation (MAPD90–MAPD30) recorded from the ischemia/reperfusion zone (apical) in the Sham+vehicle group and the ischemia/reperfusion (IR)+vehicle group. *P<0.05 vs. Sham+vehicle. (**B**) Epicardial MAPDs and triangulation recorded from the ischemia/reperfusion zone in the Sham+L-768,673 group and the IR+L-768,673 group. *P<0.05 vs. Sham+L-768,673.

expression of KCNQ1 and KCNE1 mRNA [8,9]. However, the effect of transient and chronic ischemia on the expression of KCNQ1 and KCNE1 proteins has not been determined.

Therefore, the first objective of this study was to evaluate the pattern of I_{Ks} changes during cardiac ischemia and reperfusion, and to determine the function of the repolarization reserve in the

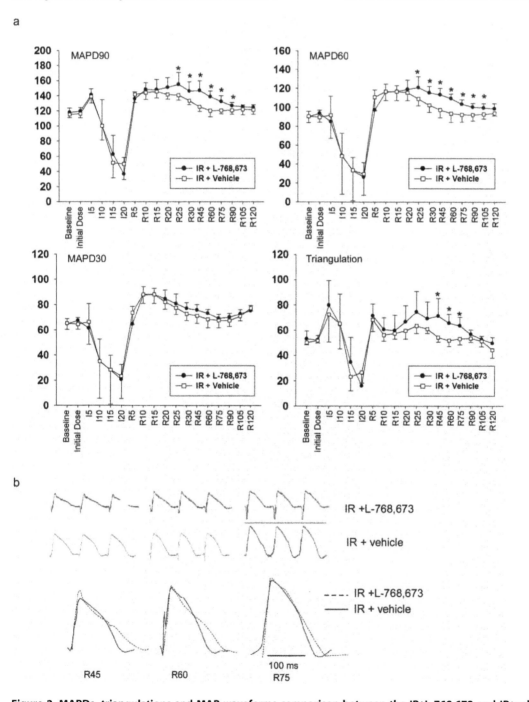

Figure 2. MAPDs, triangulations and MAP waveforms comparison between the IR+L-768,673 and IR+vehicle groups. (**A**) Epicardial MAPDs and triangulation recorded from the ischemia/reperfusion zone (apical) in the IR+L-768,673 group and the IR+vehicle group. Triangulations of the IR+L-768,673 group were increased compared with those of the IR+vehicle group by 31.1%, 26.5%, and 19.3% at R45, R60, and R75 respectively. Results are mean ± standard deviation (STD). * P<0.05 vs. IR+vehicle. (**B**) Comparison of monophasic action potential (MAP) waveforms between the IR+L-768,673 and IR+vehicle groups at R45, R60, and R75.

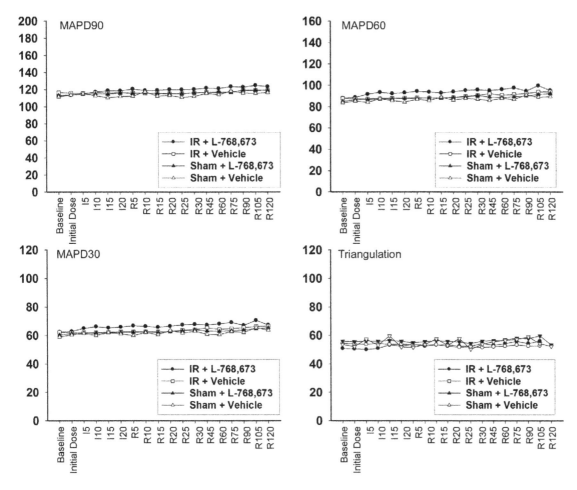

Figure 3. Epicardial MAPD90/60/30 and triangulation (MAPD90 - MAPD30) recorded from the remote zone (basal). Results were means ± STD. There were no significant differences between groups.

prevention of ventricular arrhythmias. In addition, the influence of transient and chronic ischemia on I_{Ks} channel subunit expression and the related electrophysiological outcomes were evaluated.

Results

Effect of L-768,673 on ischemia/reperfusion-induced MAP changes

In comparison with the Sham+vehicle group, occlusion of the coronary artery greatly shortened the MAP durations at 90%, 60%, and 30% repolarization (MAPD90, MAPD60, and MAPD30) of the ischemic epicardium in the IR+vehicle group; it also caused a decrease in triangulation due to an abrupt shortening of the MAPDs (Figure 1A). When the coronary perfusion was restored, the MAPDs all rebounded and exceeded the baseline value, before they gradually returned to baseline levels with continued reperfusion (Figure 1A). The same phenomena were observed in the IR+L-768,673 group when compared with the Sham+L-768,673 group (Figure 1B).

In the interval between reperfusion for 25 min (R25) and R90, the MAPD90 and MAPD60, but not the MAPD30, of the ischemia/reperfusion zone were significantly prolonged in the IR+L-768,673 group, when compared with the IR+vehicle group (Figure 2A). This denoted that in the presence of L-768,673, the

reperfusion-induced prolongation of both the MAPD90 and MAPD60 was more evident and the return of the MAPD90 and MAPD60 to baseline was delayed; however, the MAPD30 did not show the same trend. This deviation led to an increase of triangulation (MAPD90–MAPD30) in the interval between R45 and R75, compared with the IR+vehicle group (Figure 2A). The MAP waveform of the IR+L-768,673 group was characteristic of a slowing of the fast repolarization (Figure 2B). Whereas, remote zone MAPDs recorded in all of the four groups exhibited mild, insignificant fluctuations (Figure 3).

The main effects of L-768,673 on MAPD90, MAPD30 and triangulation were further examined (Table 1). It was found that with the exclusion of the influence of ischemia/reperfusion, L-768,673 exerted independent impact on MAPD90 only at the time points R30, R45, R60, and R75, on triangulation only for the time points R45, R60, and R75; whereas, it exerted no independent impact on MAPD30. This finding perfectly demonstrated that I_{Ks} currents activated slowly and peaked during the late phase 3 and that blockade of I_{Ks} influenced only MAPD90, a surrogate of MAPD, with no effect on MAPD30, which represented the early phase of repolarization (phase 2 to the beginning of phase 3). The reperfusion after transient ischemia and I_{Ks} blockade by L-768,673 had a synergistic effect on prolongation of the MAPD90 and on the increase of triangulation in the interval between R45 and R75.

Table 1. The P value of main effects and interaction effects of I/R or sham operation and L-768,673 or vehicle on MAPD and triangulation.

Time point	MAPD90			MAPD30			Triangulation		
	I/R	L-768,673	Interaction	I/R	L-768,673	Interaction	I/R	L-768,673	Interaction
Baseline	0.714	0.353	0.929	0.210	0.900	0.980	0.094	0.178	0.887
Initial dose	0.272	0.109	0.838	0.101	0.123	0.432	0.262	0.301	0.402
I5	0.000*	0.572	0.857	0.700	0.843	0.500	0.005*	0.622	0.534
I10	0.055	0.861	0.826	0.001*	0.946	0.960	0.126	0.852	0.794
I15	0.000*	0.477	0.355	0.000*	0.917	0.869	0.000*	0.414	0.147
I20	0.000*	0.435	0.206	0.000*	0.720	0.858	0.000*	0.299	0.051
R5	0.000*	0.848	0.126	0.097	0.313	0.158	0.000*	0.348	0.980
R10	0.000*	0.187	0.901	0.000*	0.590	0.372	0.205	0.279	0.665
R15	0.000*	0.633	0.870	0.000*	0.449	0.449	0.540	0.848	0.575
R20	0.000*	0.058	0.368	0.000*	0.431	0.747	0.021*	0.177	0.561
R25	0.000*	0.111	0.053	0.000*	0.241	0.757	0.004*	0.344	0.088
R30	0.000*	0.021*	0.164	0.000*	0.262	0.100	0.001*	0.078	0.528
R45	0.000*	0.002*	0.021*	0.000*	0.065	0.478	0.038*	0.011*	0.044*
R60	0.001*	0.001*	0.009*	0.000*	0.096	0.564	0.246	0.003*	0.009*
R75	0.012*	0.007*	0.052	0.008*	0.248	0.831	0.422	0.010*	0.021*
R90	0.411	0.087	0.411	0.004*	0.150	0.689	0.145	0.195	0.523
R105	0.343	0.663	0.242	0.000*	0.257	0.988	0.000*	0.798	0.431
R120	0.349	0.108	0.916	0.000*	0.661	0.291	0.000*	0.026	0.993

I/R = Ischemia/reperfusion, interaction = interaction effect of ischemia/reperfusion and L-768,673, Triangulation = MAPD90–MAPD30.
$P < 0.05$ highlighted by *.

Influence of ischemia/reperfusion and L-768,673 on ventricular arrhythmias

A comparison of the occurrence of ventricular tachycardia, ventricular fibrillation, and total premature ventricular beats (PVB) did not show any significant differences between the groups (Table 2). The whole reperfusion period was then stratified by the presence or absence of a significant difference in triangulation between the IR+L-768,673 and the IR+vehicle groups into three consecutive intervals. Intervals 1, 2 and 3 corresponded to the interval from the initiation of reperfusion to R30, the interval from R30 to R75, and the interval from R75 to R120 respectively. PVBs in the IR+L-768,673 group were found to be significantly increased (4.6-fold) in Interval 2, compared with those in the IR+vehicle group, as shown in Table 2. This finding was in agreement with the significant triangulation synergistically induced by reperfusion and I_{Ks} blockade.

Effect of transient and chronic ischemia on MAPD shortening induced by epinephrine

The adrenergic stimulation triggered by bolus injection of epinephrine consisted of an increase heart rate (HR), acceleration and shortening of the MAPD90, MAPD60, and MAPD30 (Table 3). Concomitantly, the increase in MAP triangulation made the ventricles more vulnerable to ventricular arrhythmias, which partially explained why adrenergic stimulation induced ventricular arrhythmias in a normal heart. Moreover, the shortening of the peri-infarct epicardial MAP30 in the Infarct (2-d) group was as prominent as in other groups, whereas the peri-infarct epicardial MAPD90 of this group was only minimally changed. As a result, triangulation of the peri-infarct epicardium increased to the greatest extent in the Infarct (2-d) group (Figure 4).

Table 2. Ventricular tachycardia (VT), ventricular fibrillation (VF), and total premature ventricular beats (PVB) of the ischemia/reperfusion (IR)+L-768,673 and IR+vehicle groups.

Group	VT[*]	VF[*, ‡]	Total PVB	PVB in Interval 1[§]	PVB in Interval 2[§]	PVB in Interval 3[§]
IR+L-768,673	4/8	9/15	67 (14, 714.5)	10.5 (5.75, 30.0)	14.0 (9.5, 74.0)[**]	2.0 (0.0, 20.0)
IR+vehicle	1/8	9/15	60.5 (30.5, 131.5)	57.5 (16.8, 520.3)	2.5 (0.5, 10.0)	0 .0 (0.0, 2.0)

*All of the VTs and VFs occurred within 30 min of reperfusion.
‡Animals that developed sustained VF were included in the analysis of VF, but were excluded from the analysis of other electrophysiological data.
§Intervals 1, 2 and 3 were the interval from the initiation of reperfusion to R30, the interval from R30 to R75, and the interval from R75 to R120 respectively.
PVB data is expressed as median (25th percentile, 75th percentile). **$P < 0.05$ vs. IR+vehicle. The median was increased by 4.6-fold in Group IR+L-768,673. No significant differences between VT, VF, total PVB, PVB in Interval 1 and PVB in Interval 3 were detected between the groups.

Table 3. Comparison of MAP data recorded at the peri-infarct zone and heart rate (HR) in animals subjected to ischemia and healing, infarction, or sham operation.

Peri-infarct zone	Healing (2-d) (n = 6)	Infarct (2-d) (n = 8)	Sham (2-d) (n = 7)	Healing (5-d) (n = 7)	Infarct (5-d) (n = 7)	Sham (5-d) (n = 8)
First operation						
HR $_{pre-op}$ (bpm)	294±8	306±13	292±6	293±7	297±9	287±13
MAPD30 $_{pre-op}$ (ms)	70.2±4.0	70.8±3.7	70.8±4.1	70.1±2.8	69.9±3.1	70.5±3.0
MAPD60 $_{pre-op}$ (ms)	98.8±3.5	101.1±3.5	100.6±4.4	99.7±3.9	99.3±4.1	100.7±3.5
MAPD90 $_{pre-op}$ (ms)	120.7±4.1	122.0±4.3	123.0±5.1	121.7±4.6	121.3±5.3	123.3±4.8
Triangulation $_{pre-op}$ (ms)	50.5±2.2	51.2±3.9	52.2±4.0	51.6±4.5	51.4±4.7	52.7±4.3
Second operation						
HR $_{post-op}$ (bpm)	300±11	292±4	309±13	298±7	294±10	295±10
MAPD30 $_{post-op}$ (ms)	66.1±6.9	66.6±4.0	67.8±3.4	68.9±3.4	70.6±5.0	69.6±3.8
MAPD60 $_{post-op}$ (ms)	92.9±8.2	95.2±3.7	96.5±5.6	97.8±3.0	100.3±3.5	99.3±3.5
MAPD90 $_{post-op}$ (ms)	118.7±4.3	123.6±3.2	118.7±4.1	120.4±2.1	125.9±3.6	120.6±2.3
Triangulation $_{post-op}$ (ms)	52.6±4.5	57.0±6.1	51.9±3.9	51.6±4.3	55.2±8.5	51.1±4.2
Epinephrine injection						
HR $_{epi\ i.v.}$ (bpm)	382±14*	382±11*	378±11*	363±8*	366±6*	370±9*
HR acceleration (%)	27.3	30.8	22.3	21.8	24.5	25.4
MAPD30 $_{epi\ i.v.}$ (ms)	52.3±3.9*	36.2±6.6*	45.4±5.9*	54.1±3.8*	52.5±5.4*	50.4±4.9*
MAPD60 $_{epi\ i.v.}$ (ms)	73.8±6.9*	73.2±13.4*	64.3±6.2*	77.1±7.3*	74.4±6.1*	71.9±5.8*
MAPD90 $_{epi\ i.v.}$ (ms)	90.7±4.8*	114.3±9.4*#	90.9±7.4*	92.3±6.4*	94.0±2.6*	90.5±5.8*
Triangulation $_{epi\ i.v.}$ (ms)	38.3±4.0*	78.1±11.3*#	45.5±6.9*	38.2±5.3*	41.5±7.6*	40.1±5.1*
MAPD90 shortening (ms)	28.0±7.7	10.6±7.2#	28.9±8.3	28.1±5.0	31.9±2.2	30.1±5.6

Pre-op corresponds to data recorded at the first operation; post-op to data at the second operation; epi i.v. to data at the peak stimulation of epinephrine. Triangulation = MAPD90−MAPD30; MAPD90 shortening = MAPD90$_{post-op}$−MAPD90$_{epi\ i.v.}$; HR, heart rate; adr, epinephrine; bpm, beats per minute; i.v., intravenous injection.
*P<0.05 vs. post-op;
#P<0.05 vs. infarct (2-d).

Influence of transient and chronic ischemia on adrenergic stimulation-induced ventricular arrhythmias

Ventricular fibrillation was not induced in any of the animals subjected to transient or chronic ischemia, or in any of the corresponding control animals, when they were challenged with adrenalin. There were five episodes of ventricular tachycardia, which lasted for a total duration of 49 s, all of which occurred in 2/8 animals in the Infarct (2-d) group, although nonparametric statistical analysis showed no significance (Table 4). However, the Infarct (2-d) group was shown to be more vulnerable to ventricular arrhythmias than any of the other groups after pooling together total ventricular ectopy, with the exception of runs of ventricular tachycardia (Figure 5A).

Effect of transient and chronic ischemia on expression of I$_{Ks}$ subunits

KCNQ1 mRNA expression remained unchanged in both the peri-infarct zone and the remote zone in our RT-PCR experiments (Figure 5B). However, KCNQ1 protein expression showed a different pattern in the peri-infarct zone under different ischemic protocols. KCNQ1 protein expression was greatly downregulated in the peri-infarct zone following ischemia for 2 d, and its expression in the peri-infarct zone increased again by approximately 2-fold by day 5. Transient ischemia was associated with a milder, but significant, impact on KCNQ1 protein expression, although no differences were identified between the Healing (2-d) and Healing (5-d) groups (Figure 5C). The steep downregulation of KCNQ1 protein expression (approximately 80%) might have severely compromised the repolarization reserve of the peri-infarct zone cardiomyocytes, which would in turn have led to an increased incidence of ventricular arrhythmias and greater triangulation of MAP in the Infarct (2-d) group under adrenergic stimulation. If the loss of the KCNQ1 protein subunit failed to exceed a certain threshold (for example, approximately one-third of the normal range shown in this study), the repolarization reserve was still able to function well and could at least compensate for a single factor that compromised other outward currents (that is, in this study, adrenergic stimulation inhibiting I$_{Kr}$). Not surprisingly, the effect on KCNQ1 protein expression following transient or chronic ischemia in the remote zone was negligible, which was consistent with the unaffected MAPs in this zone.

KCNE1 mRNA levels were analyzed by RT-PCR; no significant differences were identified between groups (data not shown). Unfortunately, KCNE1 protein bands were very weak, which was consistent with the known low level expression of this protein in the rabbit [10]; therefore, conclusions regarding the protein expression levels of this subunit were not definitive.

Discussion

Repolarization reserve and ischemia/reperfusion-related ventricular arrhythmias

Even though it is widely acknowledged that the complications of cardiac ischemia, such as ATP deficiency, elevation of [K$^+$]o, local acidosis, and lysophosphatidylcholine accumulation [11], amongst others lead to ischemia-induced arrhythmias and cardiac injury,

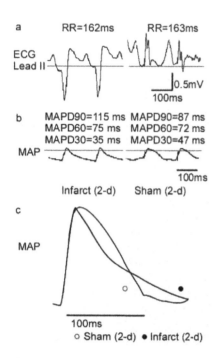

Figure 4. Comparison of waveforms between the Sham (2-d) and Infarct (2-d) groups after bolus injection of epinephrine. The only morphological differences in peri-infarct MAP were identified in the Infarct (2-d) group. **(A)** ECG Lead II waveforms showing that both groups had a comparable degree of heart rate increase. **(B)** MAP recorded at the peri-infarct epicardial zone showing that after the adrenergic challenge, the MAP of the Infarct (2-d) group had a dramatic shortening of MAPD30, whereas the MAPD90 was only minimally changed. **(C)** Direct overlapping of MAP showing that the MAP of the Infarct (2-d) group demonstrates more prominent triangulation.

the effect of ischemia and subsequent reperfusion on cardiac repolarization ion current has not been extensively explored. It has been shown that activation of I_{KATP} by low levels of ATP played an important role in the decrease in APD during ischemia [12]. On the other hand, the outward currents responsible for repolarization under normal conditions (for example I_{K1}) were inhibited by low intracellular ATP levels [13]. With the restoration of blood flow, ischemic components were gradually cleared from the local milieu, which also brought about a subsequent transmembrane ion current variation that remains to be further elucidated.

The prolongation of MAPD in the early phase of reperfusion, which was reported previously by Bes et al. and Ducroq et al. *in vitro* [6,7], was confirmed in our study *in vivo*. The careful use of controls in this study also demonstrated that blockade of I_{Ks} by L-768,673 prolonged both the MAPD90 and MAPD60 in the interval between R30and R90, which provided evidence of the increased contribution of the I_{Ks} current in repolarization

currents. As previously demonstrated [2], blockade of I_{Ks} failed to lengthen normal ventricular muscle APD. In contrast, under conditions of ischemia and reperfusion, the independent effect of L-768,673 on MAPD90 prolongation at R30, R45, R60, and R75 revealed that the contribution of I_{Ks} to repolarization was markedly increased in this period. A similar increase in the contribution of I_{Ks} during this period was also shown by the synergistic effect of both ischemia/reperfusion and L-768,673 on MAPD90 prolongation at R45 and R60. Therefore, it may be inferred that I_{Ks} serves as an important repolarization reserve current and becomes the main repolarization current rather than I_{Kr} in early reperfusion. The administration of L-768,673 in this situation led to an increase in ventricular arrhythmias, which was a consequence of impairment of the repolarization reserve.

Triangulation and predisposition to ventricular arrhythmias

The association between proarrhythmic effects and action potential prolongation may not be causal. MAPD90 is primarily the sum of the plateau and the fast repolarization phase of the action potential; therefore, MAPD90 can be lengthened by prolonging the plateau or by prolonging the fast repolarization phase, referred to as delaying or slowing of the fast repolarization respectively. The latter, described as triangulation of the action potential, is a reliable biomarker for proarrhythmia that was first described in 2001 by Hondeghem et al. in an automated Langendorff-perfused isolated rabbit heart preparation [14]. It is important to stress that lengthening of the MAPD90 without triangulation is not proarrhythmic, but rather antiarrhythmic [15].

Triangulation resulted from a reduction in outward repolarizing currents and/or an increase in depolarizing inward currents during fast repolarization; in MAP recordings, dispersion of repolarization may also contribute to triangulation. These conclusions have been previously confirmed with numerous experimental protocols performed on isolated tissues, perfused hearts, and experimental animals by other researchers [15,16,17,18,19,20].

Triangulation was found to be increased in the interval between R45 and R75 in the IR+L-768,673 group; within this period, there was also a statistically significant synergistic effect of ischemia/reperfusion and L-768,673 on the increase in triangulation. Both these observations were consistent with the increased incidence of ventricular arrhythmias. In the transient and chronic ischemia protocol, increased triangulation of the peri-infarct epicardium under adrenergic stimulation in the Infarct (2-d) group was also observed, which increased the propensity for ventricular arrhythmias.

It has recently been reported that sarcoplasmic reticulum calcium (Ca^{2+}) handling alteration resulted in a decrease in phase 2 of the action potential and was the key determinant of action potential triangulation in mice [21]. This may be largely due to the absence of I_{Ks} in species such as the rat and mouse [22], in which the APD is much shorter than in bigger animals such as the guinea pig, rabbit,

Table 4. Comparison of episodes of ventricular tachycardia within 10 min of bolus injection of epinephrine.

Ventricular Tachycardia	Healing (2-d)	Infarct (2-d)	Sham (2-d)	Healing (5-d)	Infarct (5-d)	Sham (5-d)
Incidence	0/6	2/8	0/7	0/7	0/7	0/8
Episodes	0	5	0	0	0	0
Sum of duration(s)	0	49	0	0	0	0

No significant differences were identified between the groups; however, the runs of ventricular tachycardia occurred exclusively in the 2-d infarct group.

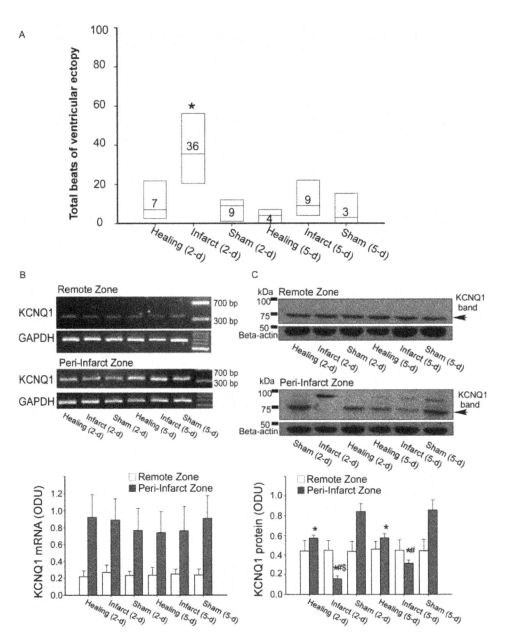

Figure 5. Comparison of ventricular premature beats and KCNQ1 expression between groups. (A) Comparison of the total premature ventricular beats (PVBs) between the groups within 10 min after bolus injection of epinephrine. Results are presented in a box plot format (n = 6–8) where boxes indicate the 25–75% interval along with the median of the data. * P<0.05 vs. the other groups. **(B)** Reverse transcription-polymerase chain reaction (RT-PCR) of KCNQ1 mRNA levels. Top: Examples of KCNQ1 mRNA with samples harvested from the peri-infarct zone and remote zone of the Healing (2-d; n = 6), Infarct (2-d; n = 8), Sham (2-d; n = 7), Healing (5-d; n = 7), Infarct (5-d; n = 7), and Sham (5-d; n = 8) groups of rabbit hearts. Bottom: mean KCNQ1 mRNA band intensities. **(C)** Western blot analysis of membrane-associated KCNQ1 protein levels. Top: Representative immunoblot results showing membrane KCNQ1 protein (~75 kDa) with samples harvested from the peri-infarct zone and remote zone of the six groups of rabbit hearts. Bottom: mean membrane KCNQ1 protein band intensities. * P<0.05 vs. Sham (2-d) and Sham (5-d) respectively; # P<0.05 vs. Healing (2-d) and Healing (5-d) respectively; $ P<0.05 vs. Infarct (5-d).

dog, and humans. Transient outward potassium current (I_{to}) and Ca^{2+} handling were found to be the main current that determined action potential in these species. However, the importance of sarcoplasmic reticulum Ca^{2+} handling in action potential triangulation of large animals still needs to be carefully evaluated.

KCNQ1 expression and cardiac ischemia

There have been a limited number of reports regarding the effect of ischemia on I_{Ks} amplitude and KCNQ1 expression. Selected

examples of other animal models of heart disease, for which remodeling of I_{Ks} has been described and for which information on the underlying changes in channel subunit expression was available, are listed in Table 5. This comparison illustrates that an apparently similar phenotypic change can have divergent molecular mechanisms. To date, neither KCNQ1 nor KCNE1 protein expression levels under conditions of ischemia have been reported.

In this study, membrane KCNQ1 protein expression was severely depressed by chronic ischemia and moderately downreg-

Table 5. Divergent molecular mechanisms for potassium channel remodeling in animal models of heart disease.

Species/Region	Etiology	Functional changes	Molecular changes at the protein level		Molecular changes at the mRNA level		Reference No.
			KCNQ1	KCNE1	KCNQ1	KCNE1	
Rabbit/ventricle	AV block with ventricular pacing						
	Tachycardia	↓	↓	↓*	↓	↓	[24]
	Bradycardia	↓	↓	↓*	↓	↓	[24]
Rabbit/ventricle	Pacing-induced heart failure	↓	-	ND	-	-	[39]
Dog/ventricle	AV block-induced hypertrophy	↓	↓	↓	↓	↓	[40]
Dog/ventricle	Chonic ICM by microembolizations	↓	↓‡	↓	ND	ND	[41]
Dog/ventricle	Myocardial infarction	↓	ND	ND	↓	↓	[8]

AV, atrioventricular; ICM, ischemic cardiomyopathy; ND, not determined; -, no change.
*Weak bands limited the reliability of the measurement.
‡KCNQ1.2, a truncated isoform of canine KCNQ1, was increased and may suppress I_{Ks} in a dominant-negative fashion.

ulated by transient ischemia (20 min ischemia in our protocol). However, KCNQ1 protein expression did recover to some extent by d5 after chronic ischemia, and no significant difference was observed between cardiac KCNQ1 protein expression at d2 and d5 after transient ischemia. As a pore-forming subunit of the I_{Ks} channel, decreased KCNQ1 protein levels could lead to a rapid decrease in I_{Ks} current, which has been well documented in human Romano-Ward Syndrome (LQT1 subtype) gene research [23] and in ion channel subunit remodeling research in animals exposed to long term arrhythmias [24]. Consistent with previous studies, our results confirmed the strong relationship between low KCNQ1 protein levels and diminished repolarization reserve, which resulted in triangulation of the action potential and an increased incidence of ventricular arrhythmias after adrenergic stimulation. The fact that only a dramatic decrease in KCNQ1 protein levels was associated with increased arrhythmic incidence provided evidence that downregulation of the I_{Ks} channel subunit may be complicated by multiple compensatory mechanisms in the cardiomyocyte, such as potent repolarization reserve comprised of various potassium channels, diminished Ca^{2+} current minimizing Ca^{2+} overload, which were not addressed in our experiments [25].

No significant changes in KCNQ1 or KCNE1 mRNA expression levels were identified. The reasons for the discrepancy between observed changes in KCNQ1 protein levels and unchanged mRNA expression levels in this study are unclear, but several explanations can be offered. Firstly, changes in protein expression levels may fall behind changes in mRNA expression levels for a period of time that ranges from minutes to days. In this

and previous studies, limited time points were chosen, which may prevent the detection and interpretation of dynamic changes in chemical biomarker levels. Secondly, changes in mRNA expression levels may not reflect changes in the functional protein subunit levels, because infarction may affect many processes, which include protein translation, subunit modification, assembly, processing, and trafficking. Known KCNQ1 subunit modifications to date include classical phosphorylation and dephosphorylation [26,27], glycosylation and deglycosylation [28,29], and most recently, ubiquitylation [30]. This discrepancy provides a clue that post-translational mechanisms may play a more important role in I_{Ks} subunit suppression.

Limitation of study

In addition to APD and triangulation, other variables had been identified in the MAP waveform that predict the pro-arrhythmic effect of drugs or pathophysiological conditions in a comprehensive manner under different experimental protocols. Among them, triangulation, reverse use dependence, instability and dispersion of ventricular repolarization, together with the cardiac wavelength are powerful proarrhythmic predictors [31]. APD and triangulation were applied in this study to identify the association between ventricular arrhythmias and repolarization reserve compromise; other as yet unidentified predictors may also play an important role. Subunit interactions, whose importance in ion channel function regulation is well-established [32], were not addressed in the current study due to low KCNE1 protein expression level. The roles of other ion channels in cardiac ischemia-reperfusion induced ventricular arrhythmias were not exhaustively covered

Table 6. Details of PCR.

Gene		Primer sequences (5'–3')	PCR product length (bp)	Annealing temperature (°C)	Cycles
KCNQ1	Forward	GCCGCAGCAAGTATGTCG	317	58.6	33
	Reverse	CCTTCTCAGCAGGTACACGA			
KCNE1	Forward	CCGTGATGCCCTTTCTGACC	263	62	34
	Reverse	GTACGCCCTGTCTTTCTCCTG			
GAPDH	Forward	GATCCATTCATTGACCTCCACTA	683	58.6	30
	Reverse	CACCACCTTCTTGATGTCGTC			

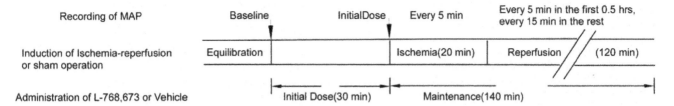

Figure 6. Study protocol 1 of experiments. Monophasic action potentials were recorded after the equilibration at both the middle of the infarct zone and the unaffected zone of the epicardium. For L-768,673, The infusion rate of the initial dose was 0.5 μg/kg/h for 30 min, and the maintenance rate was 0.25 μg/kg/h for two hours. MAP duration data were expressed as MAPD90/60/30$_{Baseline, Initial Dose, I5, I10, I15, I20, R5, R10, R15, R20, R25, R30, R45, R60, R75, R90, R105, R120}$, which stood for MAPD90/60/30 recorded at baseline, after initial dose, at ischemia for 5 min, 10 min, 15 min, 20 min and at reperfusion for 5 min, 10 min, 15 min, 20 min, 25 min, 30 min, 45 min, 60 min, 75 min, 90 min, 105 min, 120 min, respectively.

in this study, even if control groups had been well set up in the protocols.

Conclusions

The results of this study highlight the importance of maintaining an intact repolarization reserve for the prevention of ventricular arrhythmias both in cardiac ischemia/reperfusion and in the infarcted heart under adrenergic challenge. I_{Ks} served as a protective current in securing action potential repolarization, and the reduction of I_{Ks} that resulted from downregulation of the I_{Ks} channel subunit protein contributed to ventricular arrhythmias.

Materials and Methods

Animal preparation

All animal experiments were approved by the Animal Care Committee of Sun Yat-sen University, Guangzhou, China, and all investigations conformed to the Guide for the care and Use of Laboratory Animals published by the United States National Institutes of Health. New Zealand white rabbits (1.5–2.0 kg) of either sex were purchased from the Provincial Medical Laboratory Animal Center (Guangzhou, China).

In vivo model of rabbit coronary artery occlusion/reperfusion

In a modification of a previously published procedure [33], Rabbits were anesthetized by subcutaneous administration of ketamine (40 mg/kg body weight) and Xylazine (8 mg/kg body weight). An endotracheal tube was inserted and used for ventilation with room air at 38 strokes per min and a stroke volume of 7 ml/kg with a positive end-expiratory pressure of 2 KPa applied. Body temperature was maintained by an appropriate heating lamp. Arterial blood pressure was recorded by left jugular artery intubation. The heart was exposed by performing a midline thoracotomy. A ligature was placed around the left circumflex coronary artery at a distance of 10 mm from its origin at the coronary groove. The ends were exteriorized and

passed through a tapered polyethylene tube. After the animal had been allowed to stabilize for 15 min, coronary artery occlusion was achieved by pressing the tube against the heart muscle while pulling on the ligature, followed by clamping the tube with a hemostat; this was accompanied by immediate pallor of the left ventricular free wall, a marked drop in blood pressure, and immediate ST segment elevation in the ECG waveform. Reflow was initiated by releasing the ligature, which was accompanied by immediate hyperemia of the left ventricular free wall as well as a marked increase of blood pressure.

Electrophysiological parameters

ECG Lead II was recorded continuously with subcutaneous needle electrodes. A spring-loaded epicardial Ag-AgCl electrode was made as described previously [34]. Epicardial monophasic action potentials (MAPs) were recorded at various locations in the ventricular epicardium using the electrode at specific time points intermittently throughout the experiment. All data were recorded using a TME BL420 multichannel recorder (TME Technology, Chengdu, China). The diagnoses of ventricular arrhythmias were made in accordance with the Lambeth convention [35]. The MAP parameters measured included: monophasic action potential duration (MAPD) at 30%, 60%, and 90% of repolarization (MAPD30, MAPD60, and MAPD90, respectively). Each parameter was average of at least 5 measurements. The slowing of repolarization in MAP was assessed quantitatively by triangulation, which was calculated as the difference between MAPD90 and MAPD30 in milliseconds (MAPD90 - MAPD30).

Drugs

An appropriate portion of L-768,673, a highly selective I_{Ks} blocker that has been extensively studied in *in vitro* and *in vivo* models [36,37,38], was first dissolved in 100% ethanol at a concentration of 1 mg/ml, followed by suspension in 0.9% saline to yield a final concentration of 5 mg/l. Then the formulation was dosed via the left marginal vein with an initial dose of 1 μg/kg for 30 min (to ensure complete drug equilibration) while a maintain-

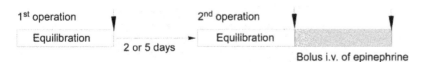

Figure 7. Study protocol 2 of experiments. Monophasic action potentials were recorded after the equilibration at both the peri-infarct zone and the unaffected zone of the epicardium during each open chest operation and at the time point of peak adrenergic excitation. MAP duration data were expressed as MAPD90/60/30$_{pre-op, post-op, epi i.v.}$ which stood for MAPD90/60/30 recorded at first operation, at second operation, and after the bolus intravenous injection of epinephrine, respectively.

ing dose of 0.5 µg/kg for 2 h [37,38]. Control group animals were dosed with an equal volume of vehicle solution, i.e. 100% ethanol dissolved in 0.9% saline at a concentration of 0.5% (v/v).

Reverse transcription-polymerase chain reaction

Total RNA was isolated from samples with TRIzol reagent (Invitrogen Corporation, Carlsbad, CA, USA), followed by chloroform extraction and isopropanol precipitation. cDNA was synthesized by reverse transcription. PCR was performed using the cDNA templates in a reaction buffer containing a corresponding primer (Table 6) and Taq DNA polymerase (Invitrogen Corporation). The PCR products were then separated using agarose gel electrophoresis. The bands were visualized under ultraviolet light following ethidium bromide staining. PCR product integrity was quantitated using the UVItec gel system (UVItec Limited, Cambridge, United Kingdom) and were normalized using the corresponding GAPDH data.

Immunoblot analysis

Membrane fractions were prepared using the BioVision Plasma Membrane Protein Extraction Kit. Protein samples were separated with 8% SDS-PAGE using a minigel system (Bio-Rad Laboratories, Hercules, CA, USA). Proteins were transferred onto an Immobilon-P polyvinylidene fluoride membrane (0.45 µm pore size; Millipore Corporate, Billerica, MA, USA) in 25 mM Tris base, 200 mM glycine, and 20% methanol using the Mini Trans-Blot transfer apparatus (Bio-Rad Laboratories, Hercules, CA, USA). Following the transfer, the membranes were incubated for 2 h at 4°C in blocking buffer (PBS containing 5% nonfat milk powder and 0.1% Tween 20). The membrane was incubated for 18 h at 4°C in blocking buffer containing primary antibody. Antibodies against KCNQ1 (sc-10646; goat) and KCNE1 (sc-16796; goat) were purchased from Santa Cruz Biotechnology, Santa Cruz, CA, USA. After membranes were washed, the bound antibody was detected using horseradish peroxidase-conjugated donkey anti-goat IgG secondary antibody (Santa Cruz Biotechnology, Santa Cruz, CA, USA) in blocking buffer for 1 h, followed by detection with the BeyoECL Plus detection system (Catalog # P0018). The immunoblots were exposed on Fuji film. Band signals were detected and quantified with laser scanning and Image J software. The immunoblot band intensity values reported herein correspond to background-subtracted optical density units (ODUs) normalized to β actin signal intensity for the same sample.

Study protocol 1

In protocol 1, which was based on a 2×2 factorial design, 42 animals were randomized to receive either 20 min of left circumflex coronary artery occlusion followed by 120 min of reperfusion (IR) or a sham operation for the same duration (Sham), with either intravenous administration of L-768,673 or a similar volume of the vehicle. The initial sample sizes of the four groups were as follows: IR+L-768,673, n = 15; IR+vehicle, n = 15; Sham+L-768,673, n = 6; Sham+vehicle, n = 6 (Figure 6). In accordance with the Lambeth conventions [35], seven animals in both the IR+vehicle group and the IR+L-768,673 group that developed sustained ventricular fibrillation were censored in the analysis of electrophysiological data because of the potentially unpredictable manifestations thereafter.

Study protocol 2

In protocol 2, 56 animals were randomly divided into the following six groups: Healing (2-d) group (n = 10); Infarct (2-d) group (n = 10); Sham (2-d) group (n = 8); Healing (5-d) group (n = 10); Infarct (5-d) group (n = 10); and Sham (5-d) group (n = 8). The induction of ischemia and reperfusion were performed in a manner identical to the first protocol. Infarction was induced by direct tightening of the ligature. Several animals were excluded from the analysis because of the development of sustained ventricular fibrillation: in the Healing (2-d) group, 4/10; in the Infarct (2-d) group, 2/10; in the Healing (5-d) group, 3/10; and in the Infarct (5-d) group, 3/10.

The number of surgical survivors were 6/10 animals in the Healing (2-d) group; 8/10 from the Infarct (2-d) group; 7/8 from the Sham (2-d) group; 7/10 from the Healing (5-d) group; 7/10 from the Infarct (5-d) group; and 8/8 from the Sham (5-d) group. Following surgery, the surviving animals were housed in cages for 2 d or 5 d. At the end of the protocol, the chests of the anesthetized animals were reopened, and the animals received a 40 µg/kg intravenous bolus of 0.01% (w/v) epinephrine [16]. Monophasic action potentials (MAPs) in both the peri-infarct epicardial zone and the intact epicardial zone were recorded during each operation and after the administration of epinephrine stimulation (Figure 7). Cardiac tissues were harvested and distinguished as peri-infarct zone and intact zone or the counterpart in control groups.

Data analysis and statistics

All quantitative data with normal distributions were expressed as means ± STD. Other data without normal distributions were expressed as medians with 25th and 75th percentile. Means were compared between groups with two-way ANOVA, followed by the SNK-t post hoc test. The main and interaction effects of operation (ischemia/reperfusion or sham operation) and drug treatment (L-768,673 or vehicle) were analyzed by two-way ANOVA using a General Linear Model.

The presence of any life-threatening ventricular arrhythmias (e.g., ventricular fibrillation, ventricular tachycardia) between groups were assessed with the Fisher's exact test. The number of premature ventricular beats between groups were expressed as median with 25th and 75th percentile and were compared by using the K independent nonparametric test, followed by two independent Kruskal-Wallis nonparametric tests.

Values of P<0.05 indicated statistical significance. All statistical tests were performed using SPSS statistics 17.0 (GraphPad Software Inc., San Diego, CA, USA).

Acknowledgments

The L-768,673 compound used in this study was provided by Merck & Inc Co., Whitehouse Station, NJ, USA.

Author Contributions

Conceived and designed the experiments: X. Guo X. Gao YW LP YZ SW. Performed the experiments: X. Guo X. Gao YW LP YZ SW. Analyzed the data: X. Guo X. Gao YW LP YZ SW. Contributed reagents/materials/analysis tools: X. Guo X. Gao YW LP YZ. Wrote the paper: X. Guo X. Gao YW LP YZ SW.

References

1. Roden DM, Yang T (2005) Protecting the heart against arrhythmias: potassium current physiology and repolarization reserve. Circulation 112: 1376–1378.
2. Lengyel C, Iost N, Virag L, Varro A, Lathrop DA, et al. (2001) Pharmacological block of the slow component of the outward delayed rectifier current (I(Ks)) fails to lengthen rabbit ventricular muscle QT(c) and action potential duration. Br J Pharmacol 132: 101–110.
3. Volders PG, Stengl M, van Opstal JM, Gerlach U, Spatjens RL, et al. (2003) Probing the contribution of IKs to canine ventricular repolarization:

key role for beta-adrenergic receptor stimulation. Circulation 107: 2753–2760.

4. Jost N, Virag L, Bitay M, Takacs J, Lengyel C, et al. (2005) Restricting excessive cardiac action potential and QT prolongation: a vital role for IKs in human ventricular muscle. Circulation 112: 1392–1399.

5. Carmeliet E (1999) Cardiac ionic currents and acute ischemia: from channels to arrhythmias. Physiol Rev 79: 917–1017.

6. Ducroq J, Rouet R, Salle L, Puddu PE, Repesse Y, et al. (2006) Class III effects of dofetilide and arrhythmias are modulated by [K+]o in an in vitro model of simulated-ischemia and reperfusion in guinea-pig ventricular myocardium. Eur J Pharmacol 532: 279–289.

7. Bes S, Vandroux D, Tissier C, Devillard L, Brochot A, et al. (2005) Direct, pleiotropic protective effect of cyclosporin A against simulated ischemia-induced injury in isolated cardiomyocytes. Eur J Pharmacol 511: 109–120.

8. Jiang M, Cabo C, Yao J, Boyden PA, Tseng G (2000) Delayed rectifier K currents have reduced amplitudes and altered kinetics in myocytes from infarcted canine ventricle. Cardiovasc Res 48: 34–43.

9. Dun W, Boyden PA (2005) Diverse phenotypes of outward currents in cells that have survived in the 5-day-infarcted heart. Am J Physiol Heart Circ Physiol 289: H667–673.

10. Zicha S, Moss I, Allen B, Varro A, Papp J, et al. (2003) Molecular basis of species-specific expression of repolarizing K+ currents in the heart. Am J Physiol Heart Circ Physiol 285: H1641–1649.

11. Watanabe I, Kanda A, Engle CL, Gettes LS (1997) Comparison of the effects of regional ischemia and hyperkalemia on the membrane action potentials of the in situ pig heart. Experimental Cardiology Group, University of North Carolina at Chapel Hill. J Cardiovasc Electrophysiol 8: 1229–1236.

12. Ganitkevich V, Reil S, Schwethelm B, Schroeter T, Benndorf K (2006) Dynamic responses of single cardiomyocytes to graded ischemia studied by oxygen clamp in on-chip picochambers. Circ Res 99: 165–171.

13. Shieh RC, John SA, Lee JK, Weiss JN (1996) Inward rectification of the IRK1 channel expressed in Xenopus oocytes: effects of intracellular pH reveal an intrinsic gating mechanism. J Physiol 494(Pt 2): 363–376.

14. Hondeghem LM, Carlsson L, Duker G (2001) Instability and triangulation of the action potential predict serious proarrhythmia, but action potential duration prolongation is antiarrhythmic. Circulation 103: 2004–2013.

15. Martin RL, Su Z, Limberis JT, Palmatier JD, Cowart MD, et al. (2006) In vitro preclinical cardiac assessment of tolterodine and terodiline: multiple factors predict the clinical experience. J Cardiovasc Pharmacol 48: 199–206.

16. Viitasalo M, Paavonen KJ, Swan H, Kontula K, Toivonen L (2005) Effects of epinephrine on right ventricular monophasic action potentials in the LQT1 versus LQT2 form of long QT syndrome: preferential enhancement of "triangulation" in LQT1. Pacing Clin Electrophysiol 28: 219–227.

17. Milberg P, Eckardt L, Bruns HJ, Biertz J, Ramtin S, et al. (2002) Divergent proarrhythmic potential of macrolide antibiotics despite similar QT prolongation: fast phase 3 repolarization prevents early afterdepolarizations and torsade de pointes. J Pharmacol Exp Ther 303: 218–225.

18. Milberg P, Fleischer D, Stypmann J, Osada N, Monnig G, et al. (2007) Reduced repolarization reserve due to anthracycline therapy facilitates torsade de pointes induced by IKr blockers. Basic Res Cardiol 102: 42–51.

19. Lu HR, Vlaminckx E, Van Ammel K, De Clerck F (2002) Drug-induced long QT in isolated rabbit Purkinje fibers: importance of action potential duration, triangulation and early afterdepolarizations. Eur J Pharmacol 452: 183–192.

20. Champeroux P, Viaud K, El Amrani AI, Fowler JS, Martel E, et al. (2005) Prediction of the risk of Torsade de Pointes using the model of isolated canine Purkinje fibres. Br J Pharmacol 144: 376–385.

21. Valverde CA, Kornyeyev D, Ferreiro M, Petrosky AD, Mattiazzi A, et al. (2010) Transient Ca2+ depletion of the sarcoplasmic reticulum at the onset of reperfusion. Cardiovasc Res 85: 671–680.

22. Liu GX, Zhou J, Koren G (2008) Single-channel properties of I K,slow1 and I K,slow2 in mouse ventricular myocytes. Pflugers Arch 456: 541–547.

23. Chouabe C, Neyroud N, Guicheney P, Lazdunski M, Romey G, et al. (1997) Properties of KvLQT1 K+ channel mutations in Romano-Ward and Jervell and Lange-Nielsen inherited cardiac arrhythmias. Embo J 16: 5472–5479.

24. Tsuji Y, Zicha S, Qi XY, Kodama I, Nattel S (2006) Potassium channel subunit remodeling in rabbits exposed to long-term bradycardia or tachycardia: discrete arrhythmogenic consequences related to differential delayed-rectifier changes. Circulation 113: 345–355.

25. Aggarwal R, Boyden PA (1995) Diminished Ca2+ and Ba2+ currents in myocytes surviving in the epicardial border zone of the 5-day infarcted canine heart. Circ Res 77: 1180–1191.

26. Potet F, Scott JD, Mohammad-Panah R, Escande D, Baro I (2001) AKAP proteins anchor cAMP-dependent protein kinase to KvLQT1/IsK channel complex. Am J Physiol Heart Circ Physiol 280: H2038–2045.

27. Chen L, Kurokawa J, Kass RS (2005) Phosphorylation of the A-kinase-anchoring protein Yotiao contributes to protein kinase A regulation of a heart potassium channel. J Biol Chem 280: 31347–31352.

28. Freeman LC, Lippold JJ, Mitchell KE (2000) Glycosylation influences gating and pH sensitivity of I(sK). J Membr Biol 177: 65–79.

29. Chang JS, Wendt T, Qu W, Kong L, Zou YS, et al. (2008) Oxygen deprivation triggers upregulation of early growth response-1 by the receptor for advanced glycation end products. Circ Res 102: 905–913.

30. Jespersen T, Membrez M, Nicolas CS, Pitard B, Staub O, et al. (2007) The KCNQ1 potassium channel is down-regulated by ubiquitylating enzymes of the Nedd4/Nedd4-like family. Cardiovasc Res 74: 64–74.

31. Hondeghem LM (2008) Use and abuse of QT and TRIaD in cardiac safety research: importance of study design and conduct. Eur J Pharmacol 584: 1–9.

32. Jespersen T, Grunnet M, Olesen SP (2005) The KCNQ1 potassium channel: from gene to physiological function. Physiology (Bethesda) 20: 408–416.

33. Morales C, Gonzalez GE, Rodriguez M, Bertolasi CA, Gelpi RJ (2002) Histopathologic time course of myocardial infarct in rabbit hearts. Cardiovasc Pathol 11: 339–345.

34. Franz MR (1991) Method and theory of monophasic action potential recording. Prog Cardiovasc Dis 33: 347–368.

35. Walker MJA (1988) The lambeth conventions: guidelines for the study of arrhythmias in ischaemia, infarction, and reperfusion. Cardiovasc Res. pp 447–455.

36. Guerard NC, Traebert M, Suter W, Dumotier BM (2008) Selective block of IKs plays a significant role in MAP triangulation induced by IKr block in isolated rabbit heart. J Pharmacol Toxicol Methods 58: 32–40.

37. Lynch JJ, Jr., Houle MS, Stump GL, Wallace AA, Gilberto DB, et al. (1999) Antiarrhythmic efficacy of selective blockade of the cardiac slowly activating delayed rectifier current, I(Ks), in canine models of malignant ischemic ventricular arrhythmia. Circulation 100: 1917–1922.

38. Salataa JJ, Selnickb HG, Lynch JJ, Jr. (2004) Pharmacological modulation of I(Ks): potential for antiarrhythmic therapy. Curr Med Chem 11: 29–44.

39. Rose J, Armoundas AA, Tian Y, DiSilvestre D, Burysek M, et al. (2005) Molecular correlates of altered expression of potassium currents in failing rabbit myocardium. Am J Physiol Heart Circ Physiol 288: H2077–2087.

40. Ramakers C, Vos MA, Doevendans PA, Schoenmakers M, Wu YS, et al. (2003) Coordinated down-regulation of KCNQ1 and KCNE1 expression contributes to reduction of I(Ks) in canine hypertrophied hearts. Cardiovasc Res 57: 486–496.

41. Liu XS, Jiang M, Zhang M, Tang D, Clemo HF, et al. (2007) Electrical remodeling in a canine model of ischemic cardiomyopathy. Am J Physiol Heart Circ Physiol 292: H560–571.

3

Age and Ovariectomy Abolish Beneficial Effects of Female Sex on Rat Ventricular Myocytes Exposed to Simulated Ischemia and Reperfusion

Jenna L. Ross[1], Susan E. Howlett[1,2]*

1 Department of Pharmacology, Dalhousie University, Halifax, Nova Scotia, Canada, 2 Division of Geriatric Medicine, Dalhousie University, Halifax, Nova Scotia, Canada

Abstract

Sex differences in responses to myocardial ischemia have been described, but whether cardiomyocyte function is influenced by sex in the setting of ischemia and reperfusion has not been elucidated. This study compared contractions and intracellular Ca^{2+} in isolated ventricular myocytes exposed to ischemia and reperfusion. Cells were isolated from anesthetized 3-month-old male and female Fischer 344 rats, paced at 4 Hz (37°C), exposed to simulated ischemia (20 mins) and reperfused. Cell shortening (edge detector) and intracellular Ca^{2+} (fura-2) were measured simultaneously. Cell viability was assessed with Trypan blue. Ischemia reduced peak contractions and increased Ca^{2+} levels equally in myocytes from both sexes. However, contraction amplitudes were reduced in reperfusion in male myocytes, while contractions recovered to exceed control levels in females (62.6±5.1 vs. 140.1±15.8%; p<0.05). Only 60% of male myocytes excluded trypan blue dye after ischemia and reperfusion, while all female cardiomyocytes excluded the dye (p<0.05). Parallel experiments were conducted in myocytes from ~24-month-old female rats or 5–6-month-old rats that had an ovariectomy at 3–4 weeks of age. Beneficial effects of female sex on myocyte viability and contractile dysfunction in reperfusion were abolished in cells from 24-month-old females. Aged female myocytes also exhibited elevated intracellular Ca^{2+} and alternans in ischemia. Cells from ovariectomized rats displayed increased Ca^{2+} transients and spontaneous activity in ischemia compared to sham-operated controls. None of the myocytes from ovariectomized rats were viable after 15 minutes of ischemia, while 75% of sham cells remained viable at end of reperfusion (p<0.05). These findings demonstrate that cardiomyocytes from young adult females are more resistant to ischemia and reperfusion injury than cells from males. Age and OVX abolish these beneficial effects and induce Ca^{2+} dysregulation at the level of the cardiomyocyte. Thus, beneficial effects of estrogen in ischemia and reperfusion are mediated, in part, by effects on cardiomyocytes.

Editor: Hiranmoy Das, Ohio State University Medical Center, United States of America

Funding: This study was supported in part by grants from the Canadian Institutes for Health Research (grant # MOP 97973; http://www.cihr-irsc.gc.ca/e/193.html), the Nova Scotia Health Research Foundation (http://www.nshrf.ca/) and the Heart and Stroke Foundations of Nova Scotia and New Brunswick (http://www.hsf.ca/research/en/home). Jenna Ross was supported by a studentship from the Nova Scotia Health Research Foundation. The funders had no role in study design, data collection and analysis, decision to publish, or preparation of the manuscript.

Competing Interests: The authors have declared that no competing interests exist.

* E-mail: susan.howlett@dal.ca

Introduction

There are important sex-related differences in the pathophysiology of many cardiovascular diseases, including ischemic heart disease [1–6]. Clinical studies have established that pre-menopausal women are more resistant to ischemic heart disease than men of a similar age [7], but this female advantage disappears after the onset of menopause [8]. Furthermore, the risk of ischemic heart disease increases following bilateral ovariectomy, especially in women who have not taken exogenous hormone therapy [9]. It is well established that estrogen improves vascular function and reduces atherosclerosis, which may help reduce the risk of ischemic heart disease in younger women [10]. Beneficial effects of estrogen on cardiomyocytes themselves also may contribute, although this has not been extensively investigated [4,11]. However, whether treatment with exogenous hormones is cardioprotective is controversial [12,13], and a better understanding of mechanisms by which estrogen protects the heart in the setting of myocardial ischemia is needed.

Studies in animal models also have provided evidence for sex differences in responses to myocardial ischemia and reperfusion. Experiments in intact hearts from rats and mice have shown that young adult females exhibit better recovery of contractile function and fewer arrhythmias in reperfusion than age-matched males [14–20], although this has not been seen in all studies [21,22]. Improved functional recovery in females is accompanied by smaller infarcts, less lactate dehydrogenase (LDH) release and less inflammatory cytokine production [23–25;17,20]. Female hearts also exhibit less ischemia and reperfusion injury than males under conditions that promote Ca^{2+} loading, such as β-adrenergic stimulation or increased external Ca^{2+} [26,27]. Even when sex differences are not observed in wild type hearts, female hearts show less ischemia and reperfusion injury in transgenic models with enhanced contractility, such as overexpression of Na^+-Ca^{2+} exchanger [28], overexpression of β2-adrenergic receptors [29] or ablation of phospholamban [30]. Together, these observations indicate that ischemia and reperfusion injury is less severe in young adult females when compared to males. However, these studies used intact hearts, where estrogen receptors in both cardiomyocytes and the vasculature may modify responses to ischemia and reperfusion [11]. Whether responses of individual cardiomyocytes to myocardial ischemia is influenced by sex and whether this can help explain the resistance of female hearts to ischemia and reperfusion injury has not been investigated.

We have developed a model of ischemia and reperfusion injury in ventricular myocytes isolated from the hearts of male animals [31–33]. This model uses a simulated "ischemic" Tyrode's solution that mimics features of ischemia such as hypoxia, acidosis, lactate accumulation, hyperkalemia, hypercapnia, and substrate deprivation. When myocytes from male animals are exposed to simulated ischemia they exhibit increased intracellular Ca^{2+} levels, along with post-ischemic contractile dysfunction (stunning) and reduced viability in reperfusion [32–33]. The objectives of this study were to use this model to determine: 1) whether ventricular myocytes isolated from young adult female hearts were resistant to ischemia and reperfusion injury when compared to cells from age-matched males; 2) whether ischemia and reperfusion injury was exacerbated by the aging process in myocytes from aged females; and 3) whether cellular ischemia and reperfusion injury was enhanced by long term reduction in ovarian estrogen induced by ovariectomy (OVX). Contractile function, intracellular Ca^{2+} and cell viability were compared throughout ischemia and reperfusion in ventricular myocytes from 3-month-old rats of both sexes. Some studies also used myocytes from aged (~24-month-old) female rats and myocytes from 5–6-month-old female rats who had undergone a bilateral OVX at 3–4 weeks of age. Our results demonstrated that individual ventricular myocytes from young adult females were significantly more resistant to ischemia and reperfusion injury than cells from age-matched males. This female advantage was abolished by either advanced age or by removal of ovarian estrogen through OVX. These data indicate that beneficial actions of estrogen in myocardial ischemia are mediated, in part, by actions on the myocytes themselves.

Materials and Methods

For full details of Methods, please refer to Appendix S1.

Ethics Statement

Protocols were approved by the Dalhousie University Committee on Laboratory Animals (No. 10-029) and followed Canadian Council on Animal Care Guide to the Care and Use of Experimental Animals (CCAC, Ottawa, ON: Vol, 1, 2nd edition, 1993: Vol. 2, 1984). Sodium pentobarbital anesthesia was used and all efforts were made to reduce suffering.

Myocyte Isolation

Myocytes were isolated from 3 month old male and female Fischer 344 rats, ~24 month old females and from 5–6 month old females after OVX or sham operation at 3–4 weeks. Ventricular myocytes were isolated as described [33]. Briefly, rats were anesthetized with sodium pentobarbital (220 mg/kg, IP). The heart was perfused through the aorta with oxygenated low Ca^{2+} buffer (200 μM) followed by nominally Ca^{2+} free buffer plus collagenase and dispase II (37°C). After digestion, the ventricles were minced, stored in a high K^+ substrate-enriched buffer and filtered before use. OVX was confirmed by uterine atrophy.

Ischemia and Reperfusion

Myocytes were loaded with fura-2 AM as described [33] and superfused at 37°C with normal Tyrode's solution (in mM: 126 NaCl, 20 NaHCO₃, 0.9 NaH₂PO₄, 4 KCl, 0.5 MgSO₄,

1.8 CaCl₂, 5.5 glucose; pH 7.4, 95% O₂, 5% CO₂). Cells were paced at 4 Hz with trains of 20 (3 ms) pulses followed by a 2.5 s delay. The pacing frequency of 4 Hz was chosen to be near the physiological frequency in the rat. The 2.5 s pauses were incorporated in the protocol to observe spontaneous activity if it occurred. Control recordings were made for 15 minutes in normal Tyrode's solution, then cells were exposed ischemic Tyrode's solution for 20 minutes (in mM: 123 NaCl, 6 NaHCO₃, 0.9 NaH₂PO₄, 8 KCl, 0.5 MgSO₄, 20 Na-Lactate, and 1.8 CaCl₂; pH 6.8, 90% N₂, 10% CO₂) [31]. During ischemia, 90% N₂, 10% CO₂ was directed over the experimental chamber to reduce the pO_2 as described previously [34]. Cells were reperfused with normal Tyrode's solution for up to 30 min. Cell that exhibited hypercontracture, sarcolemmal disruption and trypan blue staining were considered not viable [35]. Recordings were made at 5 min intervals throughout the protocol, with an additional recording at 2 min of reperfusion. Time controls were exposed to normal Tyrode's solution for 65 min without ischemia.

Contractions and Ca^{2+} transients were recorded simultaneously as described [33]. Ca^{2+} levels were recorded with a DeltaRam fluorescence recording system (Photon Technology International (PTI), Birmingham, NJ) and data were acquired with Felix32 software (PTI). Fura-2 was excited at 340 and 380 nm and emission was measured at 510 nm (5 msec sampling interval). Unloaded cell shortening was measured (120 Hz) with a video edge detector (Model 105; Crescent Electronics, Sandy, UT) and CCD camera (model TM-640, Pulnix America). The ratio of fluorescence at 340 and 380 nm was converted to Ca^{2+} concentration as described previously [32,33]. Results are accurate over the range of pH values used in this study as reported previously [36] and confirmed in our earlier studies [32,33].

Analyses

Data were analyzed with Clampfit 8.2 software (Molecular Devices). The last three responses in the 20 pulse train were averaged to quantify contractions and Ca^{2+} transients once these responses had reached steady state. The incidence of spontaneous activity (beats that occurred during the 2.5 s pause) was recorded in each experiment. Alternans (alternating pattern of large and small beats during stimulation) were quantified with an alternans ratio (alternans ratio = 1 – S/L, where S = amplitude of small beat and L = amplitude of large beat) [33]. The value of "n" is the number of myocytes used. Statistical analyses were performed with either Sigmaplot 8.1 or Sigmastat 3.1 (Systat Software Inc.). Data other than cell viability and incidence are presented as the mean ± SEM. Cell viability was evaluated with a log rank test. Spontaneous activity was analyzed with a Fisher Exact test. Other analyses used a t-test or a two-way repeated-measures analysis of variance (post-hoc test = Student-Newman-Keuls or Tukey tests). Differences were significant for $p < 0.05$.

Results

Physical Characteristics of Young Adult Male and Female Rats

Selected physical characteristics of young adult male and female rats were compared as shown in Table 1. Males and females were the same age, but the males were 67% heavier than the females (Table 1). Table 1 also shows baseline peak contractions and Ca^{2+} transients recorded from male and female myocytes after 15 minutes of pacing at 4 Hz, just prior to exposure to simulated ischemia and reperfusion. Contractions were normalized to cell length, as we found that cells from females were smaller than cells from males (Table 1). Peak contractions and Ca^{2+} transients were

Table 1. Baseline Characteristics: Experiments with Young Adult and Aged Rats.

Parameter	Young Male (n)	Young Female (n)	Aged Female (n)
Age (days)	90.3±2.9† (15)	93.2±5.0† (13)	744.3±3.7 (11)
Body weight (g)	300.4±6.2 (15)	179.2±3.1*† (13)	330.4±12.8 (11)
Myocyte length (μm)	112.5±3.9 (16)	92.6±3.6*† (12)	121.3±4.7 (12)
Contraction (%)	2.7±0.6 (13)	2.6±0.5 (10)	2.4±0.4 (8)
Ca^{2+} transient (nM)	102.3±7.9 (12)	97.0±7.0 (10)	81.3±6.8 (10)

Values shown are the means ± SEM. The value of "n" shown beside each number in brackets represents the number of animals or myocytes. Values represent peak contractions (expressed as % cell length) and Ca^{2+} transients recorded prior to ischemia in myocytes paced at 4 Hz.
*Denotes significantly different from young male animal $p<0.05$.
†Denotes significantly different from aged female animal, $p<0.05$.

similar in cells from males and females under these experimental conditions (Table 1). Systolic and diastolic Ca^{2+} levels also were similar in all groups (not shown).

Responses of Isolated Ventricular Myocytes to Simulated Ischemia and Reperfusion Differ between the Sexes

To determine whether responses of individual cardiomyocytes to myocardial ischemia were influenced by the sex of the animal, contractions and underlying Ca^{2+} transients were compared throughout ischemia and reperfusion in myocytes from young adult male and female rats. Figure 1A shows Ca^{2+} transients (top) and contractions (bottom) recorded from a male myocyte at selected time points throughout an experiment. Figure 1B–C shows mean peak contractions and Ca^{2+} transients recorded from male myocytes during ischemia and reperfusion compared to responses in time controls. Data were normalized to values recorded after 15 minutes of pacing at 4 Hz to facilitate comparisons between groups. Contractions were essentially abolished by ischemia but recovered with an overshoot immediately upon reperfusion (Figure 1B). However, peak contractions remained smaller than time controls with continued reperfusion (Figure 1B). In contrast, ischemia and reperfusion had no effect on Ca^{2+} transients throughout the experiment (Figure 1C). Ischemia caused a marked increase in diastolic Ca^{2+} and this recovered upon reperfusion (Figure 1D). Reperfusion also was associated with a modest degree of hypercontracture (Figure 1E). There were no signs of spontaneous activity in ischemia or reperfusion in this group (not shown). However, Trypan blue staining revealed that 38% of male myocytes were trypan blue positive by the end of the reperfusion period. Thus, male myocytes exposed to ischemia exhibited increased diastolic Ca^{2+}, along with post-ischemic contractile dysfunction (stunning) and reduced viability in reperfusion.

Parallel ischemia and reperfusion experiments were then performed in myocytes from young adult females. Figure 2A shows representative Ca^{2+} transients (top) and contractions (bottom) in ventricular myocytes from female rats. Mean data show that contractions decreased significantly in ischemia, but recovered upon reperfusion and exceeded time controls throughout reperfusion (Figure 2B). Peak Ca^{2+} transients declined in ischemia and early reperfusion in the female group compared to time control cells (Figure 2C). Diastolic Ca^{2+} levels rose in ischemia and recovered in reperfusion (Figure 2D). Female cells

initially exhibited hypercontracture in reperfusion, but this quickly recovered with continued reperfusion (Figure 2E). Spontaneous activity did not occur in either ischemia or reperfusion (not shown). Interestingly, all myocytes from young female rats survived exposure to ischemia and reperfusion.

To determine whether responses to ischemia and reperfusion differed significantly between the sexes, contractions and underlying Ca^{2+} transients were directly compared as shown in Figure 3. Peak contractions were reduced by ischemia to a similar degree in cells from males and females (Figure 3A). However, while peak contractions were reduced throughout most of reperfusion in male myocytes, contractions in female cardiomyocytes actually fully recovered and were significantly larger than males in reperfusion (Figure 3A). Peak Ca^{2+} transients (Figure 3B) and diastolic Ca^{2+} levels (Figure 3C) were similar in male and female myocytes during ischemia and reperfusion, and the degree of hypercontracture in reperfusion did not differ between the two groups (Figure 3D). In contrast, exposure to Trypan blue revealed a significant difference in cell viability between the sexes. Although all myocytes in the young female group excluded trypan blue after exposure to ischemia and reperfusion, cell viability declined in reperfusion in the young male group and this sex difference was statistically significant ($p<0.05$). Taken together, these findings showed that myocytes from young adult females were resistant to ischemia and reperfusion injury, while myocytes from young adult males were not.

Aging Disrupts Cardiomyocyte Ca^{2+} Handling and Exacerbates Ischemia and Reperfusion Injury in Female Myocytes

The next series of experiments determined whether ischemia and reperfusion injury in myocytes from female rats was exacerbated by the aging process. Baseline physical characteristics of the aged rats are compared to the younger animals in Table 1. The aged female rats were significantly older and heavier than the young adult females (Table 1). Interestingly, ventricular myocytes from aged females were 30% longer than myocytes from younger females (Table 1). However, peak contractions and Ca^{2+} transients were similar in cells from young and aged females prior to exposure to ischemia and reperfusion (Table 1).

To determine whether ischemia and reperfusion injury in myocytes from female rats was exacerbated by aging, responses were compared in myocytes from young adult and aged female rats. Ischemia reduced peak contractions in both groups (Figure 4A). However, while contractions fully recovered upon reperfusion in the young group, contractions did not fully recover in the aged group (Figure 4A). Ca^{2+} transients were similar during most of ischemia and reperfusion in both groups (Figure 4B). Interestingly, aging augmented the rise in diastolic Ca^{2+} that occurred in ischemia (Figure 4C). The degree of hypercontracture in reperfusion was similar in the two groups (Figure 4D). However, even though all young female myocytes remained viable throughout ischemia and reperfusion, almost 30% of the aged myocytes were trypan blue positive by the end of reperfusion ($p<0.05$; Figure 4E). These results show that aging promoted Ca^{2+} loading in ischemia and abolished the beneficial effect of female sex on cell viability and contractile function in reperfusion.

As aging was associated with increased Ca^{2+} loading in ischemia, this could promote abnormal activity and spontaneous Ca^{2+} release in ischemia and reperfusion. There was no evidence of spontaneous activity in ischemia or reperfusion in myocytes from aged rats, as in the younger adult animals (data not shown). However, ischemia did induce mechanical and Ca^{2+} transient alternans in myocytes from aged female rats, but not in cell from

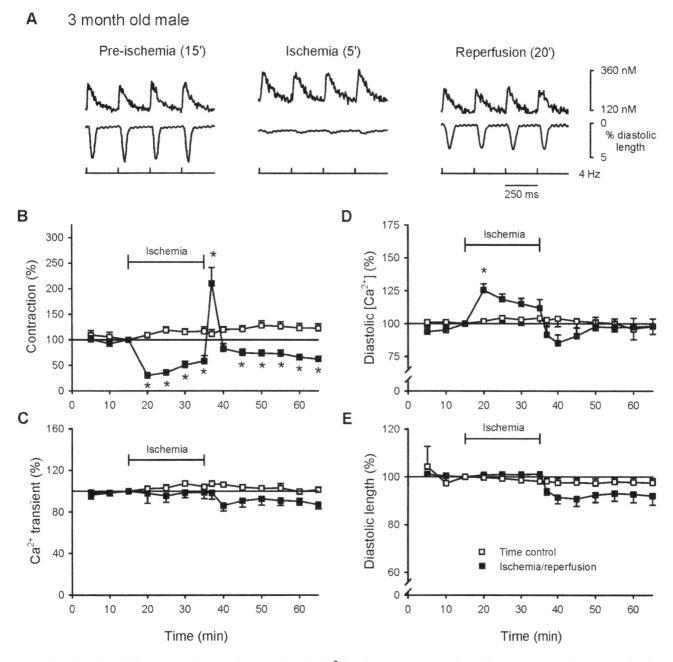

Figure 1. Ischemia inhibited contractions, enhanced diastolic Ca^{2+} loading, and promoted post-ischemic contractile dysfunction in myocytes from young adult male rats. Cells were paced at a frequency of 4 Hz for 15 minutes in normal Tyrode's buffer, exposed to simulated ischemia for 20 minutes and reperfused with normal Tyrode's for 30 minutes (filled squares). Time control cells were paced for the same length of time in normal Tyrode's buffer only (open squares). **A.** Representative examples of Ca^{2+} transients (top) and contractions (bottom) recorded prior to ischemia, after 5 minutes of exposure to ischemia and after 20 minutes of reperfusion. **B.** Mean ($\pm$ SEM) peak contractions recorded at 5 minute intervals throughout the experimental protocol. **C.** Mean amplitudes of Ca^{2+} transients recorded during these experiments. Mean levels of diastolic Ca^{2+} (**D**) and diastolic cell length (**E**) recorded throughout the protocol. In all cases, responses were normalized to values recorded after 15 minutes of stimulation, prior to exposure to ischemia. The * denotes significantly different from time control (p<0.05; n = 5 time control cells and 12 cells exposed to ischemia and reperfusion).

the younger female animals (Figure 5A). These responses were quantified with an alternans ratio as described in the methods section. Results showed mechanical (Figure 5B) and Ca^{2+} transient alternans ratios (Figure 5C) were increased dramatically in aged myocytes when compared to the younger group. Together, these results show that aging disrupted cardiomyocyte Ca^{2+} handling in myocytes from female hearts.

OVX Exacerbated Detrimental Effects of Ischemia and Reperfusion in Isolated Ventricular Myocytes

To determine whether OVX would augment ischemia and reperfusion injury at the cellular level, responses of cardiomyocytes from sham-operated and OVX female rats were compared throughout ischemia and reperfusion. Physical characteristics of the sham-operated and OVX rats used in this study are shown in

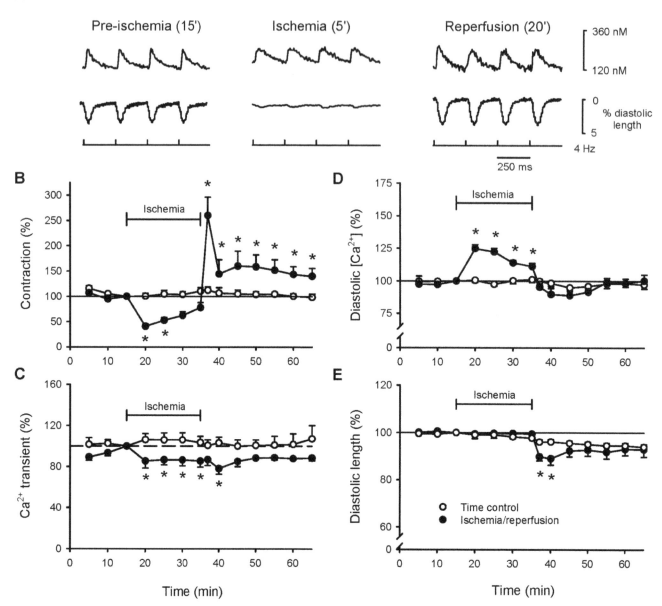

Figure 2. In contrast to males, ischemia inhibited Ca^{2+} transients and promoted recovery of contractile function in reperfusion in myocytes from young adult female rats. Myocytes were stimulated at 4 Hz for 15 minutes, exposed to ischemia for 20 minutes and reperfused for 30 minutes (filled circles). Cells that served as time controls were paced for 65 minutes without exposure to ischemia (open circles). **A.** Examples of Ca^{2+} transients (top) and contractions (bottom) recorded from female myocytes at specific times during an experiment. **B.** Mean amplitudes of contractions in females cells exposed to ischemia and reperfusion compared to time controls. **C.** Average amplitudes of Ca^{2+} transients recorded throughout the experiment. Mean levels of diastolic Ca^{2+} (**D**) and diastolic cell length (**E**) recorded throughout the experimental protocol. Responses were normalized to values recorded after 15 minutes of stimulation. The * denotes significantly different from time control (p<0.05; n = 9 time control cells and 10 cells exposed to ischemia and reperfusion).

Table 2. The sham and OVX rats were similar in age, but OVX rats were almost 30% heavier (Table 2). OVX caused significant uterine atrophy in all animals, as shown by a striking decrease in uterine wet weight (Table 2). Uterine dry weights were also significantly lower in OVX animals (values decreased from 87.9±7.5 mg in sham to 8.2±1.3 mg in OVX; p<0.05). Interestingly, peak contractions and Ca^{2+} transients were larger in cells from OVX rats when compared sham-operated controls prior to exposure to ischemia and reperfusion (Table 2). OVX

also increased diastolic Ca^{2+} under basal conditions (values increased from 105.0±5.0 in sham to 124.6±6.0 nM in OVX; p<0.05).

To determine whether OVX modified ischemia and reperfusion injury, responses were compared in myocytes from sham and OVX rats. Note that none of the OVX myocytes were viable after 15 minutes of ischemia (Figure 6A–D, arrows), so effects late in the protocol were not available. While contractions declined in ischemia in sham controls, contractions remained large in the

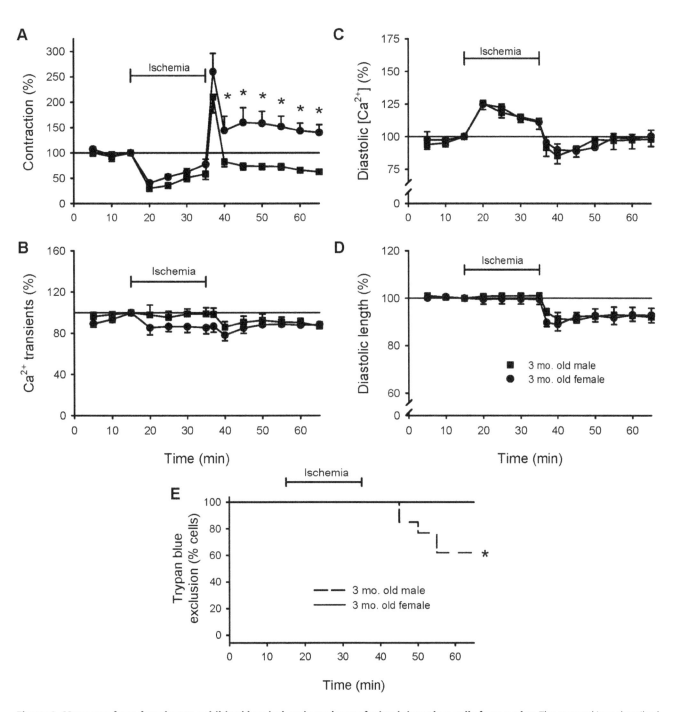

Figure 3. Myocytes from female rats exhibited less ischemia and reperfusion injury than cells from males. The protocol is as described in the legends to Figures 1 and 2. **A.** Mean magnitudes of contractions in male (filled squares) and female (filled circles) myocytes exposed to ischemia and reperfusion. **B.** Mean peak Ca^{2+} transients recorded from male and female myocytes at 5 minute intervals throughout exposure to ischemia and reperfusion. Average levels of diastolic Ca^{2+} (**C**) and resting myocyte length (**D**) recorded throughout the experimental protocol in cells from males and females. In all cases, data were normalized to values recorded after 15 minutes of stimulation. **E.** Survival curves illustrating the viability of male (dashed line) and female (solid line) cells at 5 minute intervals throughout the experimental protocol. The * denotes significantly different from young adult male value ($p < 0.05$; n = 12 male cells and 10 female cells).

initial ischemic period in OVX cells (Figure 6A). Ca^{2+} transients also increased in ischemia in OVX cells, but not in sham controls (Figure 6B). However, the increase in diastolic Ca^{2+} levels in ischemia was similar in sham and OVX myocytes (Figure 6C) and diastolic length did not differ between the two groups (Figure 6D). Figure 6E shows that OVX dramatically reduced the ability of

cardiomyocytes to tolerate ischemia. While most sham myocytes remained viable following exposure to ischemia and reperfusion, none of the OVX myocytes remained viable beyond 15 minutes of ischemia and this difference was statistically significant ($p < 0.05$). Furthermore, 71% of OVX myocytes showed spontaneous Ca^{2+} release and contractions in ischemia, as shown in the example in

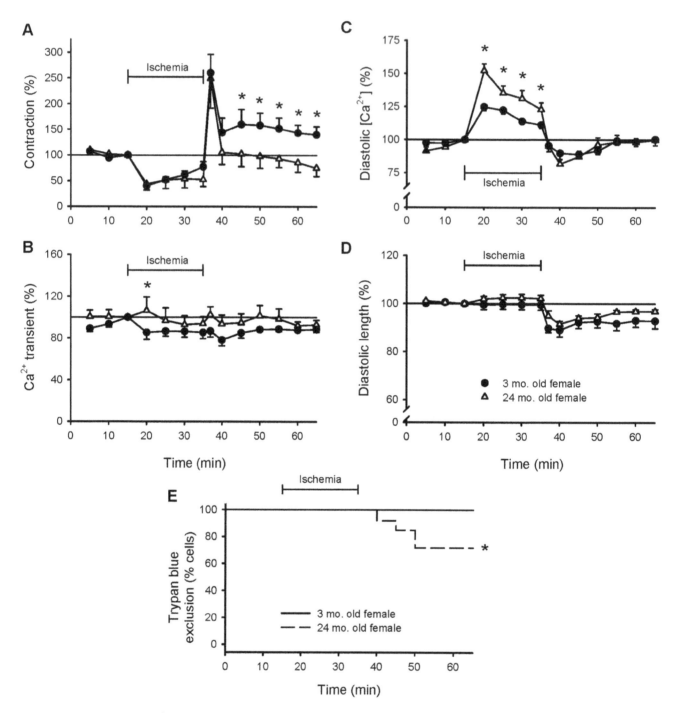

Figure 4. Aging promoted Ca^{2+} accumulation in ischemia and abolished beneficial effects of female sex on contractile function and cell viability. The experimental protocol is described in the legends to Figures 1 and 2. **A.** Mean amplitudes of contractions in young adult (filled circles) and aged female (open triangles) cells throughout exposure to simulated ischemia and reperfusion. **B.** Average peak Ca^{2+} transients recorded from young adult and aged female myocytes at 5 minute intervals throughout the experimental protocol. Mean levels of diastolic Ca^{2+} (**C**) and resting myocyte length (**D**) recorded at 5 minute intervals during the experiments in cells from young adult and aged females. All data were normalized to values recorded after 15 minutes of stimulation in the absence of ischemia. **E.** Survival curves illustrating the viability of young adult (solid line) and aged female (dashed line) cells reported at 5 minute intervals throughout the experiment. The * denotes significantly different from young adult female value (p<0.05; n = 10 young adult female cells and 8 aged female cells).

Figure 7A. By contrast, spontaneous activity did not occur in myocytes from sham-operated controls (Figure 7B). These results show that OVX disrupted Ca^{2+} homeostasis and abolished the beneficial effects of female sex on cell viability in individual cardiomyocytes.

Discussion

This study determined whether ventricular myocytes from young adult females were more resistant to ischemia and reperfusion injury than cells from males and whether ischemia

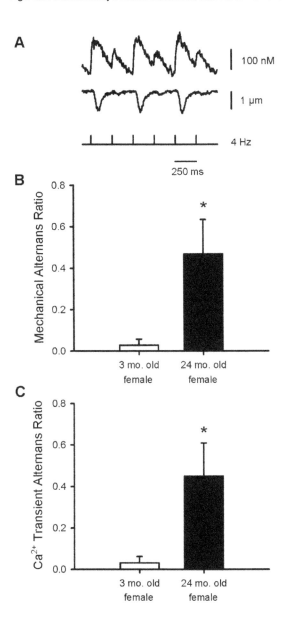

A.

| 100 nM

| 1 μm

4 Hz

250 ms

B

Mechanical Alternans Ratio

*

3 mo. old female   24 mo. old female

C

Ca²⁺ Transient Alternans Ratio

*

3 mo. old female   24 mo. old female

Figure 5. Aging was associated with the appearance of mechanical and Ca²⁺ transient alternans in ischemia in myocytes from female rats. A. Representative example of Ca²⁺ transient alternans (top) and mechanical alternans (bottom) ratios recorded in an aged female myocyte during ischemia. The occurrence of alternans was quantified as an alternans ratio with the following formula: alternans ratio = 1 - S/L, where S = the amplitude of the small beat and L = the amplitude of the large beat. Both the mechanical alternans ratio (**B**) and the Ca²⁺ transient alternans ratio (**C**) were significantly higher in myocytes from aged females than in young adult females. The * denotes significantly different from young adult female value (p<0.05; n = 10 young adult female cells and 7 aged female cells).

Table 2. Baseline Characteristics: Experiments with Sham-operated and OVX Female Rats.

Parameter	Sham-operated (n)	OVX (n)
Age (days)	165.2±7.4 (11)	179.8±9.3 (6)
Body weight (g)	182.0±5.7 (11)	234.3±7.0* (6)
Uterine wet weight (g)	0.460±0.04 (11)	0.039±0.01* (6)
Myocyte length (μm)	88.91±2.4 (7)	83.4±1.6 (7)
Contraction (%)	2.4±0.2 (7)	4.3±0.7* (7)
Ca²⁺ transient (nM)	92.5±4.7 (7)	111.0±5.1* (7)

Values shown are the means ± SEM. The value of "n" shown beside each number in brackets represents the number of animals or myocytes. Values represent peak contractions and Ca²⁺ transients (expressed as % resting cell length) recorded prior to ischemia in myocytes paced at 4 Hz.
*Denotes significantly different from sham-operated control animal, p<0.05.

reperfusion. Interestingly, age abolished the beneficial effects of female sex on cell viability and contractile function. Age also augmented the rise in intracellular Ca²⁺ levels in ischemia and this was associated with a marked increase in the occurrence of alternans. OVX also modified myocyte responses to ischemia and reperfusion. Contractions and Ca²⁺ transients were larger in cells from OVX females than in cells from sham controls in the initial ischemic period and this was accompanied by an increase in the incidence of spontaneous activity. Furthermore, none of the myocytes from OVX animals were viable by 15 minutes of ischemia. Thus, ventricular myocytes from young adult males and aged or OVX females are more susceptible to injury following ischemia and reperfusion than cells from young adult females.

To our knowledge, this is the first study to demonstrate sex differences in the responses of individual ventricular myocytes to ischemia and reperfusion injury. While myocytes from male rats exhibited a marked reduction in contractile function throughout reperfusion, cells from females recovered fully and actually exceeded values recorded in time control cells. Previous studies in Langendorff-perfused hearts have shown that contractile function recovers more fully in reperfusion in females than in males [14,16–20], although this has not been seen in all studies [22]. However, in intact hearts effects of estrogen on both the myocardium and the vasculature could contribute to cardioprotection in the setting of myocardial ischemia and reperfusion [11]. Our study is important as it shows that the improvement in recovery of myocardial contractile function in reperfusion in females is attributable, at least in part, to an increase in the ability of individual ventricular myocytes to contract.

As cardiac contractions are proportional to the magnitude of the Ca²⁺ transient [37], one explanation for the increased contractions in female myocytes during reperfusion is an increase in the size of the Ca²⁺ transient. However, our results show that this is not the case. Peak Ca²⁺ transients were not affected by ischemia and reperfusion. This result provides evidence that myofilament Ca²⁺ sensitivity increases in reperfusion in myocytes from young adult females. This contrasts with our observations in males, where reperfusion was associated with normal Ca²⁺ transients and a sustained reduction in peak contractions as shown previously [32,33]. This post-ischemic decrease in contractile function (also called stunning) is thought to be due, at least in part, to degradation of troponin I, which leads to a reduction in myofilament Ca²⁺ sensitivity [38]. Our study shows that myocytes from young females do not exhibit stunning following myocardial

and reperfusion injury in female myocytes was exacerbated by aging or by long term OVX. Results showed that responses of isolated myocytes to ischemia and reperfusion differed between the sexes. While ischemia reduced peak contractions and increased intracellular Ca²⁺ equally in myocytes from males and females, cells from males exhibited a profound reduction in post-ischemic contractile function but cells from females did not. In addition, all female myocytes remained viable during ischemia and reperfusion, but 38% of male myocytes were trypan blue positive in

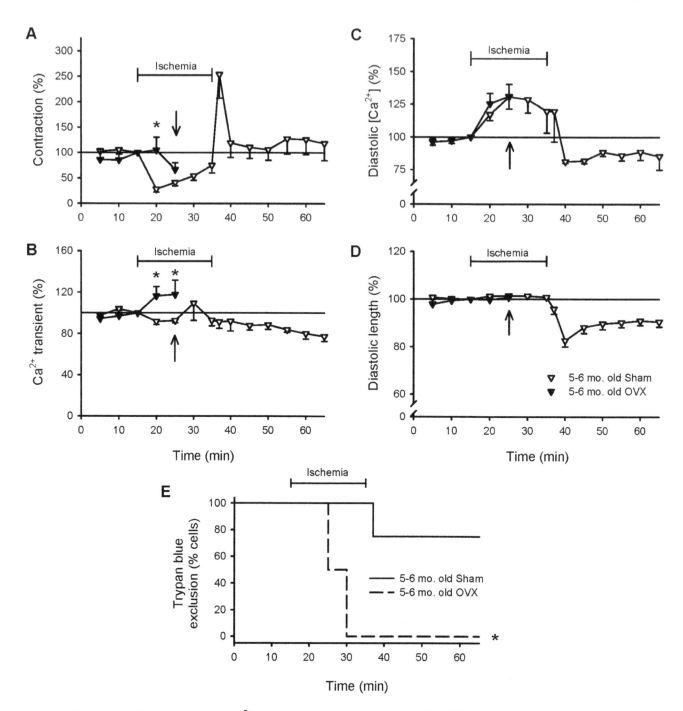

Figure 6. OVX increased contractions and Ca²⁺ transients in ischemia and none of the OVX myocytes were viable after 15 minutes of ischemia. The experimental protocol is described in the legends to Figures 1 and 2. **A**. Mean peak contractions recorded in myocytes from sham-operated (open inverted triangles) and OVX (filled inverted triangles) female rats throughout the protocol. The arrow indicates the last time point where OVX data could be collected because all OVX myocytes were trypan blue positive after 15 minutes of ischemia. **B**. Mean peak Ca²⁺ transients in sham and OVX myocytes recorded throughout the experiment. The average levels of diastolic Ca²⁺ (**C**) and diastolic cell length (**D**) in cells from sham and OVX females. Data were normalized to values recorded after 15 minutes of stimulation. **E**. Survival curves illustrating the viability of sham (solid line) and OVX female (dashed line) cells throughout the experiment. The * denotes significantly different from sham-operated control values ($p<0.05$; n = 7 sham cells and 7 OVX cells).

ischemia and suggest that the underlying mechanism is an increase in myofilament Ca²⁺ sensitivity in reperfusion.

We also found that myocytes from young female were resistant to ischemia and reperfusion injury. Although 38% of the male myocytes were trypan blue positive in reperfusion, all the myocytes

from 3 month-old female hearts resisted trypan blue stained throughout ischemia and reperfusion. This intrinsic resistance of myocytes to ischemia and reperfusion injury can explain the smaller infarcts and lower LDH release reported in female hearts following ischemia and reperfusion [17,20,23–25]. One mecha-

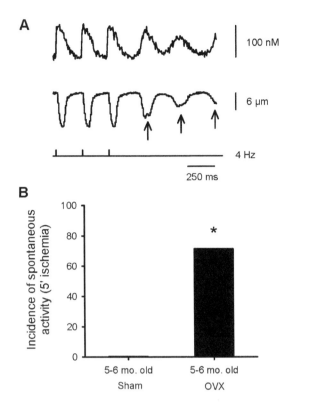

Figure 7. OVX promoted spontaneous contractions and Ca²⁺ transients in ischemia when compared to sham-operated controls. Cells were paced with trains of 20 pulses, delivered at a frequency of 4 Hz, followed by a 2.5 seconds delay to observe spontaneous activity. **A.** Representative examples of stimulated and spontaneous Ca²⁺ transients (top) and contractions (bottom) recorded in an OVX female myocyte after 5 minutes of exposure to ischemia. The first three beats are stimulated beats and the spontaneous responses are shown by the arrows. **B.** Spontaneous activity (Ca²⁺ transients and contractions) occurred in 71.4% of OVX cells. In contrast, spontaneous activity was not observed in myocytes from sham-operated animals. The * denotes significantly different from values in sham-operated females (p<0.05; n = 7 sham cells and 7 OVX cells).

nism that has been implicated in the loss of viability following ischemia and reperfusion is intracellular Ca²⁺ overload [39]. However, we found that intracellular Ca²⁺ levels rose during ischemia and declined in reperfusion to the same extent in myocytes from males and females. Thus, an important finding in our study is that the resistance of female myocytes to ischemia and reperfusion injury is not linked to sex differences in intracellular Ca²⁺ loading, because intracellular Ca²⁺ levels are similar in the two groups. Sex differences in other pathways may explain the resistance of female myocytes to ischemia and reperfusion injury. For example, sex differences in activation of apoptotic pathways and/or in the generation and regulation of reactive oxygen species may play a role in cardioprotection in the setting of ischemia and reperfusion [23,40,41].

To our knowledge, this is the first study to examine the impact of ischemia and reperfusion on Ca²⁺ homeostasis and contractile function in ventricular myocytes from aged female animals. A key finding in the present study was that age abolished beneficial effects of female sex on cell viability and contractile function in reperfusion. We found that, unlike young adult female cells, myocytes from 24 month-old females exhibited reduced cell viability and post-ischemic contractile dysfunction with no change

in peak Ca²⁺ transients in reperfusion. Previous studies reported that recovery of contractile function is impaired in aged female hearts compared to younger hearts [20,42,43]. Our data demonstrate that post-ischemic contractile in the aging female heart is due contractile dysfunction at the level of the individual myocytes. Furthermore, the data presented here demonstrate that contractile dysfunction was not due to a decrease in size of the Ca²⁺ transient available to activate contraction. Thus, the aging process abolishes beneficial effects of female sex on these indices of myocardial damage.

Aging also resulted in diastolic Ca²⁺ accumulation and the development of alternans in ischemia in female myocytes, as reported in myocytes from aged male rats [33]. Elevated levels of intracellular Ca²⁺ are implicated in many detrimental effects of ischemia and reperfusion [39]. Our observation that aged female cells accumulate substantially more Ca²⁺ in ischemia than younger cells provides a mechanism that explains the increased sensitivity of aged female hearts to ischemia and reperfusion injury [20,42,42]. The age-related decrease in activity and expression of sarco(endo)plasmic reticulum (SR) Ca²⁺-ATPase (SERCA) that has been well documented in aging male hearts [44] may also occur in aging female hearts. This would impair SR Ca²⁺ sequestration and disrupt intracellular Ca²⁺ regulation as shown in this study and previously [45]. Inhibition of SERCA in young adult hearts gives rise to cellular alternans [46], so reduced SERCA activity also may underlie the occurrence of alternans in the aging female heart.

Previous studies in rats have shown that serum estradiol levels decline by more than 60% between the ages of 3 mos and 14 mos [47,48]. This suggests that cardioprotective effects of female sex may decline with age in response to a reduction in circulating estradiol levels. Indeed, we found that removal of ovarian estrogen through OVX exacerbated adverse effects of ischemia. In contrast to sham cells, contractions showed little decline in cells from OVX animals during the initial ischemic period. Furthermore, peak Ca²⁺ transients, which were larger than sham even prior to ischemia as shown in the present study and previously [49–53], actually increased significantly upon exposure to ischemia. Ischemia also increased the incidence of spontaneous Ca²⁺ transients and contractions, and this was followed by the uptake of trypan blue dye within 15 minutes of exposure to ischemia. The larger Ca²⁺ transients and spontaneous Ca²⁺ release in observed in OVX cells in ischemia suggests that SR Ca²⁺ load is much higher in OVX myocytes than in sham controls. Indeed, we and others have shown that SR Ca²⁺ load is elevated by OVX even in the absence of ischemia [50,53]. The present study indicates that OVX promotes Ca²⁺ overload in ischemia and leads to spontaneous release of SR Ca²⁺ and ultimately a loss of cell viability.

Our results indicate that intracellular Ca²⁺ dysregulation is a major mechanism that contributes to the increased sensitivity of OVX hearts to ischemia and reperfusion injury [15,23,25,54]. Interestingly, Ca²⁺ dysregulation in OVX myocytes may help explain the increased propensity for reperfusion arrhythmias observed in aromatase knockout mice, which exhibit both estrogen suppression and testosterone elevation [14]. However, chronic aromatase deficiency also has been shown to improve cardiac functional performance and limit acute cardiomyocyte injury in reperfusion [14]. Thus, suppression of androgen-to-estrogen conversion at the tissue level also may offer inotropic benefit in the setting of myocardial ischemia and reperfusion.

In the present study, ovaries were removed at 3–4 weeks of age but the rats were 5–6 months of age when we examined responses to ischemia and reperfusion. This resulted in an OVX model characterized by long term estrogen withdrawal and the lack of exposure of the heart to normal pubertal systemic estrogen modeling. It is important to note that this model differs from the more gradual reduction in ovarian steroids that would be observed during menopause. This model also may result in hearts that are particularly susceptible to ischemia and reperfusion damage. Additional experiments with other time frames for estrogen deprivation could be explored in the future to address these issues. It is also important to note that the present study examined only acute responses of cardiomyocytes to ischemia and reperfusion. The impact of ovarian estrogen suppression on other factors that may contribute to chronic post-ischemic heart failure also would be interesting to evaluate.

We also found that both aging and OVX caused increased a large increase in body weight when compared to younger female rats. This increase in body weight would be expected to increase systemic volume load and this could promote cardiomyocyte hypertrophy. Indeed, increased volume load may contribute to the increase in cardiomyocyte length we observed in the aged group. However, cardiomyocyte length was not affected by OVX, which suggests that increased volume load does not lead to cellular hypertrophy in OVX hearts, at least over the time frame of our investigation. It is likely that an increase in adipose tissue contributes to the increase in body weight observed in aged and OVX animals, so adipose tissue is a potential non-gonadal source of estrogen in our study [55]. Nonetheless, estrogen is likely low in these models, as studies have shown that estrogen levels decline with age in the rat model [47,48] and remain lower in OVX rats than in sham animals up to 6 months after OVX [56].

Peak contractions, Ca^{2+} transients, and cell length recorded prior to exposure to ischemia and reperfusion also were examined in this study. Basal contractions and Ca^{2+} transients were larger in myocytes from OVX rats compared to sham-operated controls, as we and others have previously reported [49–53]. Basal contractions and Ca^{2+} transients also did not decline with age in female rats and aged myocytes were hypertrophied, as reported in our previous study [57]. However, the present study showed that basal contractions and Ca^{2+} transients were similar in amplitude in myocytes from 3 month-old male and female rats, when cells were

paced at 4 Hz in 1.8 mM Ca^{2+} buffer. Previous studies that have reported smaller contractions and Ca^{2+} transients in female rat cells when compared to males used slower pacing frequencies and/or lower external Ca^{2+} concentrations [58–60]. These observations suggest that sex differences in contractile function may be more prominent when Ca^{2+} loading is reduced by low pacing frequencies and/or reduced external Ca^{2+} concentrations.

In summary, the results of our study show that resistance to myocardial ischemia and reperfusion injury is present in individual ventricular myocytes from young female animals. Our study also showed that this was abolished by either advanced age or by long term removal of ovarian estrogen. Aging and OVX both caused dramatic changes in intracellular Ca^{2+} homeostasis in individual cardiac myocytes exposed to simulated ischemia. Intracellular Ca^{2+} dysregulation plays an important role in cardiovascular diseases, so our data indicate that beneficial actions of estrogen in the setting of myocardial ischemia are mediated, at least in part, by actions on Ca^{2+} handling mechanisms in the myocytes themselves. Sex hormone-regulated pathways within cardiac myocytes may be a fruitful area to explore for the identification of new targets for the treatment of ischemic heart disease in men and women.

Acknowledgments

The authors express their appreciation for excellent technical assistance provided by Dr. Jiequan Zhu, Steve Foster, Cindy Mapplebeck and Peter Nicholl. The authors also are very grateful to the late Dr. Gregory Ferrier, who was Jenna Ross's supervisor prior to his death.

Author Contributions

Conceived and designed the experiments: JLR SEH. Performed the experiments: JLR. Analyzed the data: JLR SEH. Contributed reagents/materials/analysis tools: SEH. Wrote the paper: JLR SEH.

References

1. Czubryt MP, Espira L, Lamoureux L, Abrenica B (2006) The role of sex in cardiac function and disease. Can J Physiol Pharmacol 84: 93–109.
2. Regitz-Zagrosek V (2006) Therapeutic implications of the gender-specific aspects of cardiovascular disease. Nat Rev Drug Discov 5: 425–438.
3. Murphy E, Steenbergen C (2007) Gender-based differences in mechanisms of protection in myocardial ischemia-reperfusion injury. Cardiovasc Res 75: 478–486.
4. Booth EA, Lucchesi BR (2008) Estrogen-mediated protection in myocardial ischemia-reperfusion injury. Cardiovasc Toxicol 8: 101–113.
5. Luczak ED, Leinwand LA (2009) Sex-based cardiac physiology. Annu Rev Physiol 71: 1–18.
6. Ostadal B, Netuka I, Maly J, Besik J, Ostadalova I (2009) Gender differences in cardiac ischemic injury and protection–experimental aspects. Exp Biol Med (Maywood) 234: 1011–1019.
7. Lloyd-Jones DM, Larson MG, Beiser A, Levy D (1999) Lifetime risk of developing coronary heart disease. Lancet 353: 89–92.
8. Jousilahti P, Vartiainen E, Tuomilehto J, Puska, P (1999) Sex, age, cardiovascular risk factors, and coronary heart disease: a prospective follow-up study of 14 786 middle-aged men and women in Finland. Circulation 99: 1165–1172.
9. Allison MA, Manson JE, Langer RD, Carr JJ, Rossouw JE, et al. (2008) Women's Health Initiative and Women's Health Initiative Coronary Artery Calcium Study Investigators. Oophorectomy, hormone therapy, and subclinical coronary artery disease in women with hysterectomy: the Women's Health Initiative coronary artery calcium study. Menopause 15: 639–647.
10. Blum A, Blum N (2009) Coronary artery disease: Are men and women created equal? Gend Med 6: 410–418.
11. Murphy E (2011) Estrogen signaling and cardiovascular disease. Circ Res 109: 687–696.
12. Harman SM (2006) Estrogen replacement in menopausal women: recent and current prospective studies, the WHI and the KEEPS. Gend Med 3: 254–269.
13. Rossouw JE, Anderson GL, Prentice RL, LaCroix AZ, Kooperberg C, et al. (2002) Writing Group for the Women's Health Initiative Investigators. Risks and benefits of estrogen plus progestin in healthy postmenopausal women: principal results From the Women's Health Initiative randomized controlled trial. JAMA 288: 321–333.
14. Bell JR, Porrello ER, Huggins CE, Harrap SB, Delbridge LM (2008) The intrinsic resistance of female hearts to an ischemic insult is abrogated in primary cardiac hypertrophy. Am J Physiol Heart Circ Physiol 294: H1514–H1522.
15. Lujan HL, Dicarlo SE (2008) Sex differences to myocardial ischemia and β-adrenergic receptor blockade in conscious rats. Am J Physiol 294: H1523–H1529.
16. Thorp DB, Haist JV, Leppard J, Milne KJ, Karmazyn M, et al. (2007) Exercise training improves myocardial tolerance to ischemia in male but not in female rats. Am J Physiol 293: R363–R371.
17. Wang M, Tsai BM, Kher A, Baker LB, Wairiuko GM, et al. (2005) Role of endogenous testosterone in myocardial proinflammatory and proapoptotic signaling after acute ischemia-reperfusion. Am J Physiol 288: H221–H226.
18. Wang M, Crisostomo PR, Markel T, Wang Y, Lillemoe KD, et al. (2008) Estrogen receptor beta mediates acute myocardial protection following ischemia. Surgery 144: 233–238.
19. Wang M, Wang Y, Weil B, Abarbanell A, Herrmann J, et al. (2009) Estrogen receptor beta mediates increased activation of PI3K/Akt signaling and improved myocardial function in female hearts following acute ischemia. Am J Physiol Regul Integr Comp Physiol 296: R972–R978.
20. Willems L, Zatta A, Holmgren K, Ashton KJ, Headrick JP (2005) Age-related changes in ischemic tolerance in male and female mouse hearts. J Mol Cell Cardiol 38: 245–256.

21. Lujan HL, Kramer VJ, DiCarlo SE (2007) Sex influences the susceptibility to reperfusion-induced sustained ventricular tachycardia and β-adrenergic receptor blockade in conscious rats. Am J Physiol 293: H2799–H2808.

22. Saeedi R, Wambolt RB, Parsons H, Antler C, Leong HS, et al. (2006) Gender and post-ischemic recovery of hypertrophied rat hearts. BMC Cardiovasc Disord; 6: 8.

23. Lagranha CJ, Deschamps A, Aponte A, Steenbergen C, Murphy E (2010) Sex differences in the phosphorylation of mitochondrial proteins result in reduced production of reactive oxygen species and cardioprotection in females. Circ Res 106: 1681–1691.

24. Brown DA, Lynch JM, Armstrong CJ, Caruso NM, Ehlers LB, et al. (2005) Susceptibility of the heart to ischaemia-reperfusion injury and exercise-induced cardioprotection are sex-dependent in the rat. J Physiol 564: 619–630.

25. Song X, Li G, Vaage J, Valen G (2003) Effects of sex, gonadectomy, and oestrogen substitution on ischaemic preconditioning and ischaemia-reperfusion injury in mice. Acta Physiol Scand 177: 459–466.

26. Cross HR, Murphy E, Steenbergen C (2002) Ca^{2+} loading and adrenergic stimulation reveal male/female differences in susceptibility to ischemia-reperfusion injury. Am J Physiol 283: H481–H489.

27. Gabel SA, Walker VR, London RE, Steenbergen C, Korach KS, et al. (2005) Estrogen receptor β mediates gender differences in ischemia/reperfusion injury. J Mol Cell Cardiol 38: 289–297.

28. Cross HR, Lu L, Steenbergen C, Philipson KD, Murphy E (1998) Over-expression of the cardiac Na$^+$/Ca^{2+} exchanger increases susceptibility to ischemia/reperfusion injury in male, but not female, transgenic mice. Circ Res 83: 1215–1223.

29. Cross HR, Steenbergen C, Lefkowitz RJ, Koch WJ, Murphy E (1999) Overexpression of the cardiac β2-adrenergic receptor and expression of a β-adrenergic receptor kinase-1 (βARK1) inhibitor both increase myocardial contractility but have differential effects on susceptibility to ischemic injury. Circ Res 85: 1077–1084.

30. Cross HR, Kranias EG, Murphy E, Steenbergen C (2003) Ablation of PLB exacerbates ischemic injury to a lesser extent in female than male mice: protective role of NO. Am J Physiol 284: H683–H690.

31. Cordeiro JM, Howlett SE, Ferrier GR (1994) Simulated ischaemia and reperfusion in isolated guinea pig ventricular myocytes Cardiovasc Res 28: 1794–1802.

32. Louch WE, Ferrier GR, Howlett SE (2002) Changes in excitation-contraction coupling in an isolated ventricular myocyte model of cardiac stunning. Am J Physiol Heart Circ Physiol 283: H800–H810.

33. O'Brien JD, Howlett SE (2008) Simulated ischemia-induced preconditioning of isolated ventricular myocytes from young adult and aged Fischer-344 rat hearts. Am J Physiol Heart Circ Physiol 294: H768–H777.

34. Ross JL, Howlett SE (2009) Beta-adrenoceptor stimulation exacerbates detrimental effects of ischemia and reperfusion in isolated guinea pig ventricular myocytes. Eur J Pharmacol 602: 364–372.

35. Stoddart MJ (2011) Cell viability assays: introduction. Methods Mol Biol. 2011; 740: 1–6.

36. Grynkiewicz G, Poenie M, Tsien RY (2006) A new generation of Ca^{2+} indicators with greatly improved fluorescence properties. J Biol Chem 260: 3440–3450, 1985.

37. Bers DM (2008) Calcium cycling and signaling in cardiac myocytes. Annu Rev Physiol 70: 23–49.

38. Day SM, Westfall MV, Metzger JM (2007) Tuning cardiac performance in ischemic heart disease and failure by modulating myofilament function. J Mol Med (Berl) 85: 911–921.

39. Whelan RS, Kaplinskiy V, Kitsis RN (2010) Cell death in the pathogenesis of heart disease: mechanisms and significance. Annu Rev Physiol 72: 19–44.

40. Sari FR, Watanabe K, Widyantoro B, Thandavarayan RA, Harima M, et al. (2011) Sex differences play a role in cardiac endoplasmic reticulum stress (ERS)

41. Wang F, He Q, Sun Y, Dai X, Yang XP (2010) Female adult mouse cardiomyocytes are protected against oxidative stress. Hypertension 55: 1172–1178.

42. Tomicek NJ, Miller-Lee JL, Hunter JC, Korzick DH (2011) Estrogen receptor beta does not influence ischemic tolerance in the aged female rat heart. Cardiovasc Ther doi: 10.1111/j.1755-5922.2011.00288.x.

43. McCully JD, Toyoda Y, Wakiyama H, Rousou AJ, Parker RA, et al. (2006) Age- and gender-related differences in ischemia/reperfusion injury and cardioprotection: effects of diazoxide. Ann Thorac Surg 82: 117–123.

44. Puzianowska-Kuznicka M, Kuznicki J (2009) The ER and ageing II: calcium homeostasis. Ageing Res Rev 8: 160–172.

45. Ren J, Dong F, Cai GJ, Zhao P, Nunn JM, et al. (2010) Interaction between age and obesity on cardiomyocyte contractile function: role of leptin and stress signaling. PLoS One 5: e10085.

46. Wilson LD, Wan X, Rosenbaum DS (2006) Cellular alternans: a mechanism linking calcium cycling proteins to cardiac arrhythmogenesis. Ann N Y Acad Sci 1080: 216–234.

47. Zhao W, Wen HX, Zheng HL, Sun SX, Sun DJ, et al. (2011) Action mechanism of Zuo Gui Yin Decoction's promotion on estradiol production in rats during the peri-menopausal period. J Ethnopharmacol 134: 122–129.

48. Sze SC, Tong Y, Zhang YB, Zhang ZJ, Lau AS, et al. (2009) A novel mechanism: Erxian Decoction, a Chinese medicine formula, for relieving menopausal syndrome. J Ethnopharmacol 123: 27–33.

49. Curl CL, Wendt IR, Canny BJ, Kotsanas G (2003) Effects of ovariectomy and 17 betaoestradiol replacement on [Ca^{2+}]$_i$ in female rat cardiac myocytes. Clin Exp Pharmacol Physiol 30: 489–494.

50. Kravtsov GM, Kam KW, Liu J, Wu S, Wong TM (2007) Altered Ca^{2+} handling by ryanodine receptor and Na$^+$–Ca^{2+} exchange in the heart from ovariecto-mized rats: role of protein kinase A. Am J Physiol Cell Physiol 292: C1625–C1635.

51. Wu Q, Zhao Z, Sun H, Hao YL, Yan CD, et al. (2008) Oestrogen changed cardiomyocyte contraction and beta-adrenoceptor expression in rat hearts subjected to ischaemia–reperfusion. Exp Physiol 93: 1034–1043.

52. Ma Y, Cheng WT, Wu S, Wong TM (2009) Oestrogen confers cardioprotection by suppressing Ca^{2+}/calmodulin-dependent protein kinase II. Br J Pharmacol 157: 705–715.

53. Fares E, Parks RJ, Macdonald JK, Egar JM, Howlett SE (2012) Ovariectomy enhances SR Ca^{2+} release and increases Ca^{2+} spark amplitudes in isolated ventricular myocytes. J Mol Cell Cardiol 52: 32–42.

54. Chung MT, Cheng PY, Lam KK, Chen SY, Ting YF, et al. (2010) Cardioprotective effects of long-term treatment with raloxifene, a selective estrogen receptor modulator, on myocardial ischemia/reperfusion injury in ovariectomized rats. Menopause 17: 127–134.

55. Simpson ER (2003) Sources of estrogen and their importance. J Steroid Biochem Mol Biol 86: 225–230.

56. Zhao H, Tian Z, Hao J, Chen B (2005) Extragonadal aromatization increases with time after ovariectomy in rats. Reprod Biol Endocrinol 3: 6.

57. Howlett SE (2010) Age-associated changes in excitation-contraction coupling are more prominent in ventricular myocytes from male rats than in myocytes from female rats. Am J Physiol Heart Circ Physiol 298: H659–H670.

58. Farrell SR, Ross JL, Howlett SE (2010) Sex differences in mechanisms of cardiac excitation-contraction coupling in rat ventricular myocytes. Am J Physiol Heart Circ Physiol 299: H36–H45.

59. Wasserstrom JA, Kapur S, Jones S, Faruque T, Sharma R, et al. (2008) Characteristics of intracellular Ca^{2+} cycling in intact rat heart: a comparison of sex differences. Am J Physiol Heart Circ Physiol 295: H1895–H1804.

60. Curl CL, Wendt IR, Kotsanas G (2001) Effects of gender on intracellular [Ca^{2+}]$_i$ in rat cardiac myocytes. Pflugers Arch 441: 709–716.

4

Selective Over-Expression of Endothelin-1 in Endothelial Cells Exacerbates Inner Retinal Edema and Neuronal Death in Ischemic Retina

Simon S. F. Cheung[1], Justin W. C. Leung[1], Amy K. M. Lam[1], Karen S. L. Lam[2,4], Stephen S. M. Chung[3,4], Amy C. Y. Lo[1,4¤]*, Sookja K. Chung[1,4]*

1 Department of Anatomy, The University of Hong Kong, Hong Kong, China, 2 Department of Medicine, The University of Hong Kong, Hong Kong, China, 3 Department of Physiology, The University of Hong Kong, Hong Kong, China, 4 Research Centre of Heart, Brain, Hormone and Healthy Aging, Li Ka Shing Faculty of Medicine, The University of Hong Kong, Hong Kong, China

Abstract

The level of endothelin-1 (ET-1), a potent vasoconstrictor, was associated with retinopathy under ischemia. The effects of endothelial endothelin-1 (ET-1) over-expression in a transgenic mouse model using Tie-1 promoter (TET-1 mice) on pathophysiological changes of retinal ischemia were investigated by intraluminal insertion of a microfilament up to middle cerebral artery (MCA) to transiently block the ophthalmic artery. Two-hour occlusion and twenty-two-hour reperfusion were performed in homozygous (Hm) TET-1 mice and their non-transgenic (NTg) littermates. Presence of pyknotic nuclei in ganglion cell layer (GCL) was investigated in paraffin sections of ipsilateral (ischemic) and contralateral (non-ischemic) retinae, followed by measurement of the thickness of inner retinal layer. Moreover, immunocytochemistry of glial fibrillary acidic protein (GFAP), glutamine synthetase (GS) and aquaporin-4 (AQP4) peptides on retinal sections were performed to study glial cell reactivity, glutamate metabolism and water accumulation, respectively after retinal ischemia. Similar morphology was observed in the contralateral retinae of NTg and Hm TET-1 mice, whereas ipsilateral retina of NTg mice showed slight structural and cellular changes compared with the corresponding contralateral retina. Ipsilateral retinae of Hm TET-1 mice showed more significant changes when compared with ipsilateral retina of NTg mice, including more prominent cell death in GCL characterized by the presence of pyknotic nuclei, elevated GS immunoreactivity in Müller cell bodies and processes, increased AQP-4 immunoreactivity in Müller cell processes, and increased inner retinal thickness. Thus, over-expression of endothelial ET-1 in TET-1 mice may contribute to increased glutamate-induced neurotoxicity on neuronal cells and water accumulation in inner retina leading to edema.

Editor: Ben C. B. Ko, Chinese University of Hong Kong, Hong Kong

Funding: This study was supported by the Research Grants Council of Hong Kong (RGC) HKU 7220/02M and 7313/04M. The funders had no role in study design, data collection and analysis, decision to publish, or preparation of the manuscript.

Competing Interests: The authors have declared that no competing interests exist.

* E-mail: amylo@ hku.hk (ACYL); skchung@hkucc.hku.hk (SKC)

¤ Current address: Eye Institute, The University of Hong Kong, Hong Kong, China

Introduction

Diabetic retinopathy (DR) and other ocular diseases in diabetes, such as central retinal artery occlusion (CRAO) and glaucoma, is thought to be the consequence of retinal ischemia, leading to visual impairment and blindness [1]. Retina undergoing ischemia displayed a number of pathological and cellular changes. Reactivity of glial cells are activated by up-regulated expression of glial fibrillary acidic protein (GFAP) [2], with the release of massive amounts of glutamate from injured neurons which is suggested to be neurotoxic [3]. Neuronal cell death was observed by the presence of pyknotic nuclei, especially in the cells in ganglion cell layer (GCL) [4,5,6,7,8]. Moreover, increased extracellular water transport and accumulation was present in inner retina, which is characterized by increased extracellular fluid volume, increased aquaporin-4 (AQP-4) immunoreactivity and swelling of retinal glial cells, leading to inner retinal edema [9].

Endothelin-1 (ET-1), a 21-amino acid secretory protein synthesized in vascular endothelial cells, is a potent vasoconstrictor. A possible link between elevated plasma ET-1 level and retinopathy under ischemia has been established. Administration of ET-1 into the posterior vitreous body or the optic nerve of animal models led to physiological and cellular damages of ischemic insult, including obstruction of retinal blood flow, elevated scotopic b-wave in electroretinogram and apoptosis of cells in GCL [10,11,12]. This is because the increased ET-1 concentration would elevate vitreous glutamate level [13] and augmented activities and responses to glutamate in the nuclei of the solitary tract (NTS) neurons [14], which may increase the excitotoxic effects of glutamate to neuronal cells. The hypertensive property of ET-1 was suggested to play a role in ischemic insult in retina.

In order to study the pathogenic changes of ET-1 to ischemic stress in central nervous system, a hypertensive transgenic mouse model with over-expression of ET-1 in vascular endothelial cells using Tie-1 promoter (TET-1 mice) has been generated [15]. It has been shown that a more severe neurological deficit, larger brain infarct size and infarct volume following transient middle cerebral artery occlusion (MCAO) was present in homozygous (Hm) TET-1 mice, indicating that over-expressing ET-1 in endothelial cells is deleterious on neuronal survival after ischemic conditions [16]. This transgenic mouse model has the advantage over other ischemic models of ET-1 by regulating expression of ET-1 level endogenously in a specific cell type (endothelial cells) rather than regulating its level by external administration to induce the respective effects under ischemia. The present study is to further investigate the effects of endothelial ET-1 in retinopathy after transient inner retinal ischemia and reperfusion of ophthalmic artery (OA) and central retinal artery (CRA) [17]. We hypothesize that TET-1 mice may induce more severe ischemia-related cellular damages and edema in retina after retinal ischemia induced by OA occlusion.

Materials and Methods

Ethics Statement

The use of animals in this study was conducted according to the requirements of the Cap. 340 Animals (Control of Experiments) Ordinance and Regulations, and all relevant legislation and Codes of Practice in Hong Kong. All the experimental and animal handling procedures were approved by the Faculty Committee on the Use of Live Animals in Teaching and Research in The University of Hong Kong (Permit number #634-01).

Generation of TET-1 transgenic mice

Male heterozygous (He) TET-1 mice were generated by microinjection of the ET-1 construct, which contains the mouse ET-1 cDNA with SV40 polyA driven by the Tie-1 promoter [16,18]. TET-1 mice were maintained in the F1 hybrid background (C57BL/6J×CBA). Animals were kept under controlled environmental conditions with respect to temperature (19°C), humidity (55%), and 12-hour light-dark schedule. They received sterilized water and mouse diet *ad libitum*.

Semi-quantitative reverse transcriptase-PCR (rt-PCR) of ET-1 gene

Mice at the age of 6 to 8 weeks were sacrificed, their eyes were cut underneath the optic nerve and the retinae were dissected under dissecting microscope (Stemi SV6; Carl Zeiss, Thornwood, NY), frozen in liquid nitrogen and stored in a −80°C. Retinal tissues were homogenized in 1 ml ice-cold TRI REAGENT® (Molecular Research Center, Cleveland, Ohio) and the total RNA from retina was isolated according to manufacturer's protocol. 1.5 µg of total RNA was treated with DNase I (Boehringer, Ingelheim, Germany) and reverse transcription was performed with Oligo(dT)18, Superscript™ II RNase H- reverse transcriptase (Invitrogen, Carlsbad, CA), DTT and dNTP mixture. The primer sequences and condition for rt-PCR of ET-1 has been previously mentioned [19]. The mouse GAPDH gene was co-amplified in the same reaction as internal control. The ratio of intensities of ET-1 to GAPDH genes expression of each sample was determined by densitometer.

Transient retinal ischemia induced by occlusion of ophthalmic artery

Age-matched Hm TET-1 and non-transgenic (NTg) mice at the age of 8 to 10 weeks were subjected to retinal ischemia as previously described [20,21,22,23]. In brief, animals were first anesthetized (2% halothane in 70% N_2O/30% O_2 for induction and 1% halothane in 70% N_2O/30% O_2 for maintenance) and the rectal temperature was kept at 37°C. An intraluminal insertion of a nylon microfilament was inserted into the right external carotid artery through internal carotid artery (ICA) up to the middle cerebral artery (MCA). This method could block the cerebral blood flow from the right ICA to OA and CRA, leading to ischemia of the right retina (ipsilateral side). The drop in retinal blood flow was indirectly monitored by laser Doppler flowmetry (Perimed, Järfälla, Sweden) where an optic fibre was placed on the skull to measure the relative regional blood flow in the core territory of the right middle cerebral artery in the brain. Anaesthesia was maintained for another 5 min after ischemia induction to ensure that the filament maintained its position inside the vessel. The wound was then closed and the animal was released from anaesthesia. Fifteen minutes before reperfusion, animals were anesthetized again as above during which the filament was removed at 2 hrs after ischemia induction. Reperfusion was then allowed for 22 hours. The mice were then sacrificed to enucleate the right and left eyeballs, which represented the ipsilateral (ischemic) and the contralateral (non-ischemic) side, respectively. A suture (tied onto the upper conjunctiva at the time of collection) was used for identification of orientation. This suture was then used during paraffin embedding to identify the superior retina. They were fixed in 4% paraformaldehyde overnight at 4°C, dehydrated with a graded series of ethanol, xylene and then embedded in paraffin wax. With the placement of the eyeball horizontally, the nasal and temporal parts were identified on either side of the paraffin block.

Histological and immunocytochemical techniques

Serial paraffin sections of 7 µm thick from non-ischemic and ischemic eyeballs were prepared using the microtome (Microm HM315, Germany). The sections were deparaffinized in xylene, rehydrated with a graded series of ethanol, and stained briefly with hematoxylin and eosin (Sigma-Aldrich, St. Louis, MO). To perform immunocytochemistry (ICC) of GFAP, glutamine synthetase (GS) and AQP-4, sections of ischemic and non-ischemic retinae were blocked with 1.5% normal goat serum (Vector Laboratories, San Francisco, CA) for 1 hour, followed by incubation in diluted primary antibodies overnight at 4°C. Incubation of blocking serum served as control. The primary antibodies and their concentrations were rabbit anti-GFAP (1:2000; Dako, Carpinteria, CA), rabbit anti-AQP-4 (1: 800; Chemicon International, Temecula, CA) and rabbit anti-GS (1: 300; Santa Cruz Biotechnology, Santa Cruz, CA). The sections were subsequently incubated with biotinylated goat anti-rabbit secondary antibody (Vector Laboratories), and immunoreactive signals were visualized by incubation with the avidin-biotin-peroxidase complex (Vector Laboratories) for 30 min and diaminobenzidine tetrahydrochloride (Zymed Laboratory, San Francisco, CA) for 2 min. Finally, the sections were counterstained with hematoxylin, dehydrated, cover-slipped and mounted with mounting medium.

Quantitation of cell death in retinal ganglion cell layer

Retinal sections containing the optic nerve that were stained with hematoxylin and eosin were chosen for viewing. Two images, one on either the nasal or temporal side, were taken at a region about 300 µm away from the optic nerve using the 20× objective (Olympus IX71, Olympus, Japan) as previously described [21,22,23]. Cells with pyknotic nuclei and the total number of cells in GCL in the images were counted. It was assumed that the percentage of pyknotic nuclei represented the percentage of cell loss in the GCL. The severity of cell death in GCL was classified into four levels: "severe" represented more than 80% of cells in GCL on the section had pyknotic nuclei, "moderate" represented 20% to 80% of these cells had pyknotic nuclei, less than 20% of cell death was classified as "mild", and absence of pyknotic nuclei was defined as "none". Sections from 12–14 animals in each group (n = 12–14) were analyzed.

Measurement of inner retinal thickness

Digital photographs were taken using 20× objectives from the nasal and temporal sides (about 300 μm from the optic nerve) in each of the contralateral and ipsilateral retinae. In each photo, the thickness of three regions in the retina was measured: inner nuclear layer (INL), from inner plexiform layer (IPL) to inner limiting membrane (ILM), and from INL to ILM representing the thickness of the whole retina [24]. Data from each mouse was taken by averaging two measurements from nasal and temporal sides of retina, respectively.

Statistical analysis

All data were expressed as means ± SEM. Statistical analyses were performed using one-way ANOVA with Bonferroni's post hoc tests, Fisher's exact test, Mann-Whitney Test, and Kruskal-Wallis Test by Statistical Package for the Social Sciences software (SPSS 12.0, SPSS). Difference with p value<0.05 was considered statistically significant.

Results

Up-regulated mRNA and peptide expressions of ET-1 in TET-1 mice

Total ET-1 mRNA expression in 6- to 8-week-old in Hm TET-1 mouse retina was about 2.5 times higher than that of NTg mice by semi-quantitative rt-PCR (Fig. 1), which was statistically significant (p<0.05, Kruskal-Wallis Test). This showed that over-expression of ET-1 could be observed in retina at the transcription level. Peptide expression of ET-1 was also studied in the retinal sections of 6-week-old TET-1 mouse retina by ICC using rabbit anti-ET-1 antibody. Immunopositive signal of ET-1 was localized in the nerve fibres of ILM, endothelial cells and cells in INL (Fig. 2). ET-1 peptide expression was much higher in the endothelial cells of Hm TET-1 mice when compared with that of NTg mice.

More severe cell death in retinal ganglion cell layer in TET-1 mice

Cellular morphology in retinal sections of ischemic and non-ischemic retinae of NTg and Hm TET-1 mice were examined. Similar to our previous results, there was presence of cells with pyknotic nuclei in the GCL [21,22,23]. We then strictly followed the previously published protocol in counting these cells with pyknotic nuclei and the total number of cells in the GCL. The severity of cell death in GCL was classified according to the percentage of pyknotic nuclei, which represented the percentage of cell loss in the GCL. Our quantitation showed that all contralateral retinae in NTg and Hm TET-1 mice were classified as "none". "Severe" cell death in GCL was seen in more than half (8 out of 14) of the ipsilateral retinae of Hm TET-1 mice, while the others were classified as either "moderate" (2 out of 14) or "mild" (4 out of 14). On the other hand, only 1 out of the 12 samples in the ipsilateral retina of NTg mice had "severe" cell death in GCL, while "mild" death was observed in 7 out of the 12 mice (Table 1). A significant difference in the severity of cell death in GCL

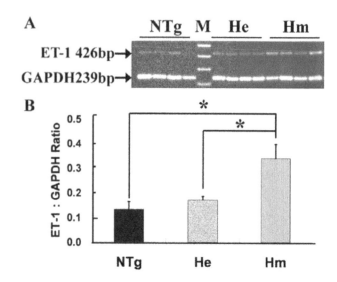

Figure 1. Semi-quantitative rt-PCR analysis showing total ET-1 mRNA expression in the retinae of non-transgenic (NTg), heterozygous (He) and homozygous (Hm) TET-1 mice. A: Ethidium bromide-stained agarose gels of rt-PCR products of ET-1, showing increased ET-1 mRNA expression in transgenic mouse retina. The molecular size marker (M) was 1 kb plus marker. B: Histograms showing the levels of ET-1 mRNA expression normalized to that of GAPDH. n = 4 for each experimental group. *: p<0.05 (Kruskal-Wallis Test).

between ipsilateral retinae of NTg and Hm TET-1 mice was observed by comparing the number of retinae with "severe" changes and with "moderate or mild" changes (p<0.05, Fisher's exact test).

Increased GFAP immunoreactivity in ischemic retina

Glial cell reactivity in the ipsilateral and contralateral retinae of NTg and Hm TET-1 mice was studied by immunocytochemical staining of GFAP (Fig. 3). In the contralateral retinae of both genotypes, GFAP was mainly expressed in the astrocytes and Müller cell endfeet in outer plexiform layer (OPL), with a few radial processes of Müller cells running proximally in IPL. The intensity of signal in Hm TET-1 and NTg mice in the contralateral retinae was similar. In the ipsilateral retinae of both genotypes, the intensity of GFAP immunoreactivity was dramatically increased in the Müller cell processes and astrocytes around the retinal capillaries when compared with their corresponding contralateral retinae. The expression was relatively stronger in the peripheral and central regions. Yet, a slightly stronger intensity

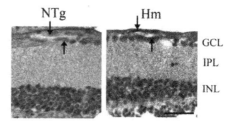

Figure 2. Immunohistochemical staining of ET-1 antibody. Immunoreactivity of ET-1 was up-regulated in the endothelial cells (arrows) of Hm TET-1 mice compared with the corresponding NTg mice. Scale bar = 25 μm.

Table 1. Severity of the presence of pyknotic nuclei in cells in ganglion cell layer (GCL) after transient inner retinal ischemia.

	None	Mild	Moderate	Severe	Non-severe (Moderate+Mild)	Total
NTg Contralateral	12	0	0	0	12	12
NTg Ipsilateral	0	7	4	1	11	12
Hm Contralateral	14	0	0	0	14	14
Hm Ipsilateral*	0	4	2	8	6	14

was observed in the ipsilateral retina of Hm TET-1 mice than that of NTg mice. This concurred with the result of more neuronal cell death observed in the ipsilateral retina of Hm TET-1 mice.

Increased glutamine synthetase immunoreactivity in the Müller cells of TET-1 ischemic retina

In the non-ischemic retinae of NTg and Hm TET-1 mice, immunoreactivity of GS was mainly present in the astrocytes, Müller cell bodies in INL and Müller cell processes from ILM to OLM (Fig. 4). The expression of GS in the peripheral and central retinal regions was similar. Slightly increased immunoreactivity was observed in the Müller cell processes in the ipsilateral retina of NTg mice when compared with the corresponding contralateral retina, as well as in the contralateral retina of Hm TET-1 mice when compared with the contralateral retina of NTg mice. A significant up-regulation of GS expression was also observed in the Müller cell processes and Müller cell bodies in the ipsilateral retina of Hm TET-1 mice when compared with the contralateral and ipsilateral retinae of NTg mice.

Increased aquaporin-4 immunoreactivity in the glial cells of TET-1 mice

Expression of a water transport protein, aquaporin-4 (AQP4), was determined for the presence of edema and water accumulation of glial cells in ischemic retina. In the contralateral retinae of both NTg and Hm TET-1 mice, positive immunoreactivity of AQP4 was found in the Müller cell processes from ILM to OLM, astrocytes around blood vessels in GCL, Müller cell bodies in INL

and astrocytic endfeet in OPL (Fig. 5). Similar findings were observed in a recent immunohistochemical study [25]. The expression of AQP4 in the peripheral and central regions was similar. Contralateral and ipsilateral retinae of NTg mice presented a similar pattern and intensity of AQP4 immunoreactivity, as well as between the contralateral retinae of NTg and Hm TET-1 mice. However, a significant up-regulation of immunoreactive signal was observed in the Müller cell processes and Müller cell bodies of the ipsilateral retina of Hm TET-1 mice compared with the corresponding contralateral retina of Hm TET-1 mice.

Increased inner retinal thickness in TET-1 mice after transient ischemia

According to our semi-quantitative observation, the major phenotype of ischemic injury in the ipsilateral retina of Hm TET-1 mice was "severe" while that of NTg mice was "mild". Therefore, representative photomicrographs from each experimental animal group were selected after careful screening for retinal thickness measurement. Similar thicknesses of INL, IPL to ILM and inner retinal layer were found between the contralateral retinae of Hm TET-1 and NTg mice (Table 2), as well as between the ipsilateral and contralateral retinae of NTg mice. On the contrary, there was a significant increase in the thickness of IPL to ILM and inner retina in the ipsilateral retina of Hm TET-1 mice when compared with the contralateral retina of Hm TET-1 mice ($p<0.05$, Mann-Whitney Test), while similar INL thickness was found between the two groups. Therefore, the increase in inner retinal thickness was solely due to the increase in the thickness from IPL to ILM.

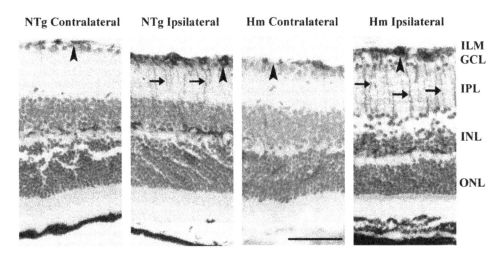

NTg Contralateral	NTg Ipsilateral	Hm Contralateral	Hm Ipsilateral	
				ILM GCL
				IPL
				INL
				ONL

Figure 3. Immunohistochemical staining of glial fibrillary acidic protein (GFAP). Compared with the contralateral retinae of NTg and Hm TET-1 mice, GFAP signal was up-regulated in the ipsilateral retinae in the astrocytes around capillaries in the inner limiting membrane (arrowheads) and the Müller cell processes in IPL (arrows). n = 5 for each experimental group. Scale bar = 50 μm.

NTg Contralateral   NTg Ipsilateral   Hm Contralateral   Hm Ipsilateral

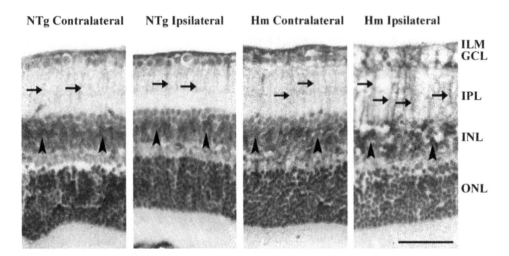

Figure 4. Immunohistochemical staining of glutamine synthetase (GS) antibody. Up-regulation of GS signal was found in the Müller cell processes in IPL (arrows) and Müller cell bodies in INL (arrowheads) in the ipsilateral retina of Hm TET-1 mice compared with the contralateral retina of Hm TET-1 mice and the ipsilateral retina of NTg mice. n = 5 for each experimental group. Scale bar = 50 μm.

Discussion

Mild inner retinal ischemia was induced by MCAO in mice with an absence [20] or a small number of apoptotic neurons [17]. As indicated by Kaja et al, this model is able to recapitulate the cellular and molecular changes in the retina after stroke. This is particularly clinically relevant since acute thrombotic/embolic stroke and transient ischemic attack in humans are often associated with temporary diminishment (ie, amaurosis fugax) or even permanent loss of vision [26].

In this study, the ischemic model induced by middle cerebral artery occlusion also resulted in a mild transient retinal ischemia with neuronal cell damage in mice with F1 hybrid background, as suggested by increased GFAP immunoreactivity in the Müller cell processes and astrocytes, and the presence of pyknotic nuclei in the cells in GCL in the NTg ipsilateral retinae. Thus, slight cellular and structural changes were present in the NTg ipsilateral retinae,

including pyknotic nuclei were present in less than 80% of cells in GCL, slightly increased GS expression in the Müller cell processes and no significant changes in AQP4 immunoreactivity and inner retinal thickness. On the contrary, more severe cellular and structural changes were observed in the ipsilateral retina of Hm TET-1 mice, including presence of pyknotic nuclei in more than 80% of cells in GCL, prominent up-regulated GS expression in Müller cell processes, up-regulation of AQP-4 immunoreactivity and significant increase in inner retinal thickness. Under these prominent cellular changes observed in the ischemic retina, we may deduce that Hm TET-1 mice with over-expression of ET-1 in endothelial cells would exacerbate the effects of neuronal cell death and retinal edema after OA occlusion. Previous studies already showed significant loss of cells in GCL layer following intraocular injection of ET-1 to the optic nerve [11,27], increased brain swelling and water contents in animals injected with ET-1 [28] and in transgenic mice with over-expressing ET-1 in

NTg Contralateral   NTg Ipsilateral   Hm Contralateral   Hm Ipsilateral

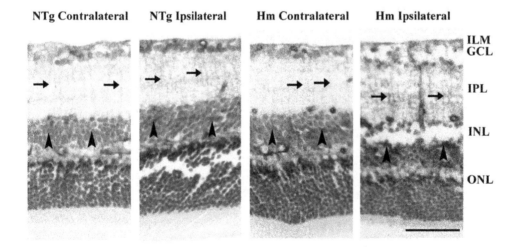

Figure 5. Immunohistochemical staining of aquaporin-4 (AQP4). Up-regulation of AQP4 signal was found in the Müller cell processes in IPL (arrows) and Müller cell bodies in INL (arrowheads) in the ipsilateral retina of Hm TET-1 mice compared with the corresponding contralateral retina, while similar intensity of AQP4 signal was present in the contralateral and ipsilateral retinae of NTg mice. n = 5 for each experimental group. Scale bar = 50 μm.

Table 2. Thicknesses of inner nuclear layer (INL), inner plexiform layer (IPL) to inner limiting membrane (ILM) and the whole inner retina (μm).

	Thickness IPL+ILM	Thickness of INL	Thickness of inner retina
NTg Contralateral	57.2±3.5	29.8±0.8	87.0±2.8
NTg Ipsilateral	61.5±3.5	30.5±1.9	92.0±5.2
Hm Contralateral	56.2±3.1	28.9±1.8	85.2±3.9
Hm Ipsilateral	71.7±3.9*	29.0±1.9	100.6±3.3*

astrocytes using GFAP promoter after transient MCAO [29], suggesting a possible correlation between induction of ET-1 to neuronal cell death and edema.

Down-regulation of GS expression has been shown in Müller cells after ischemia and reperfusion [13]. An increase in GS expression in glial cells was thus suggested to be neuroprotective with decreased glutamate neurotoxicity. However, our experimental results showed exacerbated immunoreactivity of GS in the Müller cell processes of Hm TET-1 mice, followed by more severe neuronal cell death. We propose an alternate mechanism for more severe neuronal cell death. Primary culture study on fetal murine cortical neurons showed that GS has relatively low affinity to neuronal and glial glutamate transporters, suggesting that GS may not be capable of lowering glutamate levels below the threshold of glutamate toxicity [30]. Previous studies suggested that increased ET-1 expression would up-regulate glutamate level in the vitreous after optic nerve ischemia [13], as well as the activities and responses to glutamate in NTS neurons [14], increased mRNA expression of endogenous ET-1 in TET-1 mice may enhance extracellular glutamate level in retina. During ischemic stress, the glutamate level was so high that the low-affinity GS could not reduce the glutamate level below the threshold of glutamate neurotoxicity. ET-1 itself would then impose an augmented response to glutamate-induced neurotoxicity, more pyknotic nuclei were present in the cells of GCL in Hm TET-1 ischemic retina. Further investigation is required to study the activities and roles of extracellular glutamate, GS and ET-1 to glutamate neurotoxicity in retina through the TET-1 mouse model.

AQP4 is the main water channel protein which regulates the bi-directional movement of water across membranes and involved in the maintenance of the ionic and osmotic balance [31]. Increased AQP4 expression during ischemia would promote neuronal cell swelling with over-excitation of glutamate receptors, leading to neuronal cell depolarization. Glial cell swelling occurs during reperfusion, with down-regulation of functional K^+ channels and reduced transmembrane inwardly rectifying K^+ (Kir) currents [32]. Therefore, ischemia-reperfusion process would increase extracellular fluid volume and swelling of retinal glial cells,

contributing to progressive thickening of inner retina and development of macular edema [9], which consequently contributes to photoreceptor degeneration and neuronal cell death [33]. Possible involvement of AQP4 in ET-1-induced edema has been suggested by increased brain swelling and water contents in transgenic TET-1 mice [16] and in another transgenic mouse model with over-expression of ET-1 in astrocytes using GFAP promoter [29] following transient MCAO. The results further proved that over-expression of endothelial ET-1 in Hm TET-1 mice may promote water accumulation and edema in the glial cells of inner retina, leading to more severe neuronal cell death after ischemia and reperfusion.

This study showed that the transgenic mice model with over-expression of endothelial ET-1 may enhance the effects of glutamate-induced neurotoxicity after induction of inner retinal ischemia and reperfusion with exacerbated neuronal cell death. Moreover, TET-1 mice may also contribute to increased water accumulation in the glial cells, leading to retinal edema with increased inner retinal thickness. The TET-1 mouse model after mild transient inner retinal ischemia may serve as a suitable model to study pathological changes in ischemic retinopathy simulating disease conditions like DR, glaucoma, peripheral or central ischemia which may lead to ocular ischemia or stroke, and is useful for therapeutic studies on these disorders.

Acknowledgments

The authors would like to thank Marcella Ma, Maggie Ho and Michael Koon for performing the microinjection experiment and generating the TET-1 mice as well as Janice Law and Alvin Cheung for technical advice.

Author Contributions

Conceived and designed the experiments: SSFC ACYL SKC. Performed the experiments: SSFC JWCL AKML ACYL. Analyzed the data: SSFC AKML KSLL SSMC ACYL SKC. Contributed reagents/materials/analysis tools: KSLL SSMC ACYL SKC. Wrote the paper: SSFC KSLL SSMC ACYL SKC.

References

1. Osborne NN, Casson RJ, Wood JP, Chidlow G, Graham M, et al. (2004) Retinal ischemia: mechanisms of damage and potential therapeutic strategies. Prog Retin Eye Res 23: 91–147.

2. Bringmann A, Francke M, Pannicke T, Biedermann B, Faude F, et al. (1999) Human Muller glial cells: altered potassium channel activity in proliferative vitreoretinopathy. Invest Ophthalmol Vis Sci 40: 3316–3323.

3. Gorovits R, Avidan N, Avisar N, Shaked I, Vardimon L (1997) Glutamine synthetase protects against neuronal degeneration in injured retinal tissue. Proc Natl Acad Sci U S A 94: 7024–7029.

4. Inoue-Matsuhisa E, Sogo S, Mizota A, Taniai M, Takenaka H, et al. (2003) Effect of MCI-9042, a 5-HT2 receptor antagonist, on retinal ganglion cell death and retinal ischemia. Exp Eye Res 76: 445–452.

5. Lafuente MP, Villegas-Perez MP, Selles-Navarro I, Mayor-Torroglosa S, Miralles de Imperial J, et al. (2002) Retinal ganglion cell death after acute retinal ischemia is an ongoing process whose severity and duration depends on the duration of the insult. Neuroscience 109: 157–168.

6. Nucci C, Tartaglione R, Rombola L, Morrone LA, Fazzi E, et al. (2005) Neurochemical evidence to implicate elevated glutamate in the mechanisms of high intraocular pressure (IOP)-induced retinal ganglion cell death in rat. Neurotoxicology 26: 935–941.

7. Yamamoto H, Schmidt-Kastner R, Hamasaki DI, Parel JM (2006) Complex neurodegeneration in retina following moderate ischemia induced by bilateral common carotid artery occlusion in Wistar rats. Exp Eye Res 82: 767–779.

8. Zhang Y, Cho CH, Atchaneeyasakul LO, McFarland T, Appukuttan B, et al. (2005) Activation of the mitochondrial apoptotic pathway in a rat model of central retinal artery occlusion. Invest Ophthalmol Vis Sci 46: 2133–2139.

9. Yanoff M, Fine BS, Brucker AJ, Eagle RC, Jr. (1984) Pathology of human cystoid macular edema. Surv Ophthalmol 28 Suppl: 505–511.

10. Chauhan BC, LeVatte TL, Jollimore CA, Yu PK, Reitsamer HA, et al. (2004) Model of endothelin-1-induced chronic optic neuropathy in rat. Invest Ophthalmol Vis Sci 45: 144–152.

11. Lau J, Dang M, Hockmann K, Ball AK (2006) Effects of acute delivery of endothelin-1 on retinal ganglion cell loss in the rat. Exp Eye Res 82: 132–145.

12. Takei K, Sato T, Nonoyama T, Miyauchi T, Goto K, et al. (1993) A new model of transient complete obstruction of retinal vessels induced by endothelin-1 injection into the posterior vitreous body in rabbits. Graefes Arch Clin Exp Ophthalmol 231: 476–481.

13. Kim TW, Kang KB, Choung HK, Park KH, Kim DM (2000) Elevated glutamate levels in the vitreous body of an in vivo model of optic nerve ischemia. Arch Ophthalmol 118: 533–536.

14. Shihara M, Hirooka Y, Hori N, Matsuo I, Tagawa T, et al. (1998) Endothelin-1 increases the neuronal activity and augments the responses to glutamate in the NTS. Am J Physiol 275: R658–665.

15. Koon HW (2002) Role of endothelin-1 and nitric oxide on the cardiovascular function. Hong Kong: The University of Hong Kong.

16. Leung JW, Ho MC, Lo AC, Chung SS, Chung SK (2004) Endothelial Cell-specific Over-expression of Endothelin-1 Leads to More Severe Cerebral Damage following Transient Middle Cerebral Artery Occlusion. J Cardiovasc Pharmacol 44 Suppl 1: S293–300.

17. Kaja S, Yang SH, Wei J, Fujitani K, Liu R, et al. (2003) Estrogen protects the inner retina from apoptosis and ischemia-induced loss of Vesl-1L/Homer 1c immunoreactive synaptic connections. Invest Ophthalmol Vis Sci 44: 3155–3162.

18. Koon MHW, Chung SSM, Chung SK (2002) FASEB J 15: A482.

19. Ho MC, Lo AC, Kurihara H, Yu AC, Chung SS, et al. (2001) Endothelin-1 protects astrocytes from hypoxic/ischemic injury. FASEB J 15: 618–626.

20. Block F, Grommes C, Kosinski C, Schmidt W, Schwarz M (1997) Retinal ischemia induced by the intraluminal suture method in rats. Neurosci Lett 232: 45–48.

21. Cheung AK, Lo AC, So KF, Chung SS, Chung SK (2007) Gene deletion and pharmacological inhibition of aldose reductase protect against retinal ischemic injury. Exp Eye Res 85: 608–616.

22. Li SY, Fu ZJ, Ma H, Jang WC, So KF, et al. (2009) Effect of lutein on retinal neurons and oxidative stress in a model of acute retinal ischemia/reperfusion. Invest Ophthalmol Vis Sci 50: 836–843.

23. Li SY, Yang D, Yeung CM, Yu WY, Chang RC, et al. (2011) Lycium barbarum polysaccharides reduce neuronal damage, blood-retinal barrier disruption and oxidative stress in retinal ischemia/reperfusion injury. PLoS One 6: e16380.

24. Martin PM, Roon P, Van Ells TK, Ganapathy V, Smith SB (2004) Death of retinal neurons in streptozotocin-induced diabetic mice. Invest Ophthalmol Vis Sci 45: 3330–3336.

25. Iandiev I, Pannicke T, Biedermann B, Wiedemann P, Reichenbach A, et al. (2006) Ischemia-reperfusion alters the immunolocalization of glial aquaporins in rat retina. Neurosci Lett 408: 108–112.

26. Babikian V, Wijman CA, Koleini B, Malik SN, Goyal N, et al. (2001) Retinal ischemia and embolism. Etiologies and outcomes based on a prospective study. Cerebrovasc Dis 12: 108–113.

27. Chaudhary G, Sinha K, Gupta YK (2003) Protective effect of exogenous administration of alpha-tocopherol in middle cerebral artery occlusion model of cerebral ischemia in rats. Fundam Clin Pharmacol 17: 703–707.

28. Gartshore G, Patterson J, Macrae IM (1997) Influence of ischemia and reperfusion on the course of brain tissue swelling and blood-brain barrier permeability in a rodent model of transient focal cerebral ischemia. Exp Neurol 147: 353–360.

29. Lo AC, Chen AY, Hung VK, Yaw LP, Fung MK, et al. (2005) Endothelin-1 over-expression leads to further water accumulation and brain edema after middle cerebral artery occlusion via aquaporin 4 expression in astrocytic end-feet. J Cereb Blood Flow Metab 25: 998–1101.

30. Matthews CC, Zielke HR, Wollack JB, Fishman PS (2000) Enzymatic degradation protects neurons from glutamate excitotoxicity. J Neurochem 75: 1045–1052.

31. Bringmann A, Uckermann O, Pannicke T, Iandiev I, Reichenbach A, et al. (2005) Neuronal versus glial cell swelling in the ischaemic retina. Acta Ophthalmol Scand 83: 528–538.

32. Pannicke T, Uckermann O, Iandiev I, Biedermann B, Wiedemann P, et al. (2005) Altered membrane physiology in Muller glial cells after transient ischemia of the rat retina. Glia 50: 1–11.

33. Tso MO (1982) Pathology of cystoid macular edema. Ophthalmology 89: 902–915.

5

Changes in Retinal Morphology, Electroretinogram and Visual Behavior after Transient Global Ischemia in Adult Rats

Ying Zhao², Bo Yu⁴, Yong-Hui Xiang¹, Xin-Jia Han¹, Ying Xu¹, Kwok-Fai So¹, An-Ding Xu²*, Yi-Wen Ruan¹,³*

1 Department of Central Nervous System Regeneration, Guangdong – Hongkong - Macau Institute of CNS Regeneration (GHMICR), Jinan University, Guangzhou, Guangdong, China, 2 Department of Neurology, the First Affiliated Hospital, Jinan University, Guangzhou, Guangdong, China, 3 Department of Human Anatomy, Jinan University School of Medicine, Guangzhou, Guangdong, China, 4 Department of Human Anatomy, Medical College, Shanghai University of Traditional Chinese Medicine, Shanghai, China

Abstract

The retina is a light-sensitive tissue of the central nervous system that is vulnerable to ischemia. The pathological mechanism underlying retinal ischemic injury is not fully understood. The purpose of this study was to investigate structural and functional changes of different types of rat retinal neurons and visual behavior following transient global ischemia. Retinal ischemia was induced using a 4-vessel occlusion model. Compared with the normal group, the number of βIII-tubulin positive retinal ganglion cells and calretinin positive amacrine cells were reduced from 6 h to 48 h following ischemia. The number of recoverin positive cone bipolar cells transiently decreased at 6 h and 12 h after ischemia. However, the fluorescence intensity of rhodopsin positive rod cells and fluorescent peanut agglutinin positive cone cells did not change after reperfusion. An electroretinogram recording showed that the a-wave, b-wave, oscillatory potentials and the photopic negative response were completely lost during ischemia. The amplitudes of the a- and b-waves were partially recovered at 1 h after ischemia, and returned to the control level at 48 h after reperfusion. However, the amplitudes of oscillatory potentials and the photopic negative response were still reduced at 48 h following reperfusion. Visual behavior detection showed there was no significant change in the time spent in the dark chamber between the control and 48 h group, but the distance moved, mean velocity in the black and white chambers and intercompartmental crosses were reduced at 48 h after ischemia. These results indicate that transient global ischemia induces dysfunction of retinal ganglion cells and amacrine cells at molecular and ERG levels. However, transient global ischemia in a 17 minute duration does not appear to affect photoreceptors.

Editor: Cesar V. Borlongan, University of South Florida, United States of America

Funding: This work was supported by the following grants: National Program on Key Basic Research Project of China (973 Program, 2011CB707501), the National Natural Science Foundation of China (30971530), and the Open Fund of the First Affiliated Hospital of Jinan University (2012–2014). The funders had no role in study design, data collection and analysis, decision to publish, or preparation of the manuscript.

Competing Interests: The authors have declared that no competing interests exist.

* E-mail: andingxu@gmail.com (ADX); tyiwen@jnu.edu.cn (YWR)

Introduction

The retina is a light-sensitive tissue of the central nervous system. There are several types of cells in the retina; photoreceptors (rods and cones), located close to the outer surface of the retina, receive light stimulation and convert light into electrical signals; retinal ganglion cells (RGCs), near the inner retinal surface, transmit visual signals to the visual cortex and other higher visual centers; interneurons (bipolar cells and amacrine cells), located between the photoreceptors and ganglion cells, transmit signals from the photoreceptors to the RGCs [1].

Functional signals and activities of each cell type can be recorded by the electroretinogram (ERG). From an ERG, we can observe the following waves: the a-wave (produced by photoreceptors), the b-wave (conducted by the ON-bipolar cells) [2], the oscillatory potentials (OPs, triggered by amacrine cells) [3], and the photopic negative response (PhNR, induced by RGCs) [4–7].

The visual function of the retina can be also evaluated by different behavioral methods, such as startle reflex tests [8], orientation test [9], Y-maze for visual testing [10], and the optokinetic reflex [11]. These techniques have been used to detect either eye movement or navigation ability, which is affected by vision. Recently, visual discrimination apparatus of two types was developed to assess visual function in rats. One apparatus consisted of several compartments including a curved tube, one introduction chamber, two escape alleys, three swing doors and one home cage. This apparatus was designed to train rats to distinguish two different visual stimuli [12]. The other apparatus was the black-white box which is formed by two chambers (the white and black chamber) with a door opening between them. This was employed to test the white-black visual discrimination of rats [13]. If an animal perceives light, it will escape from the white chamber to the black chamber. Because the structure of this apparatus was adequate and simpler than the other apparatus mentioned above, it was employed in the present study to detect whether transient global ischemia affects light reception.

The model of transient global ischemia is a model in which the blood supply of the brain is completely blocked for a period of time. Clinically, transient global ischemia can occur during cardiac arrest, extracorporeal circulation, asphyxiation, and complex congenital heart lesions [14,15]. During transient global ischemia, the blood supply of the retina is also completely blocked as it is derived from the internal carotid artery. It has been reported that transient global ischemia may cause sudden visual loss (amaurosis fugax) [16]. Therefore, to reveal the pathological mechanisms underlying transient global ischemia as it affects the retina will help us to understand how to protect retinal cells against ischemia.

In our previous research, we found that transient global ischemia, the 4-vessel occlusion (4-VO) model (permanent occlusion of vertebral arteries plus transient occlusion of carotid arteries), induced selective neuronal death and changes in dendritic and synaptic plasticity in the hippocampus [17–20]. However, we did not know whether retinal cells were also damaged by the same ischemic episode. In the present study we therefore used the same 4-VO model to investigate the impact of ischemia on the retina. In addition, we combined immunohistochemistry, ERG recording and visual behavior detection techniques to investigate how transient global ischemia affects different types of retinal cells and visual function.

The results showed that transient global ischemia induced a reduction in protein synthesis and the amplitudes of OPs and PhNR but did not block light perception. The structure and function of photoreceptors was also still intact.

Materials and Methods

Animals

Adult male Wistar rats (body weight 200–250 g) were used in the present study. All animal procedures were performed in strict accordance with the recommendations in the Guide for the Care and Use of Laboratory Animals of the National Institutes of Health. The protocol was approved by competent ethics committees at Jinan University. All efforts were made to minimize the suffering and number of animals used. Rats were randomly divided into five experimental groups: a control group (5 sham rats), Is (ischemia) 6 h group (5 rats sacrificed 6 h after ischemia), Is 12 h group (5 rats sacrificed 12 h after ischemia), Is 24 h group (5 rats sacrificed 24 h after ischemia) and Is 48 h group (5 rats sacrificed 48 h after ischemia). Ten rats were allocated for ERG recording. Twenty rats (10 rats in control group, and 10 rats in Is 48 h group) were employed for visual behavior detection.

Transient Global Ischemia

Transient global ischemia was induced using the 4-VO method [21] with modifications (detection of ischemic depolarization) [22]. Briefly, animals were fasted overnight (8–12 h) to produce uniform blood glucose levels. For surgery, animals were anesthetized with 10% chloral hydrate (0.4 ml/100 g; 27500, HaoMa, Guangzhou, China) by intraperitoneal injection. A silicone tube was placed loosely around each carotid artery to allow subsequent occlusion of the vessels. The animals were then placed in a stereotaxic frame and the bilateral vertebral arteries were electrocauterized. A microelectrode filled with 2M KCl was inserted into the hippocampus (2.5 mm below the brain surface) to record ischemic depolarization (ID) with an amplifier (Neuroprobe 1600, A-M System, Carlsberg, MA, USA). ID is defined as the direct current potential (DCP) from an amplifier shifted from zero to approximately −20 mV after ischemia. The duration of ID was determined by measuring the period from the beginning of the DCP reaching −20 mV to the point where the potential started at 0 mV (repolarization) after reperfusion. Transient global ischemia was produced by occluding both common carotid arteries for 17.33±0.76 min to induce ID for 12.21±0.36 min. Animals were reperfused by releasing the occlusion of bilateral common carotid arteries. Rats survived for 6 h, 12 h, 24 h or 48 h after reperfusion.

Tissue Processing

Rats were anaesthetized with 10% chloralhydrate (0.4 ml/100 g). Perfusion-fixation was carried out transcardially with 0.9% normal saline (NS) followed by 4% paraformaldehye in phosphate buffer (PB, 0.15M, PH 7.4). Eyeballs were immediately removed and post-fixed in the same fixative for 2 days. Eye tissues were processed with a series of ascending alcohols; cleared in trichloromethane; then embedded in paraffin. Retina paraffin blocks were cut horizontally at 7 μm thickness using a microtome (RM2235, Leica, Wetzlar, Germany). Six nonadjacent sections through the optic disc with an interval of 70 μm were selected from each rat, and two were mounted on a glass slide coated with gelatin. Each slide contained 10 sections from five experimental groups to ensure all group sections were processed under the same conditions.

Histochemistry

Sections for hematoxylin and eosin (HE) staining were first de-waxed in xylene, rehydrated in a series of descending alcohols, rinsed in deionized distilled water (DDW), and stained with HE. Stained sections were dehydrated in a series of ascending alcohols, cleared in xylene and mounted with coverslips.

Sections for fluorescent peanut agglutinin (PNA) staining were processed based on Blanks' study [23]. Briefly, sections were de-waxed and rehydrated as described above, then rinsed in phosphate buffered saline (PBS, 0.01M, PH 7.4) followed by incubation in 0.01M PBS containing 0.1% Tween-20 for 30 min at room temperature. The sections were transferred into 50 μg/ml fluorescent-conjugated PNA (FL-1071, Vector Laboratories, Burlingame, USA) in PBS-Tween for 1 h at room temperature, then rinsed in PBS-Tween and 0.01M PBS. The sections were mounted on glass slides with coverslips coated with an anti-quenching reagent and observed with a Leica epifluorescence microscope (DM6000B, Leica, Wetzlar, Germany).

Immunofluorescence

Sections for immunofluorescence were first de-waxed in xylene and rehydrated as described above, then rinsed in 0.01M PBS. To expose the antigens, sections were placed in citrate buffer in a water bath kettle and heated to 90°C for 15 min. After cooling to room temperature, the sections were incubated in blocking solution (5% normal goat serum, 1% BSA and 0.25% Triton X-100 in 0.01M PBS) for 1 h at room temperature, then incubated with primary antibody diluted in blocking solution overnight at 4°C. The names and concentrations of the four primary antibodies are listed in Table 1. After rinsing in 0.01M PBS, the sections were incubated in fluorescent secondary antibodies at room temperature for 1 h (Table 1) followed by washes with 0.01M PBS. Afterwards, the sections were mounted with anti-quenching reagent and a coverslip. Finally the labeled tissues were observed and photographs taken using a fluorescence microscope (DM6000B, Leica, Wetzlar, Germany) with the appropriate filters.

Table 1. Information on primary and secondary antibodies.

Primary antibodies	Host	Dilution	Catalogue	Source
β3-Tubulin(TU-20)	Mouse	1:1000	4466	Cell Signaling
Calretinin	Rabbit	1:4000	AB5054	Millipore
Recoverin	Rabbit	1:1000	AB5585	Millipore
Rhodopsin	Mouse	1:1000	MAB5356	Millipore
Secondary antibodies				
Alexa Fluor 488	Goat anti-mouse	1:500	115-545-003	Europe Ltd
Alexa Fluor 488	Goat anti-rabbit	1:500	115-545-003	Europe Ltd

Cell Counts

Based on HE staining and immunofluorescence of βIII-tubulin, calretinin and recoverin, cells were quantified in the retinal ganglion cell layer (GCL) and/or inner nuclear layer (INL). Six sections of retina, through the optic disc, were selected from each rat. Two photographs were taken per section 100 μm either side of the optic disc, with a 40x objective. Because there were 5 rats in each experimental group, a total of 60 images from 30 sections were quantitatively analyzed from each group. The number of cells in a 300 μm length of the GCL and/or INL was counted from the captured images using the cell counter of the Image J software program.

Cell Layers and Thickness

Due to the condensed arrangement of cells in the inner nuclear layer (INL) and outer nuclear layer (ONL), it was difficult to quantify cells accurately. The INL and ONL in HE stained sections were analyzed by counting cell layers and measuring the thickness of the INL and ONL. The number of sections and magnification were the same as that used for cell counting. The numbers of cell layers in the INL and ONL of HE stained sections were counted directly from the captured images. The thickness of the INL and ONL were measured using Adobe Photoshop CS6 software.

Fluorescence Intensity

To detect rhodopsin immunoreactivity and fluorescent PNA staining, images were captured under the same conditions, including light exposure time and magnification. The number of captured images was the same as that used for cell quantification. Fluorescence intensity in each experimental group was analyzed with Image J software.

Electroretinography (ERG)

Rats should usually be adapted to the dark prior to ERG recordings. Based on Wang et al [24], the time for dark-adaptation in the present study was at least 70 min to reach a stable status. Following stabilization, ERGs were obtained. In brief, the control rats were anesthetized with 10% chloralhydrate (0.4 ml/100 g) and the pupils dilated with tropicamide. Recording electrodes were placed on the corneas. Two reference electrodes were inserted into subcutaneous tissue behind the ears and one ground electrode was inserted into subcutaneous tissue of the tail. The a-wave, b-wave, OPs and PhNR were recorded using a Roland Consult electrophysiological diagnostic system (Brandenburg, Germany).

Scotopic ERGs (a-wave, b-wave, OPs; 3.0 cds/m^2, white flash) were first recorded after 70 min dark adaptation. After light adaption under a continuous blue background (25 cds/m^2) for 5 min to suppress rod cell electrical activity, PhNR was recorded with red flashes (3.0 cds/m^2). Ischemic operation was performed on the control rats after ERG recording. After electrocauterizing the vertebral arteries and isolating the common carotid arteries under lighted conditions, rats were sent to a dark-adaptation room for 70 min, followed by transient occlusion of the common carotid arteries by arterial clamps (beak 8 mm) for 17.30±0.30 min. The rats were evaluated using ERG during ischemia, 1 h and 48 h after ischemia.

The measurement of different waves is illustrated in Figure 1. The amplitude of the a-wave was measured from the baseline to the peak of the a-wave, and the amplitude of the b-wave was measured from the trough of the a-wave to the peak of the b-wave. The amplitude of OPs was determined as the sum of the amplitudes of OP1, OP2, OP3, and OP4. The amplitude of PhNR was defined as the length from baseline to the first trough immediately following the b-wave. Four waves were measured using pCLAMP9.2.

Visual Behavior Detection

Visual behavior detection was conducted using a black-white box (custom-made by Metronet Technology Ltd). There were two chambers in the box: the black chamber and white chamber (Fig. 2). An aperture (10 × 12 cm) between the black and white chambers allowed rats to travel freely from one to the other. The black chamber was illuminated with infrared light, while the white chamber was illuminated by bright white light. Two cameras, installed in the two chambers separately, captured activities of the rats and were connected to a Noldus EthoVision XT 8.0 recorder and monitor.

Rats were placed into the middle of the white compartment at the start of the trial and left in the box for 15 min. The number of intercompartmental crosses, distance moved, mean velocity and the time spent in the black chamber and white chamber were recorded by the Noldus EthoVision XT 8.0 software.

Statistical Analysis

All data were analyzed with the statistical software program SPSS17.0 and were presented as mean ± SEM. One-way Analysis-of-variance (ANOVA) followed by the SNK (Student-Newman-Keuls) multiple comparison tests was used. P-values < 0.05 were considered as significant.

Results

No Changes in Cell Numbers of the GCL, INL and ONL after Ischemia

Cell layers of the retina were identified using HE staining (Fig. 3). No obvious changes in the morphology of cells in the GCL, INL and ONL of the retina were observed after ischemia. Quantitative analysis also showed no significant differences in the number of RGCs in the GCL, or the thickness and number of cell rows in the INL and ONL between the control group and ischemic groups, all $p > 0.05$ (Table 2).

Reduction of βIII-tubulin, Calretinin and Recoverin Immunoreativities after Ischemia

RGCs were identified using anti-βIII-tubulin immunostaining. βIII-tubulin positive cell bodies of RGCs in the GCL, and positive dendrites of RGCs in the INL were identified (Fig.4 A-E).

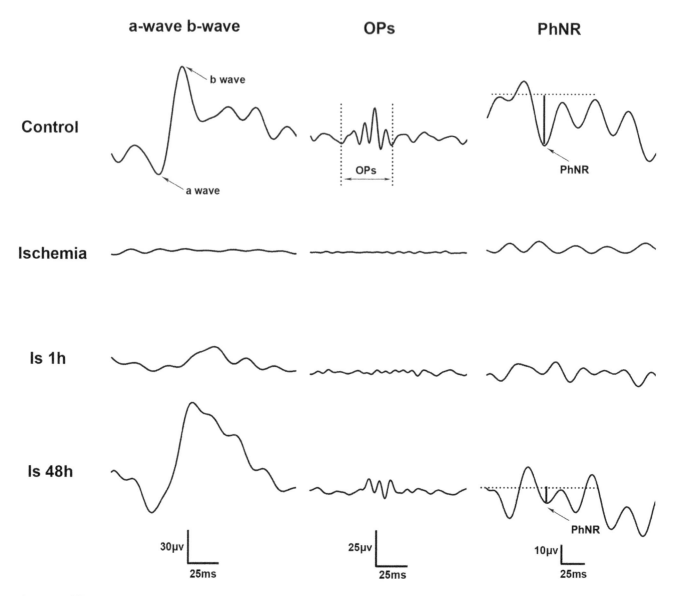

a-wave b-wave   **OPs**   **PhNR**

Control

Ischemia

Is 1h

Is 48h

Figure 1. Different waves in ERG recordings before and after ischemia. Representative dark-adapted ERG component amplitudes (a-wave, b-wave and OPs) and amplitudes of PhNR were recorded before and during ischemia, 1 h and 48 h after ischemia.

Calretinin labeling appeared in amacrine cells of the GCL and the innermost layer of the INL. Three layers of dendrites of calretinin positive cells appeared in the IPL (Fig.4 F-J). Recoverin immunoreactivity was detected in photoreceptors of the ONL and cone bipolar cells in the INL (Fig.4 K-O).

Qualitative analysis showed that the number of βIII-tubulin positive cells in the 300 μm length of the GCL was 23.72±0.31 in the control group. This number was significantly decreased in the Is 6 h (20.44±0.40), Is 12 h (20.96±0.30), Is 24 h (21.02±0.33) and Is 48 h (21.55±0.33) groups when compared with the control level, $p<0.01$(Fig. 4P). Similarly, the number of calretinin positive cells in the GCL and INL was also decreased in the Is 6 h (51.71±1.10), Is 12 h (52.11±1.02), Is 24 h (51.06±0.94) and Is 48 h (51.09±0.77) groups in comparison to the control group (55.94±0.81), $p<0.01$ (Fig. 4Q). However, the alteration patterns in recoverin immunoreactivity of the INL were slightly different from βIII-tubulin and calretinin immunoreactivities after ischemia. The number of recoverin positive cells in the control group

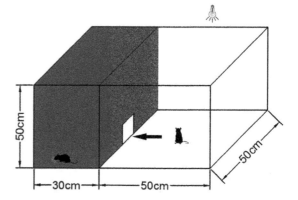

Figure 2. Schematic diagram illustrating the black-white box. The rat was placed in the middle of the white compartment at the start of the trial, and could travel freely in the white and black chambers through an aperture between the chambers.

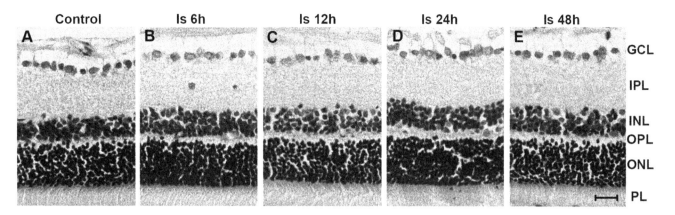

Figure 3. Photomicrograph showing HE staining of cell layers in the retina. Several layers of cells were identified from outside to inside of the retina as follows: the photoreceptor layer (PL), outer nuclear layer (ONL), outer plexiform layer (OPL), inner nuclear layer (INL), inner plexiform layer (IPL) and the ganglion cell layer (GCL). Cell bodies were seen in the GCL, INL and ONL. There were no obvious morphological changes in different groups before and after ischemia under a light microscope (A-E). Scale bar: 20 μm.

was 15.43 ± 0.36, but it reduced to 13.69 ± 0.29 at Is 6 h and 13.29 ± 0.27 at Is 12 h after ischemia, $p<0.01$. The number of recoverin positive cells then returned to the control level at Is 24 h (14.49 ± 0.31) and Is 48 h (14.57 ± 0.26), $p>0.05$ (Fig. 4R).

No Alteration of Rhodopsin Immunoreactivity and Fluorescent PNA Intensity after Ischemia

Rhodopsin was strongly expressed in the outer segment layer (PL-OS) of the retina (Fig.5 A-E). The inner segment (IS) and outer segment (OS) of cones were specifically labeled with fluorescent PNA staining in the photoreceptor layer of the retina (Fig.5 F-J). Quantitative analysis showed that there were no significant differences in either rhodopsin fluorescent intensity or PNA fluorescent intensity before and after ischemia, $p>0.05$ (Fig.5 K&L).

Different Wave Changes in ERG Recordings after Ischemia

ERG recordings were performed before ischemia, during ischemia, 1 h and 48 h after ischemia on the same rats. From figure 1, amplitudes of the a-wave, b-wave, Ops and PhNR were completely lost during ischemia. From Fig1 and Table 3, the amplitudes of the a- and b-waves at 1 h were still reduced after reperfusion when compared with the control group, $p<0.05$. The amplitudes of the a-wave and the b-wave almost recovered to the control level at 48 h after reperfusion, $p>0.05$. Although there was no significant difference between the control group and the

ischemic groups, the values of the b/a-wave ratio at 1 h and 48 h after ischemia were only half of the control level (Table 3). The amplitudes of OPs and PhNR still disappeared during and 1 h after ischemia. Although they were present 48 h after reperfusion, the OPs and PhNR amplitudes were still smaller than the control level, $p<0.01$ (Fig.1 and Table 3).

Alteration of Visual Behavioral Detection after Ischemia

Rats prefer staying in dark places. Therefore, when a rat was placed in the center of the white chamber (Fig.2 and Fig.6 B&D), it would enter the black chamber through an aperture between the white and black chamber. Rats stayed in the dark chamber for a longer time than in the white chamber in both the control group (Fig.6 A&B) and ischemic group (Fig.6 C&D). Statistically, there was no significant difference in the duration in the dark chamber between the control group (790.19 ± 23.80 s) and Is 48 h group (800.15 ± 12.37 s, $p>0.05$) (Fig.7 A). However, the distance moved in the black chamber was reduced in the Is 48 h group (1750.16 ± 180.87 cm) when compared with the control group (2930.49 ± 171.17 cm), $p<0.01$ (Fig.7 B); and in the white chamber was decreased in the Is 48 h group (500.42 ± 115.74 cm) when compared with the control group (1141.92 ± 242.67 cm), $p<0.05$ (Fig.7 C). Mean velocity at 48 h after ischemia in black chamber (2.23 ± 0.25 cm/s) were also reduced when compared to control animals (3.79 ± 0.28 cm/s), $p<0.01$ (Fig.7 D); and in white chamber was decreased in the Is 48 h group (4.38 ± 0.78 cm/s) when compared with the control group (11.19 ± 1.63 cm/s), $p<0.05$ (Fig.7 E). Finally, the number of intercompartmental

Table 2. Changes in the number, thickness and cell layers of the retina.

Groups	n	Number of cells in GCL	Thickness of INL (μm)	Number of rows in INL	Thickness of ONL (μm)	Number of rows in ONL
Control	5	27.66 ± 0.57	18.78 ± 0.42	4.58 ± 0.07	34.41 ± 0.61	9.73 ± 0.20
Is 6h	5	26.16 ± 0.54	19.00 ± 0.35	4.23 ± 0.06	33.47 ± 0.60	9.19 ± 0.17
Is 12h	5	26.74 ± 0.39	20.10 ± 0.53	4.32 ± 0.06	33.66 ± 0.68	9.46 ± 0.17
Is 24h	5	27.60 ± 0.51	18.54 ± 0.62	4.30 ± 0.06	32.17 ± 0.88	8.84 ± 0.18
Is 48h	5	27.89 ± 0.47	18.40 ± 0.34	4.17 ± 0.05	32.54 ± 0.51	9.04 ± 0.17
		$P>0.05$	$P>0.05$	$P>0.05$	$P>0.05$	$P>0.05$

All groups were compared with the control group.

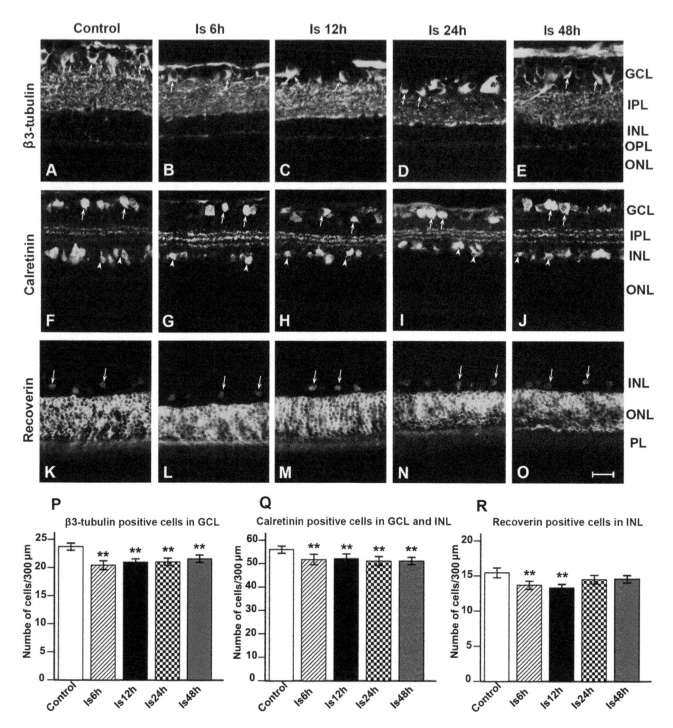

Figure 4. Immunofluorescent reactivities and cell numbers in different retinal layers. A-E: βIII-tubulin immunoreativity was observed in the somata of retinal ganglion cells (RGCs) in the ganglion cell layer (GCL) (arrows, A-E) and processes in the inner plexiform layer (IPL). F-J: Calretinin positive cells were found in the GCL (arrows, F-J) and INL (arrow heads, F-J) and three positive strata of processes appeared in the IPL. K-O: Recoverin immunoreactivity was detected in retinal photoreceptors and cone bipolar cells in the inner nuclear layer (INL) (arrows, K-O). Quantitative analysis showed that the number of βIII-tubulin positive cells in the GCL decreased from 6 h to 48 h after ischemia, $p<0.01$(P). The number of calretinin positive amacrine cells in the GCL and INL also decreased from 6 h to 48 h after ischemia, $p<0.01$ (Q). The number of recoverin positive cells in the INL was reduced at 6 h and 12 h after ischemia, $p<0.01$, but returned to control levels at 24 h after reperfusion, $p>0.05$ (R). Scale bar: 20 μm.

crosses in the control group was $6.07\pm1.02/900$ s, whereas it decreased at 48 h after ischemia $(3.42\pm0.48/900$ s), $p<0.05$ (Fig.7 F).

Discussion

In the present study, we investigated changes in different types of neurons of the retina using a combination of immunohisto-chemistry, ERG and visual behavior detection following transient

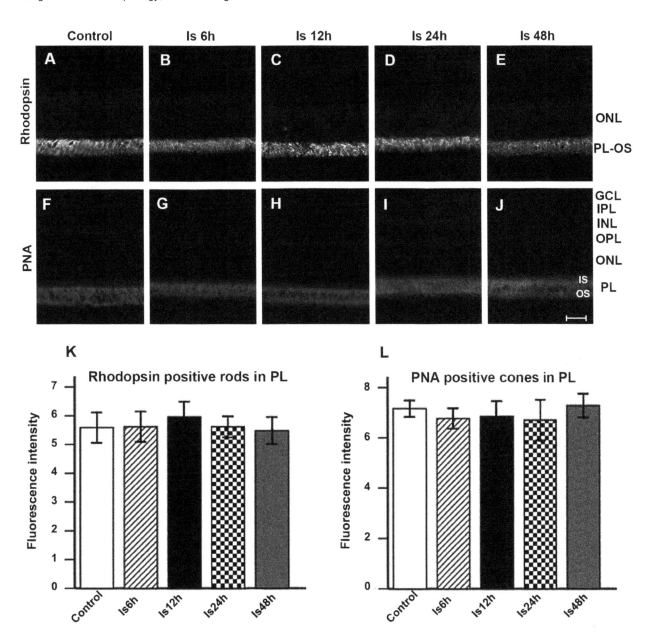

Figure 5. Rhodopsin fluorescent immunoreactivity and PNA fluorescent intensity. A-E: Rhodopsin positive cells (specific for rods) appeared in the outer segment of the photoreceptor layer of retina (PL-OS). F-J: PNA positive cells (specific for cones) were found in the inner segment (IS) and the outer segment (OS) of the photoreceptor layer (PL). Quantitative analysis showed that the fluorescence intensity of rhodopsin positive cells in the PL did not change after ischemia, $p > 0.05$ (K). The fluorescence intensity of PNA positive cells also did not change after ischemia, $p > 0.05$ (L). Scale bar: 20 μm.

Table 3. Changes in ERG recordings before and after ischemia.

Groups	n	a-wave (μV)	b-wave (μV)	b/a-wave ratio	Ops (μV)	PhNR (μV)
Control	10	28.68±2.76	52.50±4.93	2.77±1.02	42.92±2.84	24.50±3.07
Ischemia	10	disappeared	disappeared	disappeared	disappeared	disappeared
Is 1h	10	18.56±3.55*	16.25±1.31**	1.49±0.40	disappeared	disappeared
Is 48h	10	32.55±2.99	44.35±3.45	1.46±0.17	28.91±2.45**	10.40±1.84**

*: $P < 0.05$, **: $P < 0.01$, compared with the control group.

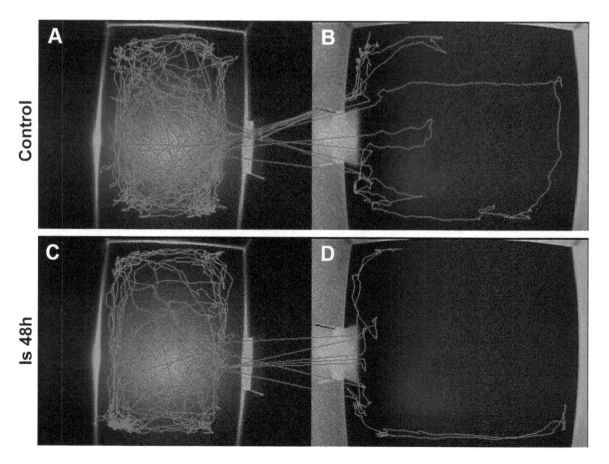

Figure 6. Behavioral detections of rats in the black-white box. The red lines represent the moving trajectory of a single rat in the two experimental groups. The representative rat in the control group spent more time traveling in the black chamber (A) than in the white chamber (B). The ischemic rat traveled in the black-white box in a similar pattern as that in the control group (C & D).

global ischemia. The results revealed varied vulnerability among different retina cell types to ischemia.

RGCs and Amacrine Cells are the Most Sensitive to Ischemia in the Retina

The severity of ischemic effects on RGCs depends on the degree and duration of ischemia. In the present study, we employed a transient global ischemia model (4-VO) without mechanical injury. Retinal ischemia was induced by permanent occlusion of the vertebral arteries plus transient occlusion of the bilateral common carotid arteries for approximately 17 min. Although we did not detect changes in the number of individual cell layers after ischemia, we found that βIII-tubulin immunoreactivity (RGCs marker) decreased from 6 h to 48 h after reperfusion. This suggests the function of RGCs was affected by the transient ischemic attack. Consistent with this, the PhNR wave was completely lost during ischemia and 1 h after reperfusion. Even at 48 h after reperfusion, the amplitude of PhNR was still not recovered, which indicated that the function of RGCs had not completely recovered by this time. ERG has been considered a more sensitive method to detect retinal injury than histology [25]. The amplitude of PhNR was considered a marker to reflect the activity of RGCs [4–7]. Based on previous studies, the amplitude of PhNR was reduced in glaucoma [6], retinal vein occlusion [7], severe diabetic retinopathy [5] and after optic nerve transection [4]. Compared to transient global ischemia, the intraocular pressure (IOP) model produced much more severe ischemic and

mechanical injury to RGCs. When the IOP was elevated to 90 to 120 mmHg for 45 to 90 min, the majority of RGCs died by 7 days or later after reperfusion [26,27]. A similar phenomenon was observed following ischemia caused by ligature of the ophthalmic vessels (LOV) [28]. Although internal carotid artery occlusion (ICAO) and occlusion of bilateral common carotid arteries (BCCAO) induced milder damage to RGCs than that induced by IOP or LOV, a longer ischemic episode (2 h in ICAO, permanent in BCCAO) also caused death of most RGCs at different stages following reperfusion [29–31].

Therefore, previous morphological studies indicated that RGCs die after severe ischemia. In the present study, morphological and ERG recording techniques showed that the function of RGCs was affected even though no changes in cell number under transient global ischemia attack were observed, which suggests RGCs are vulnerable to ischemia.

In the retina, the amacrine cell is also sensitive to ischemia. It has been reported that 30% calretinin positive amacrine cells were lost after 60 min of ischemia by elevating intraocular pressure to 100–120 mmHg, or by occlusion of the middle cerebral artery at 1–3 days reperfusion time [32]. After ligation of the internal carotid artery for 2 h, almost half of calretinin positive amacrine cells were lost 22 h following reperfusion [31]. In Dijk, et al's study, approximately 80% calretinin positive amacrine cell loss was observed at 3 days after 60 min ischemia in the IOP model [33,34]. However, Hernandez et al's study showed that calretinin

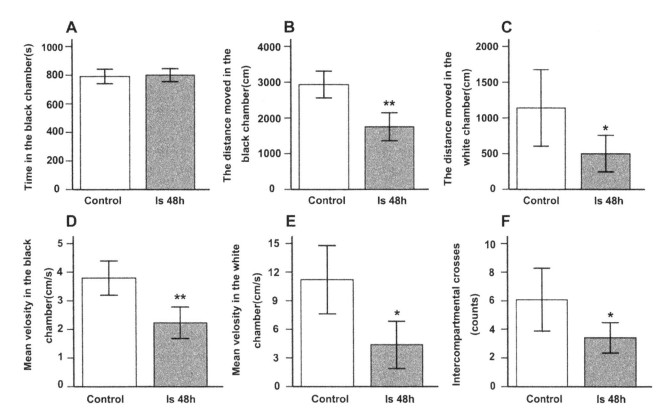

Figure 7. Statistical analysis of the parameters of behavior detection. There was no difference in the time spent in the black chamber between the control and the ischemic groups at 48 h after reperfusion, $p > 0.05$ (A). However, the distance moved in the black chamber (B, $p < 0.01$) and white chamber (C, $p < 0.05$), the mean velocity in the black (D, $p < 0.01$) and white chamber (E, $p < 0.05$), and the number of intercompartmental crosses (F, $p < 0.05$) were reduced at 48 h after reperfusion.

immunoreactivity of amacrine cells recovered at 7 days after reperfusion [35].

Compared with the above studies, amacrine cells underwent similar changes as RGCs in immunoreactivity after 17 min transient global ischemia in the present study. Approximately 10% of calretinin immunoreactive cell loss occurred from 6 h to 48 h after transient global ischemia.

In ERG studies, OPs are mainly generated by amacrine cells. It has been reported that amplitudes of OPs reduced after elevating IOP [27]. Our study has shown that transient global ischemia for 17 min completely blocked OPs during ischemia and 1 h after reperfusion. The amplitudes of OPs were still lower than the control level at 48 h after ischemia. This evidence suggests that amacrine cells are also sensitive to different types of ischemic injuries.

Bipolar Cells and Photoreceptors are Tolerant of Ischemia

Morphologically, we did not find changes in cellular layers, the thickness of the ONL, rhodopsin immunoreactivity (rods marker) or PNA fluorescent density (cones marker) before and after ischemia in the present study. These results indicate photoreceptors are most tolerant to ischemic insult. In support of this, it has been reported that the number of horizontal cells and photoreceptors of the rat retina did not change while the majority of RGCs and several subtypes of amacrine cells were lost in glaucoma models [34,36,37]. Essentially, the sensitivity to ischemia of different cell types depends on the degree and duration of ischemia. When ischemic duration is extensive, such as permanent ischemia, photoreceptor cells will eventually degenerate. Stevens and his colleagues reported that photoreceptors were lost at 3 months following permanent ligation of the bilateral common carotid artery [29].

Based on the results of ERG recordings in the present study, the a-wave disappeared during ischemia, however, it partially recovered at 1 h and completely recovered at 48 h after reperfusion. These electrophysiological results further indicate that photoreceptor cells can quickly recover after reperfusion.

Although we did not find changes in cellular layers or the thickness of the INL, the number of recoverin positive cells (cone bipolar cells) of the INL was reduced at 6 h and 12 h after reperfusion. However, this number returned to the control level 24 h after ischemia. ERG recording results from our study have also showed that the b-wave (produced by bipolar cells) disappeared during ischemia and was barely seen at 1 h following reperfusion, but it recovered by 48 h after reperfusion. The changing pattern of the b-wave after ischemia was similar to that of the a-wave, but the b/a-wave ratio decreased to almost half of the control value at 1 h and 48 h following ischemia. The b/a-wave ratio has been considered a sensitive parameter for detecting the degree of retinal injury induced by ischemia. Lower b/a-wave ratios were considered as indicators of severe injury of the retina [38,39]. It has been reported that the b-wave was totally abolished while a-wave amplitude enhanced without any histological changes of retinal neurons at day 7 following BCCAO [40]. Therefore, the results of morphology and ERG recordings in our study indicate that the function of bipolar cells was transiently affected by ischemia.

Our study has shown that RGCs and amacrine cells are most vulnerable to ischemia, while photoreceptors are most tolerant, and bipolar cells are in between. These results are consistent with those from Yamamoto and his colleagues [41]. They investigated the order of neuronal death in the retina using a BCCAO model and found that RGCs were damaged at 1 week after ischemia while INL neurons were dead at 2 months; photoreceptors were absent at 4 months after permanent BCCAO.

Ischemic Changes in Visual Behavior Detection

Although the black-white box was widely used to detect anxiety by stress [42–45], it has recently been employed to investigate visual function [13]. An animal with light perception will escape from the white chamber to the black chamber. Based on Lin's report, normal mice stayed in the black chamber for a longer time, whereas retinal degeneration *rd/rd* mice stayed in the black chamber for a shorter time because night-sensitive photoreceptors (rod cells) have been damaged. In the present study, there was no significant difference in the duration of remaining in the black chamber between the control group and ischemic group, which indicates that the animals still perceive light. However, ischemic rats showed a reduction in the distance moved and mean velocity in the black and white chamber, which may reflect a week visual acuity. In support of this, ERG results showed that the amplitudes of OPs and PhNR were reduced after ischemia. In addition, the protein synthesis of ganglion cells and amacrine cells was decreased within 2 days after ischemia in spite of an unchanging number of these cells. Therefore, transient global ischemia in a period of 17 min not only induces dysfunction in protein synthesis and electrophysiology but also in visual behavior.

Rats have a rod-dominated retina and prefer dark places where they feel more comfortable [46]. This is different with the human who is largely dependent upon cone-mediated vision. Therefore, the criteria for evaluating anxiety are different between the human and the rat. Based on previous studies, the criteria for evaluating anxiety behavior in rats includes the time within the black chamber and white chamber, the number of intercompartmental crosses, and activity in the white chamber and black chamber [42–44,47,48]. In the present study, we also explored whether transient global ischemia would induce anxiety behavior. We found that the number of intercompartmental crosses decreased in ischemic rats compared with controls, suggesting that anxiety-like behavior appears in rats after transient global ischemia. Based on Luan et al's finding that alpha/Y-like retinal ganglion cells innervate the midbrain dorsal raphe nucleus [49] and ablation of this type of RGC induced depressive-like behavior [50], it is possible that transient global ischemia induces this type of cell injury thus causing anxiety-like behavior. This behavior may indeed be due to changes in the retina that causes visual impairment but we cannot discount the possibility that anxiety-like behavior is also caused by changes to brain regions affected in this model of ischemia.

Impacts of Different Ischemia Models on the Pathology of the Retina

Different ischemic retina models were employed to investigate the impact of ischemia on the retina. A model of high IOP was used to investigate ischemic retinal autophagy [51,52]. The model by ligation of the optic nerve bundle was employed to study ischemia-induced cell mitosis in the adult rat retina [53]. The model by ligation of ophthalmic vessels (LOV) was applied to reveal ischemia-induced retinal ganglion cell death [54]. Damages to the retina in these models may be more serious than purely ischemia injury because the mechanical injury may also contribute to the retinal damage. The ischemia model by occlusion of the bilateral common carotid arteries (BCCAO) has also been employed to investigate the pathological changes of the retina in several studies [29,30,41]. All authors found a loss of retinal ganglion cells after BCCAO but due to variable chronic occlusion times they reported different latencies of ganglion cell death. The earliest time point for ganglion cell loss was 7 days after the start of occlusion as found by Yamamoto et al. The 4-VO ischemia model used in the present study produces quite different results from the BCCAO model. After approximately 17 min of complete occlusion followed by reperfusion we did not find any ganglion cell loss but a loss of immunoreactivity by some ganglion cells (and amacrine cells). Compared to the retinal ischemic models mentioned above, the 4-VO model has been employed less to observe the changes in pathology of the retina. Ozden, S. et al reported that transient global ischemia for a duration of 30 to 90 min induced the loss of ganglion cells and amacrine cells [55]. Our study showed that an approximate 17 min duration of transient global ischemia could induce changes in ERG recording and synthesis of protein of ganglion cells and amacrine cells, and anxiety-like behavior but not cell loss.

In conclusion, transient global ischemia for 17 min induced cellular, molecular and electrophysiological dysfunction of RGCs and amacrine cells within 2 days after ischemia, but did not affect photoreceptors and light perception. Bipolar cells underwent transient changes in molecular and electrophysiological levels after ischemia. The results support the idea that RGCs and amacrine cells are most vulnerable and photoreceptors are most resistant to ischemia.

Acknowledgments

We thank Dr. Gregor Campbell and Dr. Qi Cui for reviewing this manuscript and his constructive suggestions.

Author Contributions

Conceived and designed the experiments: YWR ADX. Performed the experiments: YZ BY YHX XJH. Analyzed the data: YZ BY YX YWR. Contributed reagents/materials/analysis tools: YZ YWR. Wrote the paper: YZ YWR ADX. Gave suggestions how to design the experiment, edit the results, and write the manuscript: KFS.

References

1. Masland RH (2001) The fundamental plan of the retina. Nat Neurosci 4: 877–886.
2. Kline RP, Ripps H, Dowling JE (1978) Generation of b-wave currents in the skate retina. Proc Natl Acad Sci U S A 75: 5727–5731.
3. Wachtmeister L (1998) Oscillatory potentials in the retina: what do they reveal. Prog Retin Eye Res 17: 485–521.
4. Li B, Barnes GE, Holt WF (2005) The decline of the photopic negative response (PhNR) in the rat after optic nerve transection. Doc Ophthalmol 111: 23–31.
5. Chen H, Zhang M, Huang S, Wu D (2008) The photopic negative response of flash ERG in nonproliferative diabetic retinopathy. Doc Ophthalmol 117: 129–135.
6. Viswanathan S, Frishman LJ, Robson JG, Walters JW (2001) The photopic negative response of the flash electroretinogram in primary open angle glaucoma. Invest Ophthalmol Vis Sci 42: 514–522.
7. Chen H, Wu D, Huang S, Yan H (2006) The photopic negative response of the flash electroretinogram in retinal vein occlusion. Doc Ophthalmol 113: 53–59.
8. Del Cerro M, DiLoreto D Jr, Cox C, Lazar ES, Grover DA, et al. (1995) Neither intraocular grafts of retinal cell homogenates nor live non-retinal neurons produce behavioral recovery in rats with light-damaged retinas. Cell Transplant 4: 133–139.
9. Meier P, Flister E, Reinagel P (2011) Collinear features impair visual detection by rats. J Vis 11.
10. Gianfranceschi L, Fiorentini A, Maffei L (1999) Behavioural visual acuity of wild type and bcl2 transgenic mouse. Vision Res 39: 569–574.

11. Schmucker C, Seeliger M, Humphries P, Biel M, Schaeffel F (2005) Grating acuity at different luminances in wild-type mice and in mice lacking rod or cone function. Invest Ophthalmol Vis Sci 46: 398–407.

12. Thomas BB, Samant DM, Seiler MJ, Aramant RB, Sheikholeslami S, et al. (2007) Behavioral evaluation of visual function of rats using a visual discrimination apparatus. J Neurosci Methods 162: 84–90.

13. Lin B, Koizumi A, Tanaka N, Panda S, Masland RH (2008) Restoration of visual function in retinal degeneration mice by ectopic expression of melanopsin. Proc Natl Acad Sci U S A 105: 16009–16014.

14. Madl C, Holzer M (2004) Brain function after resuscitation from cardiac arrest. Curr Opin Crit Care 10: 213–217.

15. Hogue CW, Gottesman RF, Stearns J (2008) Mechanisms of cerebral injury from cardiac surgery. Crit Care Clin 24: 83–98, viii-ix.

16. Block F, Schwarz M, Sontag KH (1992) Retinal ischemia induced by occlusion of both common carotid arteries in rats as demonstrated by electroretinography. Neurosci Lett 144: 124–126.

17. Ruan YW, Han XJ, Shi ZS, Lei ZG, Xu ZC (2012) Remodeling of synapses in the CA1 area of the hippocampus after transient global ischemia. Neuroscience 218: 268–277.

18. Ruan YW, Lei Z, Fan Y, Zou B, Xu ZC (2009) Diversity and fluctuation of spine morphology in CA1 pyramidal neurons after transient global ischemia. J Neurosci Res 87: 61–68.

19. Ruan YW, Zou B, Fan Y, Li Y, Lin N, et al. (2006) Dendritic plasticity of CA1 pyramidal neurons after transient global ischemia. Neuroscience 140: 191–201.

20. Ruan YW, Zou B, Fan Y, Li Y, Lin N, et al. (2007) Morphological heterogeneity of CA1 pyramidal neurons in response to ischemia. J Neurosci Res 85: 193–204.

21. Pulsinelli WA, Brierley JB (1979) A new model of bilateral hemispheric ischemia in the unanesthetized rat. Stroke 10: 267–272.

22. Xu ZC, Gao TM, Ren Y (1999) Neurophysiological changes associated with selective neuronal damage in hippocampus following transient forebrain ischemia. Biol Signals Recept 8: 294–308.

23. Blanks JC, Johnson LV (1983) Selective lectin binding of the developing mouse retina. J Comp Neurol 221: 31–41.

24. Wang X, Mo X, Li D, Wang Y, Fang Y, et al. (2011) Neuroprotective effect of transcorneal electrical stimulation on ischemic damage in the rat retina. Exp Eye Res 93: 753–760.

25. Osborne NN, Casson RJ, Wood JP, Chidlow G, Graham M, et al. (2004) Retinal ischemia: mechanisms of damage and potential therapeutic strategies. Prog Retin Eye Res 23: 91–147.

26. Adachi M, Takahashi K, Nishikawa M, Miki H, Uyama M (1996) High intraocular pressure-induced ischemia and reperfusion injury in the optic nerve and retina in rats. Graefes Arch Clin Exp Ophthalmol 234: 445–451.

27. Jehle T, Wingert K, Dimitriu C, Meschede W, Lasseck J, et al. (2008) Quantification of ischemic damage in the rat retina: a comparative study using evoked potentials, electroretinography, and histology. Invest Ophthalmol Vis Sci 49: 1056–1064.

28. Lafuente MP, Villegas-Perez MP, Selles-Navarro I, Mayor-Torroglosa S, Miralles de Imperial J, et al. (2002) Retinal ganglion cell death after acute retinal ischemia is an ongoing process whose severity and duration depends on the duration of the insult. Neuroscience 109: 157–168.

29. Stevens WD, Fortin T, Pappas BA (2002) Retinal and optic nerve degeneration after chronic carotid ligation: time course and role of light exposure. Stroke 33: 1107–1112.

30. Lavinsky D, Arterni NS, Achaval M, Netto CA (2006) Chronic bilateral common carotid artery occlusion: a model for ocular ischemic syndrome in the rat. Graefes Arch Clin Exp Ophthalmol 244: 199–204.

31. Li SY, Yang D, Yeung CM, Yu WY, Chang RC, et al. (2011) Lycium barbarum polysaccharides reduce neuronal damage, blood-retinal barrier disruption and oxidative stress in retinal ischemia/reperfusion injury. PLoS One 6: e16380.

32. Lee JH, Shin JM, Shin YJ, Chun MH, Oh SJ (2011) Immunochemical changes of calbindin, calretinin and SMI32 in ischemic retinas induced by increase of intraocular pressure and by middle cerebral artery occlusion. Anat Cell Biol 44: 25–34.

33. Dijk F, van Leeuwen S, Kamphuis W (2004) Differential effects of ischemia/reperfusion on amacrine cell subtype-specific transcript levels in the rat retina. Brain Res 1026: 194–204.

34. Dijk F, Kamphuis W (2004) Ischemia-induced alterations of AMPA-type glutamate receptor subunit. Expression patterns in the rat retina–an immunocytochemical study. Brain Res 997: 207–221.

35. Hernandez M, Rodriguez FD, Sharma SC, Vecino E (2009) Immunohistochemical changes in rat retinas at various time periods of elevated intraocular pressure. Mol Vis 15: 2696–2709.

36. Kwon OJ, Kim JY, Kim SY, Jeon CJ (2005) Alterations in the localization of calbindin D28K-, calretinin-, and parvalbumin-immunoreactive neurons of rabbit retinal ganglion cell layer from ischemia and reperfusion. Mol Cells 19: 382–390.

37. Chun MH, Kim IB, Ju WK, Kim KY, Lee MY, et al. (1999) Horizontal cells of the rat retina are resistant to degenerative processes induced by ischemia-reperfusion. Neurosci Lett 260: 125–128.

38. Sabates R, Hirose T, McMeel JW (1983) Electroretinography in the prognosis and classification of central retinal vein occlusion. Arch Ophthalmol 101: 232–235.

39. Johnson MA, McPhee TJ (1993) Electroretinographic findings in iris neovascularization due to acute central retinal vein occlusion. Arch Ophthalmol 111: 806–814.

40. Barnett NL, Osborne NN (1995) Prolonged bilateral carotid artery occlusion induces electrophysiological and immunohistochemical changes to the rat retina without causing histological damage. Exp Eye Res 61: 83–90.

41. Yamamoto H, Schmidt-Kastner R, Hamasaki DI, Parel JM (2006) Complex neurodegeneration in retina following moderate ischemia induced by bilateral common carotid artery occlusion in Wistar rats. Exp Eye Res 82: 767–779.

42. Timothy C, Costall B, Smythe JW (1999) Effects of SCH23390 and raclopride on anxiety-like behavior in rats tested in the black-white box. Pharmacol Biochem Behav 62: 323–327.

43. Smythe JW, Murphy D, Timothy C, Costall B (1997) Hippocampal mineralocorticoid, but not glucocorticoid, receptors modulate anxiety-like behavior in rats. Pharmacol Biochem Behav 56: 507–513.

44. Smythe JW, Bhatnagar S, Murphy D, Timothy C, Costall B (1998) The effects of intrahippocampal scopolamine infusions on anxiety in rats as measured by the black-white box test. Brain Res Bull 45: 89–93.

45. Bradley BF, Bridges NJ, Starkey NJ, Brown SL, Lea RW (2011) Anxiolytic and anxiogenic drug effects on male and female gerbils in the black-white box. Behav Brain Res 216: 285–292.

46. Neitz J, Jacobs GH (1986) Reexamination of spectral mechanisms in the rat (Rattus norvegicus). J Comp Psychol 100: 21–29.

47. Shumyatsky GP, Tsvetkov E, Malleret G, Vronskaya S, Hatton M, et al. (2002) Identification of a signaling network in lateral nucleus of amygdala important for inhibiting memory specifically related to learned fear. Cell 111: 905–918.

48. Lagouge M, Argmann C, Gerhart-Hines Z, Meziane H, Lerin C, et al. (2006) Resveratrol improves mitochondrial function and protects against metabolic disease by activating SIRT1 and PGC-1alpha. Cell 127: 1109–1122.

49. Luan L, Ren C, Lau BW, Yang J, Pickard GE, et al. (2011) Y-like retinal ganglion cells innervate the dorsal raphe nucleus in the Mongolian gerbil (Meriones unguiculatus). PLoS One 6: e18938.

50. Ren C, Luan L, Wui-Man Lau B, Huang X, Yang J, et al. (2013) Direct Retino-Raphe Projection Alters Serotonergic Tone and Affective Behavior. Neuropsychopharmacology.

51. Russo R, Berliocchi L, Adornetto A, Varano GP, Cavaliere F, et al. (2011) Calpain-mediated cleavage of Beclin-1 and autophagy deregulation following retinal ischemic injury in vivo. Cell Death Dis 2: e144.

52. Mi XS, Feng Q, Lo AC, Chang RC, Lin B, et al. (2012) Protection of retinal ganglion cells and retinal vasculature by lycium barbarum polysaccharides in a mouse model of acute ocular hypertension. PLoS One 7: e45469.

53. Stefansson E, Wilson CA, Schoen T, Kuwabara T (1988) Experimental ischemia induces cell mitosis in the adult rat retina. Invest Ophthalmol Vis Sci 29: 1050–1055.

54. Vidal-Sanz M, Lafuente MP, Mayor S, de Imperial JM, Villegas-Perez MP (2001) Retinal ganglion cell death induced by retinal ischemia. neuroprotective effects of two alpha-2 agonists. Surv Ophthalmol 45 Suppl 3: S261–267; discussion S273–266.

55. Ozden S, Kildaci B, Muftuoglu S, Cakar N, Yildirim C (2001) Effect of trimetazidine on retinal ischemia/reperfusion injury in rats. Ophthalmologica 215: 309–317.

6

Remote Ischemic Preconditioning (RIPC) Modifies Plasma Proteome in Humans

Michele Hepponstall[1,2,3,4], Vera Ignjatovic[1,3], Steve Binos[4], Paul Monagle[1,3], Bryn Jones[1,2], Michael H. H. Cheung[1,2,3], Yves d'Udekem[1,2], Igor E. Konstantinov[1,2,3]*

1 Haematology Research, Murdoch Childrens Research Institute; Melbourne, Victoria, Australia, 2 Cardiac Surgery Unit and Cardiology, Royal Children's Hospital; Melbourne, Victoria, Australia, 3 Department of Paediatrics, The University of Melbourne; Melbourne, Victoria, Australia, 4 Bioscience Research Division, Department of Primary Industries, Melbourne, Victoria, Australia

Abstract

Remote Ischemic Preconditioning (RIPC) induced by brief episodes of ischemia of the limb protects against multi-organ damage by ischemia-reperfusion (IR). Although it has been demonstrated that RIPC affects gene expression, the proteomic response to RIPC has not been determined. This study aimed to examine RIPC induced changes in the plasma proteome. Five healthy adult volunteers had 4 cycles of 5 min ischemia alternating with 5 min reperfusion of the forearm. Blood samples were taken from the ipsilateral arm prior to first ischaemia, immediately after each episode of ischemia as well as, at 15 min and 24 h after the last episode of ischemia. Plasma samples from five individuals were analysed using two complementary techniques. Individual samples were analysed using 2Dimensional Difference in gel electrophoresis (2D DIGE) and mass spectrometry (MS). Pooled samples for each of the time-points underwent trypsin digestion and peptides generated were analysed in triplicate using Liquid Chromatography and MS (LC-MS). Six proteins changed in response to RIPC using 2D DIGE analysis, while 48 proteins were found to be differentially regulated using LC-MS. The proteins of interest were involved in acute phase response signalling, and physiological molecular and cellular functions. The RIPC stimulus modifies the plasma protein content in blood taken from the ischemic arm in a cumulative fashion and evokes a proteomic response in peripheral blood.

Editor: Yao Liang Tang, University of Cincinnati, United States of America

Funding: This project was funded by the National Health and Medical Research Council (NHMRC) grant (# 628756) and NHMRC postgraduate scholarship (# 1017734). Yves d'Udekem is a Career Development Fellow of The National Heart Foundation of Australia (CR 10M 5339). This study was supported by the Victorian Government's Operational Infrastructure Support Program. The funders had no role in study design, data collection and analysis, decision to publish, or preparation of the manuscript.

Competing Interests: The authors have declared that no competing interests exist.

* E-mail: igor.konstantinov@rch.org.au

Introduction

Ischemic preconditioning is a potent innate mechanism observed in many species whereby cells develop tolerance to ischemia-reperfusion (IR) injury when exposed to controlled periods of transient, sub-lethal ischemia prior to a prolonged ischaemia [1,2]. However, *local* ischemic preconditioning is not clinically applicable to most patients. During the past decade, a simple technique of preconditioning has been developed with the potential for rapid translation into clinical practice [3].

Remote ischemic preconditioning (RIPC) is a phenomenon where brief episodes of ischemia of one tissue (e.g., skeletal muscle) protect against IR injury in an organ at a *remote* location [4]. RIPC has great potential for clinical application as it can be applied non-invasively using a standard blood pressure cuff to induce cycles of IR to skeletal muscle [3,5]. We have previously demonstrated that brief episodes of limb ischemia protected the donor heart after transplantation [6], providing multi-organ protection against cardiopulmonary bypass-induced tissue injury [7] and effective protection during evolving myocardial infarction [8]. We have also demonstrated that IR and RIPC induced a genomic response in the myocardium and circulating leukocytes of experimental animals and in humans [9–11]. Additionally, we observed that

RIPC decreased expression of kinin receptors [12], neutrophil adhesion and also modified the functional responses of human neutrophils [13]. We have also applied RIPC to clinical practice and demonstrated, in a randomized controlled trial, the benefits of the RIPC in children undergoing cardiac surgery [14]. A recent large randomized controlled trial further demonstrated a beneficial effect of the RIPC, as a complement to angioplasty, on myocardial salvage in patients with acute myocardial infarction [5].

Although the clinical benefits of RIPC are apparent, the mechanism underlying this protection remains unknown. Others and we have previously suggested the existence of a blood-borne effector of the RIPC stimulus that is transferred from the transiently ischemic limb to remote organs rendering them resistant to prolonged ischemia [6,15]. Furthermore, it appears that transient limb ischemia not only remotely preconditions through a humoral mechanism, but also that plasma transfer from the ischemic limb of one species may protect against IR injury in other species [15].

It is intuitive to believe that the observed changes in gene expression in response to the RIPC [9,10] will result in changes protein expression. However, the proteomic response to RIPC has not been studied to date. The purpose of this study was to determine 1) if the plasma from the transiently ischemic limb has a modified proteomic profile, 2) if the proteomic changes are cumulative with each subsequent episode of transient ischemia, and 3) if the RIPC stimulus evokes a global proteomic response early and late after the induction of the transient limb ischemia.

Materials and Methods

This study was approved by the Royal Children's Hospital Ethics in Human Research Committee (#29007) and written informed consent was obtained from the participants. Five healthy adult male volunteers 36.2 ± 6.3 (mean $\pm$ SD), not on any medications were fasted overnight and underwent the RIPC protocol. The protocol consisted of 4 cycles of 5 minutes of ischemia alternating with 5 minutes of reperfusion. Ischemia was induced by inflating a standard blood pressure cuff to a pressure exceeding systolic, as previously described [14]. Venous blood samples were collected from the same arm at 6 time-points: baseline, at the beginning of each period of re-perfusion and then at 15 minutes and 24 hours following application of the RIPC stimulus. Blood samples were collected in S-Monovette® tubes (Sarstedt, Australia), containing 1 volume of citrate per 9 volumes of blood. The samples were centrifuged at 3000 rpm for 10 min at $10°C$ (Megafuge 1.0R, Heraeus), the plasma was collected and stored at $-80°C$. The samples were then analysed using two methods described below (**Figure 1**).

Two-Dimensional Difference in Gel Electrophoresis (2D-DIGE) and Mass Spectrometry

The analysis was conducted on 30 individual samples (6 samples from 5 individuals).

Albumin and IgG depletion was performed using the albumin IgG depletion kit (GE Healthcare, Australia). The remaining proteins were precipitated using acetone precipitation, as specified in the depletion kit and resuspended in buffer containing 7 mol/L urea, 2 mol/L thiourea, 4% 3-[3-cholaamidopropyl]-1-propane-sulfonate and 30 mmol/L Tris. The protein content of each sample was quantified using the Bradford assay (Bio-Rad, Hercules, CA, USA) and bovine serum albumin standards [16].

The internal standard, consisting of an equal amount of each of the 30 samples, was labelled with Cyanine 2 (Cy2) fluorescent dye (GE Healthcare, Australia) and run on each gel to control for gel-to-gel variation. Each sample was randomised to be labelled with either Cy 3 or Cy5 dye and then randomized to 15 gels. The Cy2, Cy3 and Cy5 samples (50 mg of sample/400 pmol of Cy dye) for each gel were pooled and loaded onto the Immobilized pH Gradient (IPG) strip. One 24 cm, pH 3–11 strip per gel was rehydrated with 15 ml IPG buffer and 3 ml DeStreak solution (GE Healthcare, Australia). Proteins were separated based on isoelectric point (first dimension) and molecular weight (second dimension) using previously published methodology [16]. Gels were scanned using the Typhoon Trio variable mode imager (GE Healthcare, Australia) [16]. Data obtained from the scanning were quantified using DeCyder software version 6.5 (GE Healthcare, Australia). The Differential In-gel analysis (DIA) was used to optimize spot detection. The Biological Variation Analysis (BVA) module was used for analysis of each sample according to the corresponding time point. The filtering parameters were set to determine protein spots that had a p-value of <0.05 and a 1.5-fold change in abundance between the time points.

Proteins of interest were excised from the gels robotically using the Ettan Spot-picker (GE Healthcare, Australia) and prepared for in-gel trypsinolysis as previously described [16]. Gel plugs were consecutively washed with 25 mM NH_3HCO_3 followed by 50% v/v acetonitrile for 15 min each. Following dehydration by incubation at $37°C$ for 30 min, gel plugs were incubated with

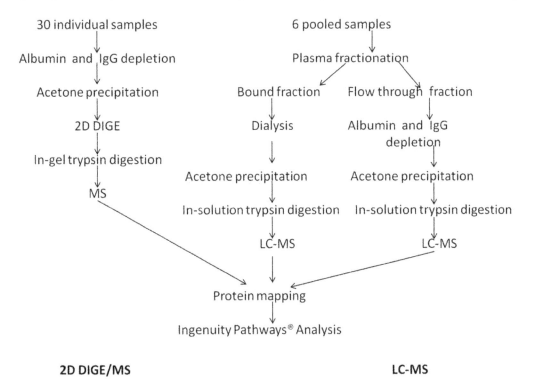

Figure 1. Two complementary proteomic methods used to assess RIPC induced changes in the plasma proteome. 2D DIGE-2Dimensional Difference in gel electrophoresis, LC– Liquid chromatography, -MS-mass spectrometry.

Table 1. Significantly changed proteins 2D DIGE/MS.

Accession number	Protein	Protein score°	p-value (t-test)	Average ratio	Main function
gi 178751	α2-antiplasmin precursor	64	0.046	1.37	Serine protease inhibitor
gi 4557321	Apolipoprotein A-1*	197	0.045	−1.21	Lipid transport
gi 8101268	Complement C3	393	0.0047	1.46	Immune response
gi 223002	Fibrin beta*	294	0.028	1.18	Haemostasis
gi 223170	Fibrinogen gamma*	198	0.018	1.24	Haemostasis
gi 8853069	Vitronectin precursor	120	0.014	−1.32	Cell adhesion

*Proteins that were also found to change significantly using LC-MS.
°The protein score indicates the confidence with which the proteins identified match the NCBInr human protein database. Only scores greater than 40 were considered to match with sufficient confidence. Average ratio indicates the degree of difference in the abundance between two protein spot groups. Values below zero indicate a down-regulation, whereas, values greater than zero indicate up-regulation.

modified porcine trypsin in 25 mM NH_3HCO_3 (Promega) (pH 9, 37°C, 15 h). Trifluoroacetic acid (0.5% w/v) was subsequently added to neutralise the trypsin. The digested proteins were concentrated directly onto a thin layer affinity matrix solution of α-cyano-4-hydroxycinnamic acid for analysis by MALDI-TOF MS. The MS reflector mode was used to generate a protein mass fingerprint for the identification of each protein (4700 Proteomics Analyzer, Applied Biosystems, USA), operating at a resolution of 10,000–15,000 FWHM (Full Width at Half Maximum). Reordered in positive reflector mode at a laser intensity of 2950, spectra were acquired at 200 Hz using a YAG laser (335 nm). A mass filter that excluded matrix cluster ions and trypsin autolysis peaks was applied. Ten of the most intense peptide ions were selected for further MS analysis (MS/MS). All MS/MS data from the TOF-TOF was acquired using a default 1 kV method at laser energy 3000–3500. The PMF and MS/MS data were combined and submitted for database searching as described in the protein mapping section below. Protein identity was listed for samples that gave a significant (P<0.05). A peptide mass tolerance of 100 ppm and up to 1 missed cleavage allowed when searching against all databases.

pH3　　　　　　　　　　　　　　**pH11**

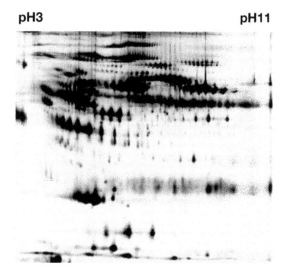

Figure 2. The protein pattern from a representative 2D-DIGE gel of human plasma proteins. pH 3 to pH 11 - left to right.

Liquid Chromotography (LC) and Mass Spectrometry

This method was applied to better assess the heparin-bound proteins. The analysis was conducted on 6 pooled samples from 5 individuals taken at 6 time points. Plasma fractionation was performed using the ÄKTA^{TM} Fast Protein Liquid Chromatography (Amersham Pharmacia Biotech AB, Uppsala, Sweden). The plasma proteins were separated into two fractions, based on their affinity to heparin [17]. One fraction contained proteins that bind heparin (*bound fraction*) and the other fraction contained those that do not bind heparin (*flow through fraction*) [17]. Plasma samples were diluted 1:3 in 50 mMTris-HCl, 0.1 M NaCl pH 7.5 (Kjellberg 2006) and passed through a 0.22 μM spin filter (Agilent Technologies, Australia) by centrifugation for 5 min. The samples were then fractionated in duplicate runs by injecting 400 μL of the sample into the AKTA system, through a 1 mL Hi-Trap Heparin column (GE healthcare, Australia) at a flow rate of 1 ml/min for 5 mins to collect the flow through fraction. The bound fraction was then eluted off the column under high salt conditions with 50 mM Tris-HCl, 3.0 M NaCl pH 7.5 for 13 mins (Kiellberg 2006). Between each sample run, the column was re-equilibrated with 50 mMTris-HCl, 0.1 M NaCl pH 7.5 for 7 minutes. Samples from the *bound* fraction were dialysed against phosphate buffered saline to reduce the salt concentration in preparation for acetone precipitation. Dialysis was performed for 48 hours with a change of buffer at 24 hours, with 25 mm×16 mm cellulose dialysis tubing (Sigma Aldrich, St Louis, USA) [18].

Albumin and IgG were depleted from the *flow through fraction* using the Albumin and IgG removal kit (GE Healthcare, Australia). This was performed to increase the probability of detecting low abundance proteins that are not bound to heparin. The *bound fraction* was not subjected to this depletion protocol as albumin and IgG do not bind to heparin and are therefore not present in this fraction.

Both the *bound fraction* and the *flow through fraction* underwent acetone precipitation and quantification [16]. In-solution trypsin digestion was performed and samples prepared for MS using a standard protocol where four volumes of ice cold acetone were added to the samples and precipitation was carried out overnight at −20°C. Protein pellets were obtained by centrifugation at 13 000 g for 20 mins at 8°C and were resuspended in 6M Urea, 100 mM Tris buffer. The protein content of each sample was quantified using the Bradford assay (Bio-Rad, Hercules, CA, USA) by comparing against a standard curve of bovine serum albumin concentration [19]. In-solution trypsin digestion was performed on 50 μg of protein from each sample. The samples were reduced

Table 2. Significantly changed proteins using LC-MS.

Protein	Cluster number*	Accession number	Protein	Protein score	Main function
1	03064; 03114	gi152207506	Alpha-1-antitrypsin	50.52	Major plasma protease inhibitor
2	0355; 01053; 01172; 01516; 01772; 02364; 02525; 02607; 02613; 02623; 02632; 03082; 03101; 03169; 03213	gi3212456	Albumin	1409.65	Maintenance of osmotic pressure (carrier protein)
3	03271; 03316; 03379	gi4502027	Albumin pre-proprotein	3915.51	Albumin synthesis
4	0851	gi4502067	Alpha-1-microglobulin/Bikunin precursor	760.52	Trypsin inhibitor
5	02542; 02625	gi2098275	Amyloidogenic Transthyretin Variants	717.28	Molecular Transport
6	1075	gi999513	Antithrombin Iii Complex Chain A,	1280.26	Protease inhibition
7	00345; 00421; 00991; 01738; 02127; 02426; 03248; 03288; 03368	gi90108664	Apolipoprotein A-I	221.85	Lipid Transport
8	01759; 00319; 01798; 02803; 03173	gi24987503	Apolipoprotein A-Ii	605.36	Lipid Transport
9	03249	gi619383	Apolipoprotein D	476.73	Lipid Transport
10	0822	gi6573461	Apolipoprotein H	1950.32	Lipid Transport
11	03243	gi4262120	Beta-globin	119.95	Haemoglobin synthesis
12	0393	gi218511956	Complement C1r	591.36	Immune response
13	1014; 0920	gi81175238; gi1314244	Complement C4B	2498.95	Immune response
14	0868	gi21730336	Complement C8 gamma	564.78	Immune response
15	1056; 0797; 0524; 0480; 0412; 0 230; 0102; 0681	gi119625338	Fibrin beta	321.18	Haemostasis
16	0781; 0400	gi223170	Fibrinogen gamma	395.17	Haemostasis
17	1015; 0927; 0853	gi109658664	Fibronectin 1	2796.95	Endothelial cell activation
18	1072; 0237	gi4504165	Gelsolin precursor	1365.75	Actin binding
19	01892; 02104	gi169791771	Haemoglobin	470.28	Oxygen binding
20	01942	gi63080988	Haemoglobin alpha-2 globin mutant	470.28	Oxygen binding
21	00935	gi47679339	Haemoglobin beta	110.75	Oxygen binding
22	03201; 02348; 02396	gi4826762; gi229323; gi296653	Haptoglobin	653.78	Haemoglobin binding
23	02059	gi45580723	Haptoglobin 2-alpha	400.55	Acute phase response
24	01237	gi119589124	Hemopexin, isoform	504.33	Heme binding
25	0900; 0793	gi4504489	Histidine-rich glycoprotein precursor	1076.52	Protein binding
26	01381	gi229536	Immunoglobulin A Light chain	439.93	Acute phase response
27	02489; 03175	gi8569502	Immunoglobulin G-1 (Fc Fragment)	1139.00	Acute phase response
28	01081; 01369	gi184747	Immunoglobulin G-1 heavy chain constant region	353.79	Acute phase response
29	02730	gi25987833	Immunoglobulin G-2 heavy chain constant region	427.39	Acute phase response
30	02372	gi311771988	Immunoglobulin G-Aptamer Complex	570.83	Acute phase response
31	0653; 00247	gi2414492	Immunoglobulin heavy chain constant region	275.38	Acute phase response
32	0937	gi553485	Immunoglobulin kappa chain variable region	117.71	Acute phase response
33	0777	gi3328006	Immunoglobulin light chain variable region	92.82	Acute phase response
34	1049; 0875; 0770; 03057	gi166007160	Immunoglobulin M	840.10	Acute phase response
35	0884; 0779; 0218	gi4467842	Immunoglobulin M heavy chain	105.89	Acute phase response
36	0942; 0925; 0421; 0356; 0344	gi55958063	Inter-alpha (globulin) inhibitor H2	1816.20	Protease inhibition
37	1024; 0892; 0871; 0801; 0762; 0662	gi225311	Lipoprotein B100	5942.27	Lipid transport

Table 2. Cont.

Protein	Cluster number*	Accession number	Protein	Protein score	Main function
38	0374	gi156616294	N-acetylmuramoyl-L-alanine amidase precursor	705.96	Peptidoglycan biosynthesis
39	0465	gi160877748	Neuropilin-1 B1 Domain In Complex With A Vegf-Blocking Fab, Chain L	909.96	Protein signalling
40	0994; 0889; 0632; 0348; 0168	gi8569387	P14-Fluorescein-N135q-S380c-Antithrombin-Iii, Chain I	1280.26	Protease inhibition
41	0519	gi229528	Protein Len, Bence-Jones	687.73	Immune response
42	03436	gi229526	Protein Rei, Bence-Jones	558.14	Immune response
43	01545	gi223069	Protein Tro alpha 1 H	707.61	Immune response
44	00132; 00479; 01819; 00088; 00270; 00395; 00603; 00910; 00978; 01032; 01972; 01602; 01127; 01975; 02244; 03107; 3362	gi110590597; gi194383506; gi110590599	Transferrin	3130.44	Iron binding
45	01415	gi1881852	Sry-related HMG box gene	101.3	DNA binding
46	02051; 02692	gi18655424	Vitamin D Binding Protein	994.05	Vitamin D sterol transport
47	03398	gi139641	Vitamin D-binding protein precursor	1023.55	Vitamin D sterol transport
48	02516	gi4699583	Zinc-Alpha-2-Glycoprotein	145.06	Lipid transport

Cluster number refers to the number alocated to each peptide fragment in the Genedata software. Accession number refers to the corresponding protein from the NCBInr human protein database. Protein score is a score assigned by the Proteome Discoverer software to indicate the confidence with which the proteins identified match the NCBInr human protein database. Only Protein scores greater than 40 were considered to match with sufficient confidence.
*- Each cluster number equals a unique piptide identified for the particular protein.

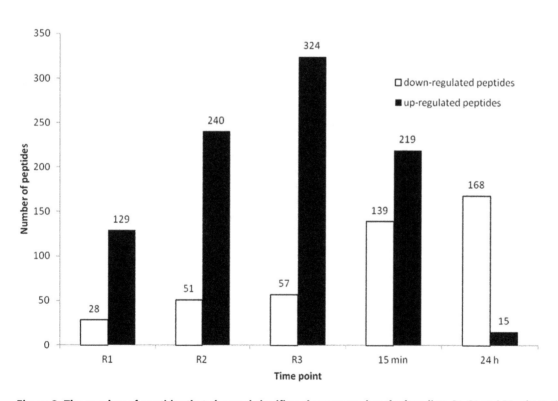

Figure 3. The number of peptides that changed significantly compared to the baseline. R1, R2 and R3 refer to the blood samples taken immediately after the first, second and third period of transient limb ischemia catching the blood coming from the ischemic arm at the beginning of each cycle of reperfusion (R), demonstrating a cumulative proteomic response to the RIPC stimulus. The remaining two samples were taken from the same arm at 15 minutes and 24 hours after completion of the RIPC stimulus, demonstrating an early and late global proteomic response to the RIPC stimulus.

Table 3. Differentially expressed proteins coming from the ischemic arm demonstrating up regulation and down regulation.

Proteins up regulated	Proteins down regulated
α2-antiplasmin precursor	Alpha-1-microglobulin/Bikunin precursor
Albumin	Antithrombin Iii Complex, Chain A
Albumin pre-proprotein	Apolipoprotein H
Alpha-1-antitrypsin	Complement C1r
Amyloidogenic Transthyretin Variants	Complement C4B
Apolipoprotein A-I	Complement C8 Gamma
Apolipoprotein A-Ii	Gelsolin precursor
Apolipoprotein D	Histidine-rich glycoprotein precursor
Beta-globin	Immunoglobulin heavy chain constant region
Fibrin beta	Immunoglobulin light chain variable region
Fibronectin 1	Immunoglobulin M
Haemoglobin	Immunoglobulin M heavy chain
Haemoglobin alpha-2 globin mutant	N-acetylmuramoyl-L-alanine amidase precursor
Haemoglobin beta	Neuropilin-1 B1 Domain In Complex With A Vegf-Blocking Fab, Chain L
Hemopexin, isoform	P14-Fluorescein-N135q-S380c-Antithrombin-Iii Chain I,
Haptoglobin	Protein Len, Bence-Jones
Haptoglobin 2-alpha	Vitronectin precursor
Immunoglobulin A Light chain	
Immunoglobulin G-Aptamer Complex	
Immunoglobulin G-1 (Fc Fragment)	
Immunoglobulin G-1 heavy chain constant region	
Immunoglobulin G-2 heavy chain constant region	
Immunoglobulin kappa chain variable region	
Inter-alpha (globulin) inhibitor H2	
Lipoprotein B100	
Protein Rei, Bence-Jones	
Protein Tro alpha 1 H	
Sry-related HMG box gene	
Transferrin	
Vitamin D Binding Protein	
Vitamin D-binding protein precursor	
Zinc-Alpha-2-Glycoprotein	

with 10 mM dithiothreitol for one hour, followed by alkylation with 55 mM iodoacetamide for one hour. The concentration of urea was reduced to <1M by diluting the sample with 0.4M Tris buffer at pH 7.8. Sequencing grade porcine trypsin (Promega, Madison, WI, USA) was added at a ratio of 1:20 and trypsin digestion then carried out overnight at 37°C. The reaction was stopped by titration with concentrated acetic acid until the pH was lower than pH 6.

Following trypsin digestion, samples were passed through Oasis HLB extraction cartridges (Waters, Ireland) preconditioned with methanol and equilibrated with 2% acetonitrile and 0.1% Trifluroacetic acid (TFA). Bound peptides were first eluted with 80% acetonitrile containing 0.1% TFA, followed by 100% acetonitrile and 0.1% TFA. The combined eluant was lyophilised by freeze drying, after which each was reconstituted in 200 μL of 0.1% formic acid in preparation for mass spectrometry.

LC MS/MS was carried out on a LTQ Orbitrap Velos (Thermo Scientific, West Palm Beach, FL, USA) equipped with a nanoelectrospray interface coupled to an Ultimate 3000 RSLC

nanosystem (Dionex, Sunnyvale, CA, USA). The nanoLC system used an Acclaim Pepmap nano-trap column (Dionex – C18, 100 Å, 75 μm×2 cm) and an Acclaim Pepmap RSLC analytical column (Dionex - C18, 100 Å, 75 μ m×15 cm). Typically for each LCMSMS experiment 1 μl of each peptide preparation, equating to 250 ng total peptide, was loaded onto the enrichment (trap) column followed by separation and elution of peptides from the analytical column employing a gradient from 3% to 45% acetonitrile over 90 minutes. The LTQ-Orbitrap Velos mass spectrometer was operated in the data dependent mode with nano ESI spray voltage of +1.6 kv, capillary temperature of 250°C and S-lens RF value of 60%. All spectra were acquired in positive mode with full scan MS spectra scanning from m/z 300–2000 in the flight time mode at 60,000 resolution after accumulating to a target value of 1.00e6 with maximum accumulation of 500 ms. The 8 most intense peptide ions with charge states ≥2 were isolated at a minimum threshold value of 2000 and fragmented by low energy collision induced dissociation (CID) with normalized collision energy of 35, activation Q of 0.25 and activation time of

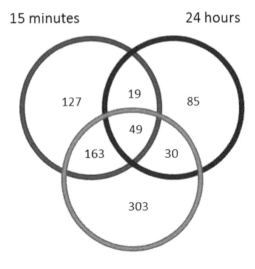

15 minutes   24 hours

127   19   85

49

163   30

303

RIPC stimulus

Figure 4. Venn diagram demonstrating the number of peptides that changed significantly during transient limb ischemia (combining all R1, R2, and R3 reperfusion periods), as well as at 15 minutes and 24 hours after the RIPC stimulus, compared with the baseline sample.

10 ms. A dynamic exclusion of 1 repeat over 10 sec with exclusion duration of 15 sec was set. At all times, monoisotopic precursor selection was enabled. Each sample was run in triplicate with 2 blank injections between each triplicate set to minimize the effect of sample carryover [20]. Data processing was carried out using Expressionist Refiner MS (Genedata, Basel, Switzerland) to align MS data, carry out noise reduction, and for peak extraction (clustering). Clustering of MS/MS spectra was employed to identify the spectra of the same peptide (from triplicate runs) and to replace them with a single representative spectrum. Once clustered, peak area intensity measurements of precursor ions were extracted and analysed for statistical relevance using Genedata Analyst to compare each of the 3 samples collected post ischemia and 15 minutes and 24 hours thereafter with the baseline sample. Subsequently, peptides showing up or down-regulated expression (p<0.001 above a computer generated false discovery rate) across the time-points were collated into lists for identification using a targeted MS/MS approach. For biomarker discovery using targeted mass spectrometry analysis, the mass spectrometer was operated in the data-dependant mode as described above with the following modifications. The 10 most intense peptide ions with charge states ≥ 2 were isolated at a minimum threshold value of 2000 from an assigned parent list. A dynamic exclusion of 4 repeats over 30 sec with exclusion duration of 15 sec was set.

The MS data was loaded onto Proteome Discoverer 1.2 software suite (Thermo Scientific, West Palm Beach, FL, USA) and submitted to Mascot v.2.2.04 (Matrix Science, London, UK) www.matrixscience.com) to match against the National Centre for Biotechnology Information (NCBInr), Bethesda, US database. An initial filter of precursor mass was set between 300 to 6000 Da. The peptide mass tolerance was set to 20 ppm and 0.8 Da for MS/MS fragmentation ions Searches were carried out on the latest version of the NCBInr human database (National Centre for Biotechnology Information, Bethesda, US). Enzyme specificity was trypsin with a maximum of 2 missed cleavages. Cysteine carbaidomethylation (+57.0215 Da) and methionine oxidation

(+15.9949 Da) were set as the fixed and variable modification respectively for all searches. ESI-FTICR was set as the default instrument search setting. All the spectra were searched against the decoy database to achieve a targeted false discovery rate of 1%. Only those peptides that matched the database with medium (FDR <0.05) or high confidence (FDR <0.01), ie protein score greater than 40, with spectra that matched the original data analysis for fragmentation pattern, retention time and mass to charge ratio were considered when assigning a positive match. Individual MS/MS spectra from the targeted runs within a precursor tolerance of 2 ppm and maximum R/T difference of 1.5minutes were merged (clustered) into single representative spectrum.

Results

Using the 2D DIGE (**Figure 2**) with individual plasma samples, 33 spots were determined to have changed significantly in response to RIPC, p<0.05. From these protein spots, 6 proteins were successfully identified by MS and are presented in **Table 1**.

Using LC-MS analysis, 806 peptides were differentially expressed compared with the baseline sample (p<0.001), and of these, 133 (16.5%) peptides were successfully mapped to 48 known proteins in the NCBInr database (**Table 2**). The remaining peptides could not be matched to proteins currently available in the database.

The number of up-regulated peptides increased with reperfusion (**Figure 3**), and the number of up-regulated peptides peaking at 324 peptides following the third cycle of ischemia. Similarly, the number of down-regulated peptides increased steadily throughout the RIPC protocol, with the highest number of down-regulated peptides observed 24 hours following application of the RIPC stimulus.

The number of peptides that changed significantly compared to the baseline sample during the RIPC protocol as well as at 15 minutes and 24 hours after the RIPC stimulus is presented in **Figure 4**. Proteins that were differencially expressed at the various timepoints are shown in **Table 3, 4 and 5**.

Three of the proteins were identified using both experimental approaches. These proteins were fibrin beta, fibrinogen gamma and apolipoprotein A. The main pathway involved in the RIPC response was acute phase response signalling.

Discussion

A multi-organ protection by RIPC can be transferred to the target organs via humoral factors in plasma [6,15]. Those factors may or may not be proteins. However, proteomic changes in plasma are an important component of the inflammatory response to IR injury. Thus, it appeared logical to examine proteomic changes in plasma induced by transient limb ischemia.

To the best of our knowledge, this is the first study to examine the global proteomic changes in plasma induced by brief forearm ischemia. Arrell et al., demonstrated in a rabbit model that pharmacologically induced preconditioning evoked proteomic changes in the myocardium [21]. Although proteomic changes in the target organ are of great interest, we focused on describing proteomic changes in plasma, in light of evidence that transfer of plasma from the transiently ischemic limb induced RIPC in the target organs [15].

Proteomic evaluation of plasma is challenging due to the high abundance proteins that obscure lower abundance proteins [22,23]. We depleted two most abundant proteins – albumin and IgG. Although we attempted to deplete the samples of these high abundance proteins, residual albumin and IgG were still

Table 4. Differentially expressed proteins in response to the RIPC stimulus demonstrating up regulation and down regulation during the early response (15 min).

Proteins up regulated	Proteins down regulated
Albumin	Alpha-1-microglobulin/Bikunin precursor
Albumin pre-proprotein	Antithrombin Iii Complex, Chain A
Alpha-1-antitrypsin	Apolipoprotein H
Amyloidogenic Transthyretin Variants	Complement C4B
Apolipoprotein A-I	Complement C8
Apolipoprotein A-Ii	Complement C1r
Apolipoprotein D	Gelsolin precursor
Beta-globin	Histidine-rich glycoprotein precursor
Complement C3	Immunoglobulin heavy chain constant region
Fibrinogen gamma	Immunoglobulin light chain variable region
Fibrin beta	Immunoglobulin kappa chain variable region
Fibronectin 1	Immunoglobulin M
Haemoglobin	Immunoglobulin M heavy chain
Haemoglobin alpha-2 globin mutant	Lipoprotein B100
Hemopexin, isoform	N-acetylmuramoyl-L-alanine amidase precursor
Haptoglobin	Neuropilin-1 B1 Domain In Complex With A Vegf-Blocking Fab, Chain L
Haptoglobin 2-alpha	P14-Fluorescein-N135q-S380c-Antithrombin-Iii, Chain I
Haemoglobin beta	Protein Len, Bence-Jones
Immunoglobulin A Light chain	
Immunoglobulin G-Aptamer Complex	
Immunoglobulin G-1 (Fc Fragment)	
Immunoglobulin G-1 heavy chain constant region	
Immunoglobulin G-2 heavy chain constant region	
Inter-alpha (globulin) inhibitor H2	
Protein Rei, Bence-Jones	
Protein Tro alpha 1 H	
Sry-related HMG box gene	
Transferrin	
Vitamin D Binding Protein	
Vitamin D-binding protein precursor	
Zinc-Alpha-2-Glycoprotein	

present. Since neither albumin nor IgG binds to heparin, further separation by fractionation based on the ability to bind to heparin was helpful. Thus, we used two different, but complementary methodological proteomic approaches in order to better define the proteomic changes in plasma. Fractionation and LC permitted a better evaluation of the heparin bound fraction and effectively cleared the albumin and IgG to further unmask lower abundance proteins. By analysing both fractions, we ensured that the majority of the plasma proteome was assessed.

The results of this study demonstrated that plasma proteome changes occurred during the RIPC and were cumulative with each episode of IR. The number of peptides in plasma coming from the ischemic arm increased with each episode of transient arm ischemia. These peptides were predominantly up-regulated (**Figure 3**). In contrast, at 15 minutes and 24 hours after the RIPC stimulus the peptides were predominantly down-regulated. The latter finding is consistent with our previous genomic study

that demonstrated predominant down-regulation of pro-inflammatory gene expression early and late after the RIPC stimulus [9].

We identified 51 proteins which were differentially expressed in response to the RIPC protocol compared to baseline when the results of the two approaches were combined. The proteins identified, play a role in a range of cellular functions including immune response, haemostasis, haemoglobin binding and synthesis, protease inhibition, acute phase response, iron binding, lipid transport, oxygen binding, heme binding, vitamin D transport, protein binding, maintenance of osmotic pressure, trypsin inhibition, molecular transport and protein signalling, endothelial cell activation, actin binding, peptidoglycan biosynthesis and DNA binding. This suggests that the mechanisms involved in RIPC may involve a complex interaction of multiple redundant pathways such that there is regulation of cells surviving or yielding to ischemic damage. Many proteins identified in our study are biomarkers of cardiovascular disease [24].

Table 5. Differentially expressed proteins in response to the RIPC stimulus demonstrating up regulation and down regulation during the late response (24 h).

Proteins up regulated	Proteins down regulated
Amyloidogenic Transthyretin Variants	Albumin
Apolipoprotein A-Ii	Albumin pre-proprotein
Apolipoprotein D	Alpha-1-antitrypsin
Fibrinogen gamma	Alpha-1-microglobulin/Bikunin precursor
Fibrin beta	Antithrombin-Iii Complex, Chain A,
Hemopexin, isoform CRA_a	Apolipoprotein H
Haptoglobin 2-alpha	Apolipoprotein A1
Immunoglobulin A Light chain	Complement C4B
Protein Rei, Bence-Jones	Complement C8
Protein Tro alpha 1 H	Complement C1r
Sry-related HMG box gene	Fibronectin 1
Transferrin	Gelsolin precursor
Zinc-Alpha-2-Glycoprotein	Histidine-rich glycoprotein precurso
	Haemoglobin
	Immunoglobulin heavy chain constant region
	Immunoglobulin light chain variable region
	Immunoglobulin G-1 (Fc Fragment)
	Immunoglobulin G-1 heavy chain constant region
	Immunoglobulin G-2 heavy chain constant region
	Immunoglobulin kappa chain variable region
	Immunoglobulin M
	Immunoglobulin M heavy chain
	Inter-alpha (globulin) inhibitor H2
	Lipoprotein B100
	N-acetylmuramoyl-L-alanine amidase precursor
	Neuropilin-1 B1 Domain In Complex With A Vegf-Blocking Fab, Chain L,
	P14-Fluorescein-N135q-S380c-Antithrombin-Iii, Chain I
	Protein Len, Bence-Jones
	Vitamin D Binding Protein
	Vitamin D-binding protein precursor

Alpha-1-antitrypsin is one such protein that has been shown to contribute to protection of the kidney in a mouse model of IR injury through the initiation of the acute phase response to injury and exerting anti-apoptotic and anti-inflammatory effects [25]. We found this protein to be up regulated during the RIPC protocol as well as 15 minutes later consistent with its known role as an initiator of the acute phase response during injury. Haptoglobin is another acute phase protein with apparent involvement in IR injury. The level of haptoglobin is decreased during IR injury and normalized by preconditioning, attenuating the IR injury [26]. We found consistently higher levels of haptoglobin at all time points analysed compared to baseline.

Apolipoproteins were shown to be predominantly up-regulated during the RIPC stimulus as well as during the early and late after it. Apolipoproteins prevent endothelial dysfunction and inhibit lipid oxidation in models of myocardial and renal IR injury [27,28] and may play a role in protection against IR injury. In particular, apolipoprotein A1 is involved in IR injury and has anti-inflammatory activity [28]. Apolipoprotein A1 protected against IR injury through suppression of intercellular adhesion molecule-1

and p-selectin expression, thus, decreasing neutrophil adhesion and subsequent tissue injury that resulted in improved cardiac contractility. It also reduced release the of creatnine kinase, tumor necrosis factor-alpha and other inflammatory cytokines and myeloperoxidase serum levels post ischemic insult [28–30]. Arrhythmias (ventricular tachycardia and ventricular fibrillation) associated with IR can be attenuated by lipoproteins [31].

Two complement proteins (C1r and C8) were down-regulated in our study during and after the RIPC stimulus. This is consistent with previous studies that demonstrated the gene expression of these proteins to be down regulated in the myocardium of rabbits in vivo [32] and in isolated rabbit hearts [33] in response to a preconditioning stimulus.

Haemostatic proteins have also been implicated in ischemic preconditioning [34]. They activate fibrinolysis and reduce inflammation through mechanisms involving fibrinogen gamma [34]. In addition, fibrin beta decreases myocardial infarct size, scar formation, inflammation and the levels of cytokines (interleukin 1 beta, tumor necrosis factor-alpha and interleukin 6) in plasma [35]. Intravenous administration of fibrin-derived peptides is cardioprotective and reduces infarct size in rodents and pigs and appears to be as effective as preconditioning [35,36]. Administration of fibrin beta to humans is reported to be safe with potential to protect against IR injury [36].

Transferrin was up-regulated during and after the RIPC. Although the exact involvement of transferrin in protection against IR injury is unknown, transferrin regulates production of reactive oxygen species via iron regulation and appears to have a protective role in IR injury [37,38].

Although our analysis revealed proteins that are known to have a role during IR injury, there were also proteins whose role during IR injury is unknown. Our discussion is therefore centered on the proteins with known involvement in the IR injury. We were unable to obtain MS/MS data for all peptides that were changed significantly and these peptides require further analysis. The analysis involved matching peptide sequences against the sequence data of known proteins in the NCBInr human database. It is possible that there are proteins that have not been mapped in this database and therefore the origin of some of the detected peptides is not known. Peptides not identified in existing database searches may reflect programmed frame shifts or DNA sequencing errors [39].

A few studies suggested that a blood borne factor thought to be responsible for the ability of RIPC serum to transfer protection appears to have a molecular weight below 30 kDa [40–43]. Recently, Shimizu et al [40] demonstrated for the first time that transient limb ischemia liberates protective factors with molecular masses below 15 kDa, resistant to freezing and thawing, which is hydrophobic and not easily denatured. Serejo et al [42] have recently reported that the blood effluent from preconditioned rat hearts which was dialyzed to retain molecules above a molecular mass of 3500 Da had protective properties. On the other hand, Lang et al [43] reported that no differentially abundant proteins from RIPC with a known signalling function could be found above molecular mass of 8 kDa, the lower molecular mass limit of their proteomic study. Interestingly, Serejo et al [42] concluded that their finding "excludes the participation of adenosine (267.24 Da), opioids (500–800 Da), bradykinin (1060.22 Da), and other substances with molecular weights below the dialysis cutoff (3.5 kDa) as putative mediators of preconditioning". These results still remain controversial and should be interpreted cautiously. At the present study, we found that some plasma proteins with molecular mass below 30 kDa coming from ischemic arm were up-regulated, for example, amiloidogenic transthyretin varients (15887 Da), apolipoprotein D (21276 Da), beta globin (2104 Da), haemoglobin alpha 2 (15258 Da), haemoglobin beta (15998 Da), vitamin D binding protein (2905 Da), while complement 8 gamma

(22277 Da) was down-regulated. Proteomic assessment of the plasma taken from ischemic arms needs further scrutiny.

In the current study, the global proteomic responses to the RIPC stimulus reflected the genomic responses to the RIPC stimulus demonstrated in our previous study [9], in which there was a predominance of down-regulation of gene expression both early (at 15 minutes) and late (at 24 hours) after transient limb ischemia. We observed an increased number of down-regulated proteins in the early and even more so, during the late response to the RIPC stimulus.

Further research needs to be carried out to identify the pathways implicated in the RIPC response as well to identify the peptides and other metabolites that may be involved. This could be achieved by further depleting plasma of high abundance proteins to investigate those found in plasma at lower abundance. Furthermore, a proteomic assessment of plasma dialysate might be useful to assess the proteins with molecular weight of less than 15–30 kDa. If an effector of the RIPC stimulus is identified and its potency is properly enhanced, the application of such augmented RIPC could be immense, including all fields of cardiac surgery, organ transplantation, protection against stroke and post-cardiopulmonary bypass renal failure.

The study was designed to assess a global proteomic response to the RIPC and not to determine the proteins that may confer the protection. As such the study did not specifically assess the protein of low molecular weight.

Conclusions

In summary, the results of this study demonstrate that the RIPC stimulus evokes a global proteomics response early and late, with predominant decrease in protein expression. There was an overall trend of up-regulation of protein expression in blood taken from the transiently ischemic limb during the RIPC protocol and this increase in the number of up-regulated peptides was cumulative with each cycle of the IR of the limb.

Acknowledgments

The authors acknowledge the support of Ms Robyn Summerhayes, Dr Nori Oka and Dr Matt Liava'a and Ms Chantal Attard during the processing of the samples.

Author Contributions

Conceived and designed the experiments: VI IK MH SB. Performed the experiments: VI MH SB. Analyzed the data: MH SB. Contributed reagents/materials/analysis tools: VI SB. Wrote the paper: MH IK. Participated in study design and manuscript editing: PM MC BJ Yd'U.

References

1. Murry CE, Jennings RB, Reimer KA (1986) Preconditioning with ischemia: a delay of lethal cell injury in ischemic myocardium. Circulation 74: 1124–1136.
2. Kanoria S, Jalan R, Seifalian AM, Williams R, Davidson BR (2007) Protocols and mechanisms for remote ischemic preconditioning: a novel method for reducing ischemia reperfusion injury. Transplantation. 84: 445–458.
3. Kharbanda RK, Nielsen TT, Redington AN (2009) Translation of remote ischaemic preconditioning into clinical practice. Lancet.374: 1557–1565.
4. Gho BC, Schoemaker RG, van den Doel MA, Duncker DJ, Verdouw PD (1996) Myocardial protection by brief ischemia in noncardiac tissue. Circulation. 94: 2193–2200.
5. Botker HE, Kharbanda R, Schmidt MR, Bottcher M, Kaltoft AK, et al. (2010) Remote ischaemic conditioning before hospital admission, as a complement to angioplasty, and effect on myocardial salvage in patients with acute myocardial infarction: a randomised trial. Lancet. 375: 727–734.
6. Konstantinov IE, Li J, Cheung MM, Shimizu M, Stokoe J, et al. (2005) Remote ischemic preconditioning of the recipient reduces myocardial ischemia-reperfusion injury of the denervated donor heart via a Katp channel-dependent mechanism. Transplantation. 79: 1691–1695.
7. Kharbanda RK, Li J, Konstantinov IE, Cheung MM, White PA, et al. (2006) Remote ischaemic preconditioning protects against cardiopulmonary bypass-induced tissue injury: a preclinical study. Heart. 92: 1506–1511.
8. Schmidt MR, Smerup M, Konstantinov IE, Shimizu M, Li J, et al. (2007) Intermittent peripheral tissue ischemia during coronary ischemia reduces myocardial infarction through a KATP-dependent mechanism: first demonstration of remote ischemic perconditioning. Am J Physiol Heart Circ Physiol.292: H1883–1890.
9. Konstantinov IE, Arab S, Kharbanda RK, Li J, Cheung MM, et al. (2004) The remote ischemic preconditioning stimulus modifies inflammatory gene expression in humans. Physiol Genomics.19: 143–150.
10. Konstantinov IE, Arab S, Li J, Coles JG, Boscarino C, et al. (2005) The remote ischemic preconditioning stimulus modifies gene expression in mouse myocardium. J Thorac Cardiovasc Surg. 130: 1326–1332.
11. Konstantinov IE, Coles JG, Boscarino C, Takahashi M, Goncalves J, et al. (2004) Gene expression profiles in children undergoing cardiac surgery for right heart obstructive lesions. J Thorac Cardiovasc Surg.127: 746–754.

12. Saxena P, Shaw OM, Misso NL, Naran A, Shehatha J, et al. (2011) Remote ischemic preconditioning stimulus decreases the expression of kinin receptors in human neutrophils. J Surg Res. 171: 311–316.

13. Shimizu M, Saxena P, Konstantinov IE, Cherepanov V, Cheung MM, et al. (2010) Remote ischemic preconditioning decreases adhesion and selectively modifies functional responses of human neutrophils. J Surg Res.158: 155–161.

14. Cheung MMH, Kharbanda RK, Konstantinov IE, Shimizu M, Frndova H, et al. (2006) Randomized controlled trial of the effects of remote ischemic preconditioning on children undergoing cardiac surgery: first clinical application in humans. J Am Coll Cardiol. 47: 2277–2282.

15. Shimizu M, Tropak M, Diaz RJ, Suto F, Surendra H, et al. (2009) Transient limb ischaemia remotely preconditions through a humoral mechanism acting directly on the myocardium: evidence suggesting cross-species protection. Clin Sci (Lond). 117: 191–200.

16. Ignjatovic V, Lai C, Summerhayes R, Mathesius U, Tawfilis S, et al. (2011) Age-related differences in plasma proteins: how plasma proteins change from neonates to adults. PLoS One. 6: e17213.

17. Kjellberg M, Ikonomou T, Stenflo J (2006) The cleaved and latent forms of antithrombin are normal constituents of blood plasma: a quantitative method to measure cleaved antithrombin. J Thromb Haemost. 4: 168–176.

18. Andrew SM, Titus JA, Zumstein L (1997) Current protocols in immunology: John Wiley and sons Inc;.

19. Stone KL, Williams KR (2002) Enzymatic Digestion of Proteins in Solution and in SDS Polyacrylamide Gels. In: Walker JM, ed. The protein protocols handbook. Totowa, New Jersey: Humana Press Inc : 511–523.

20. Ang CS, Binos S, Knight MI, Moate PJ, Cocks BG, et al. (2011) Global survey of the bovine salivary proteome: integrating multidimensional prefractionation, targeted, and glycocapture strategies. J Proteome Res. 10: 5059–5069.

21. Arrell DK, Elliott ST, Kane LA, Guo Y, Ko YH, et al. (2006) Proteomic analysis of pharmacological preconditioning: novel protein targets converge to mitochondrial metabolism pathways. Circ Res. 99: 706–714.

22. Anderson NL, Anderson NG (2002) The human plasma proteome: history, character, and diagnostic prospects. Mol Cell Proteomics. 1: 845–867.

23. Darde VM, Barderas MG, Vivanco F (2007) Depletion of high-abundance proteins in plasma by immunoaffinity subtraction for two-dimensional difference gel electrophoresis analysis. Methods Mol Biol. 357: 351–364.

24. Anderson L (2005) Candidate-based proteomics in the search for biomarkers of cardiovascular disease. J Physiol.563(Pt 1): 23–60.

25. Daemen MA, Heemskerk VH, van't Veer C, Denecker G, Wolfs TG, et al. (2000) Functional protection by acute phase proteins alpha(1)-acid glycoprotein and alpha(1)-antitrypsin against ischemia/reperfusion injury by preventing apoptosis and inflammation. Circulation.102: 1420–1426.

26. Fernandez V, Castillo I, Tapia G, Romanque P, Uribe-Echevarria S, et al. (2007) Thyroid hormone preconditioning: protection against ischemia-reperfusion liver injury in the rat. Hepatology. 45: 170–177.

27. Calabresi L, Gomaraschi M, Rossoni G, Franceschini G (2006) Synthetic high density lipoproteins for the treatment of myocardial ischemia/reperfusion injury. Pharmacol Ther.111: 836–854.

28. Gu SS, Shi N, Wu MP (2007) The protective effect of ApolipoproteinA-I on myocardial ischemia-reperfusion injury in rats. Life Sci.81: 702–709.

29. Gomaraschi M, Calabresi L, Rossoni G, Iametti S, Franceschini G, et al. (2008) Anti-inflammatory and cardioprotective activities of synthetic high-density lipoprotein containing apolipoprotein A-I mimetic peptides. J Pharmacol Exp Ther.324: 776–783.

30. Shi N, Wu MP (2008) Apolipoprotein A-I attenuates renal ischemia/reperfusion injury in rats. J Biomed Sci.15: 577–583.

31. Imaizumi S, Miura S, Nakamura K, Kiya Y, Uehara Y, et al. (2008) Antiarrhythmogenic effect of reconstituted high-density lipoprotein against ischemia/reperfusion in rats. J Am Coll Cardiol.51: 1604–1612.

32. Tanhehco EJ, Yasojima K, McGeer PL, McGeer EG, Lucchesi BR (2000) Preconditioning reduces myocardial complement gene expression in vivo. Am J Physiol Heart Circ Physiol.279: H1157–1165.

33. Tanhehco EJ, Yasojima K, McGeer PL, Washington RA, Kilgore KS, et al. (1999) Preconditioning reduces tissue complement gene expression in the rabbit isolated heart. Am J Physiol.277: H2373–2380.

34. Warzecha Z, Dembinski A, Ceranowicz P, Dembinski M, Cieszkowski J, et al. (2007) Influence of ischemic preconditioning on blood coagulation, fibrinolytic activity and pancreatic repair in the course of caerulein-induced acute pancreatitis in rats. J Physiol Pharmacol. 58: 303–319.

35. Zacharowski K, Zacharowski PA, Friedl P, Mastan P, Koch A, et al. (2007) The effects of the fibrin-derived peptide Bbeta(15–42) in acute and chronic rodent models of myocardial ischemia-reperfusion. Shock.27: 631–637.

36. Roesner JP, Petzelbauer P, Koch A, Mersmann J, Zacharowski PA, et al. (2007) The fibrin-derived peptide Bbeta15–42 is cardioprotective in a pig model of myocardial ischemia-reperfusion injury. Crit Care Med.35: 1730–1735.

37. Cairo G, Tacchini L, Recalcati S, Azzimonti B, Minotti G, et al. (1998) Effect of reactive oxygen species on iron regulatory protein activity. Ann N Y Acad Sci.851: 179–186.

38. Tacchini L, Fusar Poli D, Bernelli-Zazzera A, Cairo G (2002) Transferrin receptor gene expression and transferrin-bound iron uptake are increased during postischemic rat liver reperfusion. Hepatology. 36: 103–111.

39. Gupta N, Tanner S, Jaitly N, Adkins JN, Lipton M, et al. (2007) Whole proteome analysis of post-translational modifications: applications of mass-spectrometry for proteogenomic annotation. Genome Res.;17: 1362–1377.

40. Shimizu M, Tropak M, Diaz RJ, Suto F, Surendra H, et al. (2009) Transient limb ischemia remotely preconditions through a humoral mechanism acting directly on the myocardium: evidence suggesting croass-species protection. Clin Sci (Lond) 117: 191–200.

41. Dickson EW, Blehar DJ, Carraway RE, Heard SO, Steinberg G, et al. (2001) Naloxone blockes transferred preconditioning in isolated rabbit hearts. J Mol Cell Cardiol 33: 1751–1756.

42. Serejo FC, Rodrigues LF, da Silva Tavares KC, de Carvalho AC, Nascimento JH (2007) Myocardial injury is decreased by late remote ischaemic preconditioning and aggravated by tramadol in patients undergoing cardiac surgery: a randomised controlled trial. J Cardiovasc Pharmacol 49: 214–220.

43. Lang SC, Elsasser A, Scheler C, Vetter S, Tiefenbacher CP, et al. (2006) Myocardial preconditioning and remote renal preconditioning: identifying a protective factor using proteomic methods? Basic Res Cardiol 101: 149–158.

7

In Vivo Imaging of Brain Ischemia Using an Oxygen-Dependent Degradative Fusion Protein Probe

Youshi Fujita[1], Takahiro Kuchimaru[2], Tetsuya Kadonosono[2], Shotaro Tanaka[3], Yoshiki Hase[1], Hidekazu Tomimoto[4], Masahiro Hiraoka[5], Shinae Kizaka-Kondoh[2], Masafumi Ihara[1,6]*, Ryosuke Takahashi[1]

1 Department of Neurology, Graduate School of Medicine, Kyoto University, Sakyo-ku, Kyoto, Japan, 2 Department of Biomolecular Engineering, Tokyo Institute of Technology Graduate School of Bioscience and Biotechnology, Nagatsuta-cho, Midori-ku, Yokohama, Japan, 3 Department of Biochemistry, School of Medicine, Tokyo Women's Medical University, Tokyo, Japan, 4 Department of Neurology, Mie University Graduate School of Medicine, Mie, Japan, 5 Department of Radiation Oncology and Image-applied Therapy, Kyoto University Graduate School of Medicine, Shogoin, Sakyo-ku, Kyoto, Japan, 6 Department of Regenerative Medicine and Research, Institute of Biomedical Research and Innovation, Minatojima, Chuo-ku, Kobe, Hyogo, Japan

Abstract

Within the ischemic penumbra, blood flow is sufficiently reduced that it results in hypoxia severe enough to arrest physiological function. Nevertheless, it has been shown that cells present within this region can be rescued and resuscitated by restoring perfusion and through other protective therapies. Thus, the early detection of the ischemic penumbra can be exploited to improve outcomes after focal ischemia. Hypoxia-inducible factor (HIF)-1 is a transcription factor induced by a reduction in molecular oxygen levels. Although the role of HIF-1 in the ischemic penumbra remains unknown, there is a strong correlation between areas with HIF-1 activity and the ischemic penumbra. We recently developed a near-infrared fluorescently labeled-fusion protein, POH-N, with an oxygen-dependent degradation property identical to the alpha subunit of HIF-1. Here, we conduct *in vivo* imaging of HIF-active regions using POH-N in ischemic brains after transient focal cerebral ischemia induced using the intraluminal middle cerebral artery occlusion technique in mice. The results demonstrate that POH-N enables the *in vivo* monitoring and *ex vivo* detection of HIF-1-active regions after ischemic brain injury and suggest its potential in imaging and drug delivery to HIF-1-active areas in ischemic brains.

Editor: Maria A. Deli, Biological Research Centre of the Hungarian Academy of Sciences, Hungary

Funding: This work was supported by Grants-in-Aid for Young Scientists (B) (to YF) and for Scientific Research (B) (to MI) from the Japanese Ministry of Education, Science, and Culture and by the Global COE Program "Center for Frontier Medicine" funded by the Ministry of Education, Culture, Sports, Science, and Technology (MEXT), Japan. This study is part of a joint research program focusing on the development of technology to establish a Center of Excellence for nanomedicine and carried out by the Kyoto City Collaboration of Regional Entities for Advancing Technology Excellence assigned by the Japan Science and Technology Agency. The funders had no role in study design, data collection and analysis, the decision to publish, or manuscript preparation.

Competing Interests: The authors have declared that no competing interests exist.

* E-mail: iharama@gmail.com

Introduction

Hypoxia-inducible factor 1 (HIF-1) is activated by a variety of stimuli, including focal cerebral ischemia [1]. HIF-1 is a heterodimeric transcription factor consisting of an oxygen-regulated alpha subunit (HIF-1α) and a constitutively expressed beta subunit (HIF-1ß), which play a central role in cellular adaptation by regulating a wide array of genes in response to limited oxygen availability [2]. Under normoxia, prolyl hydroxylases (PHDs) hydroxylate specific proline residues of the oxygen-dependent degradation domain (ODD) of HIF-1α, leading to its polyubiquitination by the von Hippel–Lindau protein (VHL) and subsequent proteasomal degradation. In contrast, hypoxia abrogates prolyl hydroxylation by PHDs and, after VHL binding to HIF-1α, leads to the stabilization and accumulation of HIF-1α [3,4,5].

Oxygenation of brain tissue is impaired as a result of occlusion of a cerebral blood vessel causing subsequent irreversible infarction. The infarct core is surrounded by a hypoxic area [6], known as the ischemic penumbra [7], a region of hypoperfused, functionally impaired, but still viable tissue, in which HIF-1 activation is observed [8,9]. Therefore, the HIF-1-active region in the ischemic brain provides a suitable target for efficiently treating cerebral infarction.

We previously reported that a fusion protein containing the $ODD_{548-603}$ of human HIF-1α is efficiently degraded under normoxic conditions, via a VHL-mediated protein degradation system, in a manner similar to that of HIF-1α [10]. Using ODD-dependent degradation as a target-specific distribution and taking advantage of the capability of the protein-transduction domain (PTD) fusion protein to penetrate the cell membrane, we have developed PTD-ODD fusion proteins that specifically target HIF-1-active cancer cells *in vivo* [11–15]. We recently created a near-infrared fluorescent (NIRF)-labeled PTD-ODD-HaloTag (POH) that functions as an imaging probe specific to HIF-1-active cancer cells both *in vitro* and *in vivo* [16] (Fig. 1). Because NIRF-labeled POH (POH-N) is efficiently delivered to regions with less blood flow [11] and the PTD fusion protein can penetrate the blood–brain barrier [17], POH may be applicable to ischemic brain diseases as a specific probe for detecting HIF-1-active ischemic penumbra.

Here, we investigated the performance of POH-N as a molecular probe for imaging and targeting HIF-1-active regions in an

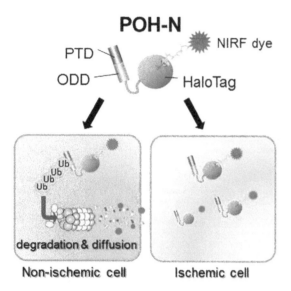

POH-N

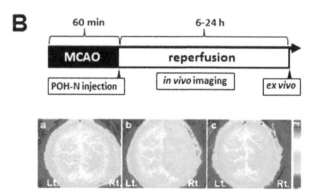

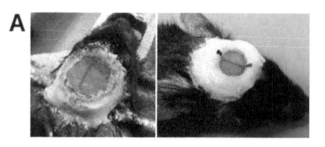

Figure 1. POH-N probe structure. Under normoxic conditions, POH-N is immediately degraded via VHL-mediated ODD, and the resultant POH-N fragments diffuse from the cells. In contrast, POH-N is more stable in HIF-1-active cells, thus creating a contrast between HIF-1-active and HIF-1-inactive cells.

Figure 2. Experimental design. (A) Cranial window in a C57/BL6 mouse. Experimental design of the closed cranial window. (B) Experimental design (upper panel). Representative two-dimensional images of cerebral blood flow measured by laser speckle perfusion imaging before MCAO (a), during MCAO (b), and after reperfusion (c) are shown in the lower panels. MCAO: middle cerebral artery occlusion.

ischemic stroke mouse model. The results demonstrate that POH-N allows *in vivo* monitoring and *ex vivo* detection of the HIF-1-active regions after ischemic brain injury.

Materials and Methods

Ethics statement

All animal experiments in this study were performed with the approval of the Animal Experiment Committees of Kyoto University, Graduate School of Medicine (Permit Number: MedKyo10202) and in strict accordance with the relevant national and international guidelines.

Animal preparation

The cranial window surgical procedure was performed for *in vivo* imaging, as previously described [18]. In brief, male C57BL/6J mice (6–7 weeks old) were anesthetized with 1.5% isoflurane in air, via a snout mask. A 6-mm-diameter hole was made using a fine drill bit in the skull. The center of the cranial window was located 2 mm posterior to the bregma on the midline. The dura mater was left intact. To cover the hole, an 8-mm cover glass (0.45–0.60-mm-thick) was sealed to the skull with histocompatible cyanoacrylate glue and dental cement, which adhered to the bone (Fig. 2A). Transient focal cerebral ischemia was induced using the intraluminal middle cerebral artery (MCA) occlusion (MCAO) technique [19]. Body temperature was maintained at 37°C using a feedback-controlled heating pad. An incision was made into the external carotid artery, and a silicon-coated 8-0 nylon mono-filament was inserted through the right internal carotid artery to occlude the MCA at its origin. After 60 min of occlusion, blood flow was restored by withdrawing the nylon suture. For generation of permanent occlusion of MCA, the nylon suture was not withdrawn. The survival rate of the MCAO/R model and the permanent MCAO model was more than 90% 24 hours after operation. Animals were assessed using laser speckle perfusion imaging (Omegazone; Omegawave Inc., Tokyo, Japan) to confirm

adequate induction of focal ischemia and successful reperfusion (Fig. 2B).

Plasmid construction and preparation of fusion proteins

The plasmid encoding the POH protein was constructed by substituting the coding sequences of procaspase-3 in PTD-ODD-procaspase-3 with HaloTag (Promega, Madison, WI), as previously described [16]. The plasmid encoding POmH containing the point substitution mutation, P564G [15], was prepared using a QuickChange XL site-directed mutagenesis kit (Stratagene, La Jolla, CA) at the proline residue corresponding to HIF-1α P564. Final cDNA constructs were inserted into the pGEX-6P-3 plasmids (GE Healthcare Bio-Science Corp., Piscataway, NJ). Fusion proteins were expressed in BL21-CodonPlus cells (Stratagene, La Jolla, CA) as GST-tagged proteins. These GST-tagged proteins were purified with a GST column and digested with precision protease (GE healthcare Bio-Science Corp., Piscataway, NJ) to remove GST tags from the fusion proteins. The final products were equilibrated in Mg^{2+}/Ca^{2+} free PBS (pH 8.0).

Preparation of the POH-N probe

We used NIRF dye IR800, as previously described [16]. The HaloTag ligand-IR800 was provided by Promega Corporation. HaloTag ligands (1 mg, 2.87 μmol; Promega, Madison, WI) in 100 μL of dimethyl formamide (DMF) were mixed with the NIRF dye and succinimidyl ester (1 mg, ~0.8 μmol; Invitrogen, Carlsbad, CA) in 1 mL of 10 mM boric acid (pH 8.5) in DMF. The reaction mixture was stirred in the dark for 12 h at room temperature. The reaction mixture was applied to a SepPak C18 reverse-phase column (Waters, Milford, MA), and the HaloTag

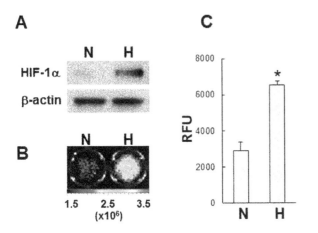

Figure 3. Stabilization of POH-N under hypoxic conditions. SH-SY5Y neuroblastoma cells cultured under normoxic (N) or hypoxic (H) conditions were treated with POH probe. (A) HIF-1α protein levels were analyzed by western blotting (a representative blot is shown). (B) The fluorescence intensity of POH probe in cells was measured. (C) Representative fluorescence images are shown. *P<0.02 (vs. normoxic condition).

ligands labeled with NIRF dye (HL-N) were resolved in 100 μL DMF. POH protein (40 μmol/L) was mixed with three volumes of HL-N (120 nmol/15 μL) in 10 mL PBS (pH 8.0) containing 100 mM Tris-HCl (pH 8.0) and 3 M $(NH_4)_2SO_4$ for 2 h. POH-N probes were subsequently purified with a PD-10 gel filtration column (GE healthcare Bio-Science Corp., Piscataway, NJ) and an Amicon-10 centrifugation column (Millipore, Billerica, MA). Purified POH-N was finally resolved in PBS (pH 8.0). Fluorescence characterizations were confirmed by SDS-PAGE fluorescence imaging. The labeling rate, calculated as described by the manufacturer, was >0.7 [16].

In vitro fluorescence measurement

SH-SY5Y neuroblastoma cells (2×10^5 cells/well) were seeded in a six-well plate (Riken Cell Bank, Tsukuba, Japan). The cells were pre-incubated under hypoxic (1% O_2) or normoxic (21% O_2) conditions for 16 h. The probe (500 nM) was then added, followed by incubation for 1 h. The cells were then washed with fresh medium, incubated for 3 h in fresh medium, and suspended in 200 μL of radioimmunoprecipitation assay (RIPA) buffer. Fluorescence was measured and imaged for 150-μL aliquots of

suspension in a 96-well plate using an Infinite® F500 microplate reader (Tecan, Durham, NC) with excitation and emission filters at 740±25 and 780±20 nm, and the IVIS®-Spectrum in vivo imaging system (Caliper Life Sciences, Alameda, CA) with excitation and emission filters at 710±15 and 800±10 nm, respectively.

Western blot analysis

To analyze cultured cells, SH-SY5Y cells were seeded in a six-well plate. The cells were pre-incubated under hypoxic or normoxic conditions for 6 h, then washed with medium, incubated for 3 h, and lysed using 200 μL of Laemmli sample buffer. Brain tissue samples were homogenized with a Dounce glass homogenizer using ice-cold RIPA buffer supplemented with protease inhibitors (Nacalai Tesque, Kyoto, Japan). Lysates were centrifuged at $10,000 \times g$ for 10 min at 4°C, and supernatants were collected. Protein concentrations were determined by the BCA protein assay (Pierce, Rockford, IL). Protein samples were electrophoresed on 10% SDS-polyacrylamide gel and transferred to PVDF membranes. The POH-N probes, β-actin and HIF-1α, were detected by a monoclonal anti-β-actin antibody (Sigma-Aldrich, St. Louis, MO) and a polyclonal anti-HIF-1α antibody (R&D Systems, Minneapolis, MN), respectively. The primary antibodies were then reacted with appropriate secondary horseradish peroxidase-conjugated antibodies (GE Healthcare Bio-Science Corp., Piscataway, NJ). Signals were detected using the chemiluminescence ECL-PLUS system (GE Healthcare Bio-Science Corp., Piscataway, NJ). Data were normalized relative to the β-actin levels and expressed as percentages of the sham-operated controls.

In vivo and ex vivo fluorescence imaging

POH probe (2 nmol) in 100 μL PBS (pH 8.0) was injected intravenously into the tail vein at 5 min, 6 hours, and 24 hours after reperfusion by the withdrawal of the nylon suture. Alternatively, POH probe (2 nmol) was injected intravenously at 60 min after permanent MCAO, without withdrawal of the nylon suture. Fluorescence images were acquired at the indicated times after injections. All fluorescence images were acquired with the IVIS®-Spectrum (Caliper Life Sciences, Alameda, CA) system, using the following parameters: excitation filter, 710±15 nm; emission filter, 800±10 nm; exposure time, 1 s; binning, small; field of view, 6×6 cm; and f-stop, 1. Some mice were sacrificed after in vivo imaging, and their brains were harvested and sliced into 3-mm-thick coronal sections. Fluorescence emissions from these brain sections were measured using the IVIS®-Spectrum

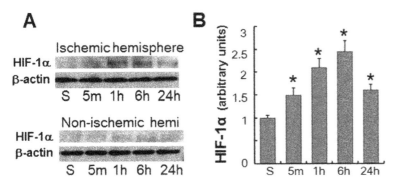

Figure 4. HIF-1α accumulation after focal brain ischemia. (A) Western blot analysis of HIF-1α in the ischemic and non-ischemic hemispheres of mice subjected to MCAO followed by reperfusion. (B) Densitometric analysis of HIF-1α protein levels in the ischemic hemispheres. Data were normalized relative to β-actin levels, and the values obtained from sham-operated controls (S) were arbitrarily defined as 1. *P<0.05 (vs. sham, n=4).

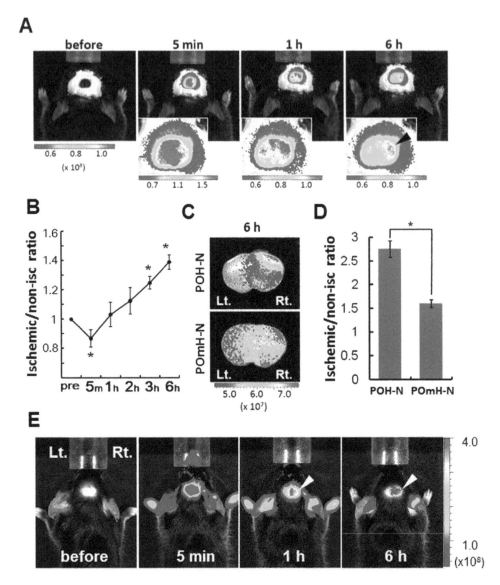

Figure 5. Imaging of HIF-1-active regions in the focal brain ischemia model. (A) Representative *in vivo* fluorescence images visualized through a cranial window before and at 5 min, 1 h, and 6 h after POH-N administration are shown. Magnified head images are shown in the lower left panels. Arrowheads indicate accumulation of the probe in the right ischemic hemisphere. (B) The relative fluorescence intensity of the ischemic hemisphere to the non-ischemic hemisphere. Fluorescence intensities were measured at the indicated times after POH-N administration. *$P < 0.05$, n = 3. (C) *Ex vivo* imaging of the coronal brain sections after POH-N injection. (D) Relative fluorescence of the ischemic hemisphere compared with the non-ischemic hemisphere at 6 h after probe administration (n = 3/group: *$P < 0.05$). Relative fluorescence values were calculated using ROIs mirrored along the midline of the cerebral hemispheres. (E) *In vivo* fluorescence images visualized without preparation of a cranial window before and at 5 min, 1 h, and 6 h after POH-N administration. Anesthetized C57BL/6J mice were shaved and depilated top of the head 24 h before experimentation. Arrowheads indicate accumulation of the probe in the right ischemic hemisphere.

system, under the same set of parameters for the excitation filter, emission filter, and exposure time. Relative fluorescence values were calculated by using regions of interest (ROIs) mirrored along the midline of the cerebral hemispheres. The contribution of the ODD domain in POH to clearance acceleration in the non-ischemic brains was examined using POmH-N, which has a point mutation corresponding to human HIF-1α (P564G) in the ODD domain and thus lacks ODD regulation [20].

Immunohistochemical analyses

Brain cryosections (10-μm-thick) were prepared using a cryostat (Leica CM3050S; Leica Microsystems, Wetzlar, Germany) and fixed in 4% paraformaldehyde. Cryosections were immunolabeled with the following primary antibodies: rabbit polyclonal anti-HIF-1α antibody (R&D Systems, Minneapolis, MN), rabbit polyclonal anti-ODD antibody [16], rabbit polyclonal anti-HaloTag antibody (Promega, Madison, WI), and rabbit polyclonal anti-HSP70 antibody (Cell Signaling Technology, Danvers, MA). Primary antibodies were applied overnight at 4°C. The sections were then incubated with biotin- or FITC-conjugated secondary antibodies. The avidin–biotin–peroxidase complex (ABC) (ABC-Elite; Vector Laboratories, Burlingame, CA) was applied, and the reaction product was visualized using diaminobenzidine (DAB). All photos were taken using a BZ-9000 microscope (Keyence, Osaka, Japan).

A

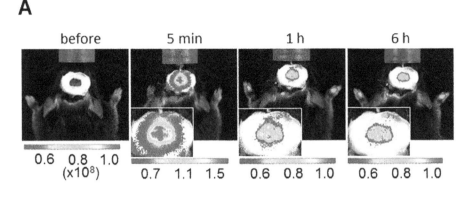

B

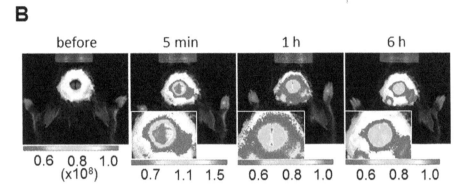

Figure 6. No clear visualization of HIF-1-active regions in the permanent brain ischemia model or with delayed injection of POH-N in the focal brain ischemia model. (A) Representative *in vivo* fluorescence images visualized through a cranial window before and at 5 min, 1 h, and 6 h after POH-N administration are shown. POH-N was injected intravenously at 60 min after permanent MCA occlusion. (B) Representative *in vivo* fluorescence images visualized through a cranial window before and at 5 min, 1 h, and 6 h following POH-N administration at 24 h after reperfusion. Magnified head images are shown in the lower left panels.

Statistical analysis

Data are presented as mean ± SEM. Statistical analyses were performed using ANOVA. Values of $P<0.05$ were considered statistically significant.

Results

Stabilization of POH-N under hypoxic conditions *in vitro*

HIF-1α protein levels increased under hypoxic conditions compared with normoxic conditions (Fig. 3A). When SH-SY5 neuroblastoma cells were treated with POH-N, significantly (*$P<0.02$) higher fluorescent signals were detected in cells cultured in hypoxic conditions compared with normoxic conditions in a manner similar to that of HIF-1α protein levels (Fig. 3B and C).

HIF-1α accumulation after focal cerebral ischemia

Quantitative western blot analysis showed that cerebral ischemia induced by transient MCAO triggered a significant (*$P<0.05$, n = 4) increase in the HIF-1α protein levels in the ischemic hemisphere (Fig. 4A and B). HIF-1α protein levels reached a peak at 6 h after 60 min MCAO in the ischemic hemisphere and declined thereafter (Fig. 4A and B).

In vivo imaging of HIF-1-active regions in an ischemic stroke model

To examine the possible application of POH-N to ischemic diseases, we administered POH-N in mice with focal cerebral

ischemia induced by transient MCAO. The fluorescent signal for POH-N was measured at the indicated times (Fig. 5A and B). Five minutes after POH-N administration, fluorescent signals were lower in the ischemic (right) hemisphere than in the non-ischemic (left) hemisphere, probably reflecting post-ischemic hypoperfusion in the ischemic hemisphere. However, at 1–6 h after POH-N administration, the fluorescence intensity increased in the ischemic hemisphere and decreased in the non-ischemic hemisphere. At 3–6 hours after POH-N administration, the relative fluorescence intensity of the ischemic hemisphere was significantly greater than the baseline, compared to that of the non-ischemic hemisphere (ischemic/non-ischemic ratio) (Fig. 5B).

ODD-dependent clearance acceleration in the non-ischemic brains

Examination of the coronal brain sections confirmed that the fluorescent signal was derived from the ischemic hemisphere, particularly in the cortical region adjacent to the striatum (infarct core), at 6 h after POH-N administration (Fig. 5C). Although the ischemic sites showed higher fluorescence intensity than the non-ischemic sites in both POH-N- and POmH-N-injected brains, the fluorescent signals in POH-N-injected brains were more restricted to the ischemic region (Fig. 5C). Furthermore, the non-ischemic sites in POH-N-injected brains showed significantly lower relative fluorescence intensities than those in POmH-N-injected brains (Fig. 5C and D). The fluorescent signal derived from the ischemic hemisphere was visualized even without cranial window (Fig. 5E).

A

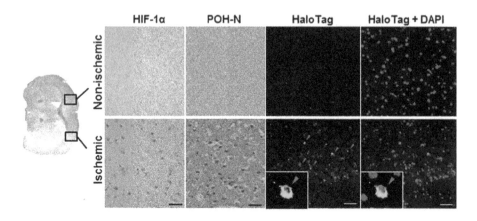

B

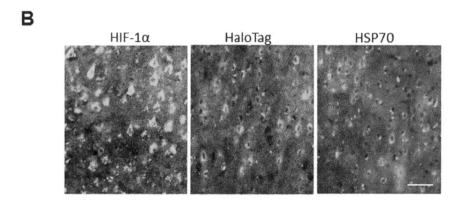

Figure 7. Immunohistochemical detection of HIF-1-active cells and POH-N probe. (A) Immunohistochemical analysis of HIF-1α, POH-N (ODD) and HaloTag (green), with or without DAPI nuclear staining (blue), at 1 day after probe administration. Panels at the bottom show magnified images. (B) Similar distributions of HIF-1α, HaloTag, and HSP70 in pyramidal neurons of the cortical layer bordering the infarct. Scale bars, 50 μm.

However, when POH-N was injected intravenously at 60 min after permanent MCAO or at 24 hours after reperfusion in the transient MCAO, fluorescence intensity was not different between the ischemic and non-ischemic hemispheres (Fig. 6A and B).

Specificity of POH-N to HIF-1α-positive cells in the ischemic brain

Occlusion of the MCA for 60 min induced reproducible ischemic infarcts in the striatum (infarct core) and cerebral cortex, as detected by histology. The specific localization of POH probe in HIF-1-active cells was examined by immunohistochemical analysis of the brain at 24 h after POH-N injection. POH protein was specifically detected in the ischemic cerebral cortex, where abundant HIF-1α-positive cells were also observed (Fig. 7). POH protein was mainly localized to the cytoplasm of cells (magnified images in Fig. 5 bottom panels), which is concordant with a previous report [16]. HIF-1α, HaloTag, and HSP70 showed similar expression patterns in cortical pyramidal neurons within the ischemic penumbra. Overall, these results demonstrate the specificity of POH to HIF-1-active ischemic, but potentially salvageable, cells.

Discussion

In vivo imaging using the POH probe was previously demonstrated to accurately identify HIF-1-active regions in a mouse cancer model [16]. The present study shows that POH-N can also detect HIF-1-active ischemic lesions in a mouse focal cerebral ischemia model. One-hour focal ischemia induced HIF-1 upregulation at 1, 6, and 24 hours post-ischemia, even after reperfusion, probably reflecting the 'no-reflow' phenomenon [21]. Although the tissue in the ischemic hemisphere may have been temporarily subject to relative hyperoxic status after reperfusion, the fluorescent POH system worked at least 24 hours post ischemia, thus enabling HIF-1 imaging. This POH fusion protein method therefore has great potential in improving the diagnosis and treatment of ischemic stroke.

The PTD-mediated delivery system has been demonstrated to enable the delivery of biologically active proteins across the blood–brain barrier. It has been shown that fusion proteins containing the PTD sequence, derived from HIV trans-activator of transcription (TAT), are delivered into the brain tissue after systemic administration [17]. To date, the efficacy of PTD fusion proteins, including the anti-apoptotic protein Bcl-xL, neurotrophic factor GDNF, and antioxidant enzyme SOD, have been demonstrated in rodent models of cerebral ischemia

[22,23,24,25]. However, many neuroprotective drugs that have shown promise in experimental animal models have failed to achieve positive results during clinical trials [26,27]. One of the reasons for such failures is that the target drug levels identified in animals cannot be tolerated by stroke patients. For example, an N-methyl-D-aspartate (NMDA) receptor antagonist has been shown to protect against ischemic stroke at plasma levels greater than 40 µg/mL in animal models; however, the highest tolerable dose in stroke patients is only half of this target level, above which neurological and psychiatric adverse effects are observed [27,28]. One potential way to circumvent such adverse effects would be to take advantage of the ODD-mediated acceleration of clearance under normoxic conditions. In our experiments, POH-N was cleared from the non-ischemic hemisphere significantly faster than POmH-N (Fig. 5). The results strongly support previous reports stating that the ODD domain contributes to the rapid clearance of POH-N from normoxic HIF-inactive tissue [16].

The ischemic penumbra, which is the functionally impaired but potentially viable tissue surrounding the infarct core, is currently considered to be the most promising target for ischemic stroke therapy. However, the accurate identification of patients exhibiting penumbral damage is not straightforward. Currently, the most widely accepted and practical method for identifying the ischemic penumbra in stroke patients is to look for an ischemic region displaying reduced perfusion on MRI but a normal signal on diffusion-weighted imaging [29]. However, several studies show that this interpretation of diffusion- and perfusion-weighted imaging may be an oversimplification [30]. Although the ischemic penumbra was originally defined on the basis of cerebral blood flow and physiological parameters [7], it can also be described in molecular terms [8] by examination of molecular layers emanating from the infarct core. Specifically, pro-apoptotic proteins and anti-apoptotic heat shock protein 70 are expressed in the layer bordering the infarct, and HIF in the layers beyond [31,32,33]. Furthermore, ischemia-induced spreading depression induces the expression of c-fos and many other immediate early genes in the outer layer [34], although such identification methods have not yet been applied in humans.

In the present study, POH-N was delivered to ischemic lesions, including peri-infarct regions (Fig. 7). This result supports the idea that the PTD allows fusion proteins to be delivered to hypoperfused tissue, most likely via diffusion, to achieve the molecular definition of an ischemic penumbra. Furthermore, POH-N significantly accumulated in the ischemic regions and was specifically detected in HIF-1-active cortical cells after focal brain ischemia (Fig. 7). We concede that this imaging technique may be deemed inferior, in terms of resolution, when compared to more established imaging techniques, such as MRI. However, such fluorescent imaging techniques may provide a useful complement to existing imaging techniques, as bedside evaluation would be available without the need of transferring stroke patients to the diagnostic radiology unit. In addition, since HaloTag ligands can be conjugated to a wide range of biomaterials, POH offers a wide range of clinical applications, including the production of imaging probes, even for MRI. Furthermore, a POH-mediated delivery system could be used to selectively target drugs to the ischemic penumbra, an area that has potential for recovery and thus may provide a target for medical interventions.

A limitation that became apparent during this study was the lack of clarity of some images of small mouse brains captured with the IVIS®-Spectrum, which hindered the clear discrimination between ischemic core and penumbra. Another limitation arose through POH-N failing to reach ischemic lesions in the permanent MCAO model. In addition, POH-N had to be injected immediately, not at 6 or 24 hours, after reperfusion to visualize HIF-1-active regions even in the transient MCAO model. Since the partial or complete recanalization rate of major vessel occlusion exceeds 50% in the tPA era [35], clinical application of this *in vivo* fluorescence imaging system should be further explored in parallel with efforts to enhance imaging sensitivity and widen the narrow time window.

Acknowledgments

We are grateful to Yumi Takahashi, Taeko Tani, and Akiko Yoshida for their skilled technical assistance, Takashi Ushiki for technical discussions, Shigeaki Watanabe (Summit Pharmaceuticals International Corporation) for providing technical support regarding IVIS, and Akira Hasegawa and Mark McDougall (Promega Corporation) for their technical advice regarding the HaloTag system. We would also like to thank Maya Uose for secretarial assistance and Ahmad Khundakar for insightful editing of the manuscript.

Author Contributions

Conceived and designed the experiments: YF T. Kuchimaru T. Kadonosono MI SKK. Performed the experiments: YF T. Kuchimaru T. Kadonosono ST YH. Analyzed the data: YF T. Kuchimaru T. Kadonosono ST SKK. Contributed reagents/materials/analysis tools: RT HT MH SKK MI. Wrote the paper: YF SKK MI.

References

1. Bergeron M, Yu AY, Solway KE, Semenza GL, Sharp FR (1999) Induction of hypoxia-inducible factor-1 (HIF-1) and its target genes following focal ischemia in rat brain. Eur J Neurosci 11: 4159–4170.
2. Semenza GL (2000) HIF-1: mediator of physiological and pathophysiological responses to hypoxia. J Appl Physiol 88: 1474–1480.
3. Kaelin WG (2005) Proline hydroxylation and gene expression. Annu Rev Biochem 74: 115–128.
4. Schofield CJ, Ratcliffe PJ (2004) Oxygen sensing by HIF hydroxylases. Nat Rev Mol Cell Biol 5: 343–354.
5. Tanimoto K, Makino Y, Pereira T, Poellinger L (2000) Mechanism of regulation of the hypoxia-inducible factor-1 alpha by the von Hippel–Lindau tumor suppressor protein. EMBO J 19: 4298–4309.
6. Marti HJ, Bernaudin M, Bellail A, Schoch H, Euler M, et al. (2000) Hypoxia-induced vascular endothelial growth factor expression precedes neovascularization after cerebral ischemia. Am J Pathol 156: 965–976.
7. Astrup J, Siesjo BK, Symon L (1981) Thresholds in cerebral ischemia—the ischemic penumbra. Stroke 12: 723–725.
8. Sharp FR, Lu A, Tang Y, Millhorn DE (2000) Multiple molecular penumbras after focal cerebral ischemia. J Cereb Blood Flow Metab 20: 1011–1032.
9. Bergeron M, Yu AY, Solway KE, Semenza GL, Sharp FR (1999) Induction of hypoxia-inducible factor-1 (HIF-1) and its target genes following focal ischaemia in rat brain. Eur J Neurosci 11: 4159–4170.
10. Harada H, Kizaka-Kondoh S, Hiraoka M (2006) Mechanism of hypoxia-specific cytotoxicity of procaspase-3 fused with a VHL-mediated protein destruction motif of HIF-1alpha containing Pro564. FEBS Lett 580: 5718–5722.
11. Harada H, Hiraoka M, Kizaka-Kondoh S (2002) Antitumor effect of TAT-oxygen-dependent degradation-caspase-3 fusion protein specifically stabilized and activated in hypoxic tumor cells. Cancer Res 62: 2013–2018.
12. Harada H, Kizaka-Kondoh S, Hiraoka M (2005) Optical imaging of tumor hypoxia and evaluation of efficacy of a hypoxia-targeting drug in living animals. Mol Imaging 4: 182–193.
13. Harada H, Kizaka-Kondoh S, Li G, Itasaka S, Shibuya K, et al. (2007) Significance of HIF-1-active cells in angiogenesis and radioresistance. Oncogene 26: 7508–7516.
14. Hiraga T, Kizaka-Kondoh S, Hirota K, Hiraoka M, Yoneda T (2007) Hypoxia and hypoxia-inducible factor-1 expression enhance osteolytic bone metastases of breast cancer. Cancer Res 67: 4157–4163.
15. Kizaka-Kondoh S, Itasaka S, Zeng L, Tanaka S, Zhao T, et al. (2009) Selective killing of hypoxia-inducible factor-1-active cells improves survival in a mouse model of invasive and metastatic pancreatic cancer. Clin Cancer Res 15: 3433–3441.
16. Kuchimaru T, Kadonosono T, Tanaka S, Ushiki T, Hiraoka M, et al. (2010) In vivo imaging of HIF-active tumors by an oxygen-dependent degradation protein probe with an interchangeable labeling system. PLoS ONE 5: e15736.

17. Schwarze SR, Ho A, Vocero-Akbani A, Dowdy SF (1999) In vivo protein transduction: delivery of a biologically active protein into the mouse. Science 285: 1569–1572.

18. Yuan F, Salehi HA, Boucher Y, Vasthare US, Tuma RF, et al. (1994) Vascular permeability and microcirculation of gliomas and mammary carcinomas transplanted in rat and mouse cranial windows. Cancer Res 54: 4564–4568.

19. Shah ZA, Namiranian K, Klaus J, Kibler K, Doré S (2006) Use of an optimized transient occlusion of the middle cerebral artery protocol for the mouse stroke model. J Stroke Cerebrovasc Dis 15: 133–138.

20. Chan DA, Sutphin PD, Yen SE, Giaccia AJ (2005) Coordinate regulation of the oxygen-dependent degradation domains of hypoxia-inducible factor 1 alpha. Mol Cell Biol 25: 6415–6426.

21. Hase Y, Okamoto Y, Fujita Y, Kitamura A, Ito H, Maki T, et al. (2012) Cilostazol, a phosphodiesterase inhibitor, prevents no-reflow and hemorrhage in mice with focal cerebral ischemia. Exp Neurol 233: 523–533.

22. Cao G, Pei W, Ge H, Liang Q, Luo Y, et al. (2002) In vivo delivery of a Bcl-xL fusion protein containing the TAT protein transduction domain protects against ischemic brain injury and neuronal apoptosis. J Neurosci 22: 5423–5431.

23. Kilic E, Dietz GP, Hermann DM, Bahr M (2002) Intravenous TAT–Bcl-Xl is protective after middle cerebral artery occlusion in mice. Ann Neurol 52: 617–622.

24. Kilic U, Kilic E, Dietz GP, Bahr M (2003) Intravenous TAT–GDNF is protective after focal cerebral ischemia in mice. Stroke 34: 1304–1310.

25. Kim DW, Eum WS, Jang SH, Kim SY, Choi HS, et al. (2005) Transduced TAT–SOD fusion protein protects against ischemic brain injury. Mol Cells 19: 88–96.

26. Fisher M, Bastan B (2008) Treating acute ischemic stroke. Curr Opin Drug Discov Devel 11: 626–632.

27. Savitz SI, Fisher M (2007) Future of neuroprotection for acute stroke: in the aftermath of the SAINT trials. Ann Neurol 61: 396–402.

28. Labiche LA, Grotta JC (2004) Clinical trials for cytoprotection in stroke. NeuroRx 1: 46–70.

29. Schlaug G, Benfield A, Baird AE, Siewert B, Lövblad KO, et al. (1999) The ischemic penumbra: operationally defined by diffusion perfusion MRI. Neurology 53: 1528–1537.

30. Kucinski T, Naumann D, Knab R, Schoder V, Wegener S, et al. (2005) Tissue at risk is overestimated in perfusion-weighted imaging: MR imaging in acute stroke patients without vessel recanalization. Am J Neuroradiol 26: 815–819.

31. Nedergaard M (1987) Neuronal injury in the infarct border: a neuropathological study in the rat. Acta Neuropathol 73: 267–274.

32. Kinouchi H, Sharp FR, Koistinaho J, Hicks K, Kamii H, et al. (1993) Induction of heat shock HSP70 mRNA and HSP70 kDa protein in neurons in the 'penumbra' following focal cerebral ischemia in the rat. Brain Res 619: 334–338.

33. Wang GL, Semenza GL (1995) Purification and characterization of hypoxia-inducible factor 1. J Biol Chem 270: 1230–1237.

34. Koistinaho J, Pasonen S, Yrjanheikki J, Chan PH (1999) Spreading depression-induced gene expression is regulated by plasma glucose. Stroke 30: 114–119.

35. Gonzalez RG (2006) Imaging-guided acute ischemic stroke therapy: From "time Is brain" to "physiology is brain". Am J Neuroradiol 27: 728–735.

8

A Cross-Sectional Study of Individuals Seeking Information on Transient Ischemic Attack and Stroke Symptoms Online: A Target for Intervention?

Anthony S. Kim[1]*, Sharon N. Poisson[1], J. Donald Easton[1], S. Claiborne Johnston[1,2]

1 Department of Neurology, University of California San Francisco, San Francisco, California, United States of America, 2 Department of Epidemiology and Biostatistics, University of California San Francisco, San Francisco, California, United States of America

Abstract

Background: Individuals with TIA/stroke symptoms often do not seek urgent medical attention. We assessed the feasibility of identifying individuals searching for information on TIA/stroke symptoms online as a target for future interventions to encourage urgent evaluation and we evaluated the performance of a self-reported risk score to identify subjects with true TIA or stroke.

Methodology/Principal Findings: We placed online advertisements to target English-speaking adults in the United States searching for TIA/stroke-related keywords. After completing an online questionnaire, participants were telephoned by a vascular neurologist to assess the likelihood of TIA/stroke. We used logistic regression and the c-statistic to assess associations and model discrimination respectively. Over 122 days, 251 (1%) of 25,292 website visitors completed the online questionnaire and 175 were reached by telephone (mean age 58.5 years; 63% women) for follow-up. Of these participants, 37 (21%) had symptoms within 24 hours, 60 (34%) had not had a medical evaluation yet, and 68 (39%) had TIA/stroke. Applying a modified $ABCD^2$ score yielded a c-statistic of 0.66, but 2 of 12 with a zero score had a TIA/stroke. Those with new symptoms were more likely to have TIA/stroke (OR 4.90, 95% CI 2.56–9.09).

Conclusions/Significance: Individuals with TIA/stroke that are seeking real-time information on symptoms online can be readily identified, in some cases before they have sought formal medical evaluation. Although a simple self-reported risk score was unable to identify a low-risk population in this selected group, this population may still present an attractive target for future interventions designed to encourage urgent medical evaluation.

Editor: Jens Minnerup, University of Münster, Germany

Funding: This study was sponsored by the National Stroke Association through a grant from Boehringer Ingelheim Pharmaceuticals, Inc. The funder had no role in study design, data collection and analysis, decision to publish, or preparation of the manuscript.

Competing Interests: The authors have declared that no competing interests exist.

* E-mail: akim@ucsf.edu

Introduction

Transient ischemic attack (TIA) is associated with a high risk of subsequent stroke, particularly in the first hours after symptom onset. [1,2] Although progress has been made to develop simple clinical scores to rapidly identify TIA patients at high risk of stroke [3] and to apply urgent interventions to prevent stroke after TIA, [4,5,6] most individuals with TIA do not seek urgent medical evaluation. [7,8].

Knowledge of TIA among the general public is poor. [9] TIA or "mini-stroke", as it is commonly known in the lay public, may not be recognized as a harbinger of stroke, particularly when symptoms are transitory or evanescent. [9,10] So even when TIA or stroke is considered as a possibility, the importance of an urgent evaluation may not be fully appreciated. Furthermore, individuals seeking appropriate evaluation may be deterred by barriers to access to healthcare providers, particularly on weekends or evenings [11] or by the prospect of lengthy or costly emergency department visits for symptoms that may be perceived of as minor or transient. [12,13] Therefore, improving early recognition of

TIA and an appreciation for the substantial risk of stroke associated with TIA may help to reduce delays in presentation for medical evaluation and create additional opportunities to prevent stroke.

Within this context, the internet has become an increasingly important source of first-line medical information [14] in part due to widespread availability and relatively low barriers to access. [15] However, despite potential advantages in terms of cost, efficiency, and reach, internet-based public health interventions to target online information-seeking behavior have been underdeveloped and understudied.

Our ultimate goal is to reduce the burden of disease from stroke by developing and refining efficient interventions to empower individuals seeking information on TIA/stroke online to seek urgent medical attention. For the present study, our primary goal was to assess the feasibility of identifying a population of individuals that are searching for information on TIA/stroke online as a potential target for future interventions to encourage appropriate urgent medical evaluation. Our main target population was subjects with TIA since these patients are at higher short-term risk of developing a stroke than patients with prevalent stroke, but since the distinction between TIA and stroke is difficult to make by both clinicians and the lay-public, we also included patients with prevalent stroke. Our secondary goal was to assess the performance of a web-based self-assessment tool based on the ABCD^2 score to identify TIA/stroke [16] in this population with the hope that this personalized information would be a more effective motivation for participants to seek appropriate medical attention than general advice on TIA.

Methods

Study Design

We conducted a cross-sectional study with recruitment, eligibility screening, enrollment, consent, and data collection activities accomplished online and with outcome assessments completed by telephone.

Instrument Development and Pre-Testing

Candidate items for the online instrument were drawn from the Questionnaire for Verifying Stroke-Free Status; [17] components of the ABCD^2 score (Age $> = 60 = 1$; Clinical Features: Speech Disturbance without weakness $= 1$, Unilateral Weakness $= 2$; Duration: 10–59 minutes $= 1$, >60 minutes $= 2$; Diabetes $= 1$); [1] and other items (frequency and timing of symptoms, suddenness of symptom onset, hypertension, and migraine history). The blood pressure item was omitted because this information would usually not be available by self-report for most participants. We pre-tested candidate items in 10 inpatients and 10 outpatients with confirmed TIA or minor stroke using semi-structured cognitive interviews to assess for comprehension and phrasing. This feedback was incorporated into the final instrument (see Text S1).

Recruitment, Screening, Consent, and Enrollment

We placed a series of advertisements using an online marketing tool (Google Adwords, Google, Mountain View, California) to target users in the United States that were searching for keywords related to "mini-stroke", "TIA", "transient ischemic attack" or that were visiting webpages with related content that were part of an online advertising network (Google Display Network; See Text S2 for a list of targeted keywords). Users that clicked on an advertisement were taken to the study homepage (http://tia.ucsf.edu/), which provided information about the research study and basic information about stroke and TIA. Users that were interested in participating in the study then completed a seven-item screening questionnaire to confirm eligibility (symptoms concerning for a transient ischemic attack or "mini-stroke" within the last 6 months; age $> = 18$; ability to read, speak, and understand English; residence in the United States; and a willingness to complete the study questionnaire and the follow-up telephone assessment.) Those who met all entry criteria were asked to provide informed consent online. Consent was confirmed using a five-item post-test of comprehension. Those who were unwilling or unable to provide consent were excluded.

Study Procedures

Participants provided contact information for the subsequent telephone assessment and then completed a 26-item questionnaire on demographic characteristics, medical history, and symptoms (See Text S3). We then scheduled a 15 minute telephone call with each participant in order to assess how likely the symptoms were due to TIA/stroke. These assessments were conducted by one of

five vascular neurologists. Each neurologist was masked to the previously submitted responses to the questionnaire. Neurologists were free to elicit any information in order to assess the likelihood of TIA/stroke including self-reported neuroimaging findings. The likelihood of TIA/stroke was rated as "definitely not", "unlikely", "probable", and "definite".

TIA was defined as an acute neurological deficit lasting less than 24 hours attributable to focal brain ischemia, without evidence of a non-ischemic etiology and stroke was defined as a new neurologic deficit lasting over 24 hours with no apparent clinical or radiologic indication of a nonvascular mimic. To assess interrater reliability, half of the participants had a second independent telephone evaluation by a separate vascular neurologist that was masked to the results of the first assessment.

Statistical Analysis

Based on questionnaire responses, we calculated a modified ABCD^2 score for each participant during the analysis phase of the study. We used logistic regression to assess univariate and multivariable associations. Cronbach's alpha was used to assess reliability across items assessing the same underlying construct (i.e. diabetes, hypertension, suddenness of symptom onset). We used a quadratic-weighted kappa to evaluate interrater agreement between the two neurologists.

Ethics Statement

The University of California San Francisco Committee on Human Research approved this study. Consent was obtained for all participants online and the Committee specifically approved this form of consent as documented in an electronic database.

Results

Recruitment and Enrollment

A total of 4,600,427 advertisements were displayed over the 122-day enrollment period which resulted in 26,602 visits (average 218 visits/day) from 25,292 unique users. Total advertising costs for the study were $8,798.74—which corresponds to $0.35 per unique visitor or $35.05 per enrollee. All fifty states were represented as assessed by an Internet Protocol address-based geolocalization algorithm.

Fully 86% percent of visitors immediately exited the website within a few seconds of arriving at the home page, which is consistent with the notion that they clearly did not qualify for the study or were not interested in enrolling. Of the 291 visitors that initiated the enrollment process, 251 (86%; 1% overall) completed the eligibility screening, online consent, and questionnaire, which is not an unexpected yield rate for internet advertisements generally since there is trivial effort and little commitment for users to click on a link to find out more information. Of these, 175 (70%) were reached by telephone for follow-up. Reasons for failing to contact participants by telephone included the following: 31 did not respond to multiple telephone calls; 14 were initially reached by telephone to confirm their participation, but did not respond to subsequent telephone calls; 6 withdrew consent when reached; and 25 listed a nonworking or incorrect telephone number.

Baseline Characteristics

The average age of participants was 59 and a majority were women (Table 1). A total of 52 participants (30%) were age 65 or older. Based on telephone area codes, participants from 40 states and the District of Columbia were represented. Vascular risk factors such as hypertension, diabetes, and a prior history of

Table 1. Characteristics of 175 users seeking information on Transient Ischemic Attack or Mini-Stroke Online.

	n = 175	
Age, mean (SD)	58.5	(12.5)
Female, n (%)	110	(63.2)
Diabetes, n (%)	33	(18.9)
Hypertension, n (%)	103	(58.9)
Prior TIA, n (%)	46	(26.3)
Prior stroke, n (%)	30	(17.1)
History of migraine, n (%)	64	(36.6)
Symptom onset, n (cumulative %)*		
within 24 hours	37	(21.8)
within 48 hours	54	(31.8)
within 1 week	88	(51.8)
within 1 month	131	(77.1)
within 6 months	170	(100.0)
Duration of symptoms, n (%)		
<10 minutes	54	(30.9)
10–59 minutes	46	(26.3)
60 or more minutes	71	(40.6)
Number of episodes within the past year, n (%)†		
1	71	(40.6)
2	29	(16.6)
3 to 5	24	(13.7)
6 to 10	18	(10.3)
11 or more	26	(14.9)
No previous episodes within the past year	104	(59.4)
Sudden onset, n (%)	102	(58.3)
Warning before episode, n (%)	33	(18.9)
Associated headache, n (%)	79	(45.1)
Speech symptoms, n (%)	95	(54.3)
Weakness, n (%)	63	(36.0)
Sensory symptoms n (%)	90	(51.4)
Double vision, n (%)	46	(26.3)
Had Not Sought Medical Attention	71	(40.6)
ABCD² score, mean (SD)‡	2.7	(1.4)

*n = 170; † n = 168; ‡ ABCD² score: age >=60 = 1 point; Clinical Features: Speech Disturbance without weakness = 1 point, Unilateral Weakness = 2 points; Duration: 10–59 minutes = 1 point, >60 minutes = 2 points; Diabetes = 1 point. The blood pressure item was excluded since this was not likely to be available by self-report.

cerebrovascular disease were common. A prior history of migraine was also frequently reported.

Reported Symptoms

Speech, motor, and sensory symptoms were commonly reported (Table 1). Double vision and associated headache were also commonly reported as well. A total of 102 (58%) participants reported that symptoms were sudden in onset (onset over seconds to minutes) and 31 (19%) reported having a warning or prodrome of impending symptoms. Some participants (71; 41%) reported symptoms that had lasted for more than an hour.

A majority of participants reported that the symptoms were new within the past year (104; 59%) but 26 (15%) reported that they had had more than 11 episodes in the past year. Most participants (131; 77%) had experienced symptoms within a month and 37 (22%) had experienced symptoms within 24 hours. A substantial number of participants (71; 41%) had not yet sought formal medical advice.

Outcomes

Based on the follow-up telephone calls, 43 (25%) participants had a probable or definite TIA, and 68 (39%) participants had a probable or definite cerebrovascular event (either stroke or TIA). There was 96% agreement between the two vascular neurologists for the diagnosis of TIA/stroke (quadratic-weighted kappa = 0.86; see Table S1) among the 84 (48%) participants that had a second independent assessment.

Assessment of ABCD² Score Components

Univariable associations between individual components of the ABCD² score and TIA/stroke are presented in Table 2. A longer duration of symptoms was significantly associated with the ultimate diagnosis of TIA/stroke (Table 2). Unilateral weakness was also associated with a nearly 2-fold higher odds of TIA/stroke (OR 1.95, 95% CI 1.08−3.68).

The mean modified ABCD² score (excluding blood pressure) was 2.7, (SD 1.4; range 0–6). The proportion of patients with a TIA or stroke stratified by risk score is shown in Figure 1. Of the 12 patients with a score of 0, two (17%) had a TIA/stroke—one participant had diplopia and unilateral facial numbness that was concerning for posterior circulation ischemia, and the other had amaurosis fugax.

Other Predictors

Participants with multiple episodes of similar symptoms within the past year were much less likely to be diagnosed with TIA/stroke (Table 2). The odds of a TIA/stroke diagnosis were nearly five times higher (OR 4.90, 95% CI 2.56−9.09) for participants with new symptoms within the last year as compared to those who had at least one previous episode of similar symptoms in the last year.

There was moderate agreement (Cronbach's alpha 0.79) among the three items on the sudden symptom onset. However, sudden symptom onset was not significantly associated with a TIA/stroke diagnosis. Those who had already sought medical advice for their symptoms were significantly more likely to have TIA/stroke (OR 2.77, 95% CI 1.38–5.59).

Multivariable Models

For Model 1, we included components of the ABCD² score except of blood pressure (Table 3). This self-reported risk score demonstrated poor discrimination for TIA/stroke (0.66, 95% CI 0.58–0.74).

For Model 2, we incorporated a categorical variable with the number of episodes of similar symptoms within the past year (Table 3). This model produced a higher c-statistic (0.76, 95% CI 0.68–0.83) for TIA/stroke. However the same two participants with a risk score of 0 described above would still have been classified in the lowest risk category.

Discussion

Using an efficient and largely automated approach, we were able to readily identify a selected group of individuals who were seeking information on recent symptoms of TIA/stroke online—

Table 2. Univariable Predictors of Cerebrovascular Outcomes Among 175 Users Searching for Information on Transient Ischemic Attack and Mini-Stroke Online.

	TIA/Stroke	
	OR (95% CI)	P
Age $\geq$ 60	1.15 (0.63,2.13)	0.65
Clinical features		
Speech disturbance	1.35 (0.73,2.50)	0.34
Unilateral weakness	1.99 (1.06,3.76)	0.03
Duration of symptoms		
less than 10 minutes	ref	
10–59 minutes	3.21 (1.35,7.61)	<0.01
60 or more minutes	3.22 (1.46,7.11)	<0.01
Diabetes	1.63 (0.76,3.51)	0.21
Male	1.23 (0.65,2.30)	0.52
Hypertension	1.00 (0.54,1.85)	0.99
Prior TIA	1.84 (0.93,3.65)	0.08
Prior stroke	0.85 (0.38,1.93)	0.70
History of migraine	1.00 (0.53,1.88)	0.99
Timing of enrollment		
within 24 hours of symptoms	ref	
within 48 hours of symptoms	1.51 (0.41,5.56)	0.54
within 1 week of symptoms	2.86 (1.01,8.06)	0.05
within 1 month of symptoms	2.37 (0.88,6.39)	0.09
within 6 months of symptoms	4.23 (1.55,11.5)	<0.01
Number of episodes within the past year		
1	ref	
2	0.26 (0.10,0.67)	<0.01
3 to 5	0.23 (0.08,0.65)	<0.01
6 to 10	0.26 (0.09,0.83)	0.02
11 or more	0.09 (0.02, 0.33)	<0.01
At least one previous episode within past year	0.20 (0.11, 0.39)	<0.01
Sudden onset	0.77 (0.42,1.43)	0.41
Warning before episode	0.89 (0.40,1.95)	0.77
Associated headache	0.85 (0.46,1.58)	0.62
Double vision	1.65 (0.84,3.27)	0.15
Sensory symptoms	1.63 (0.88,3.01)	0.12
Already sought medical attention	2.77 (1.38, 5.59)	5.59

sometimes very soon after symptom onset and often before a formal medical evaluation had been completed. Although participants in our study are unlikely to be fully representative of patients with TIA generally, or patients seeking online information on TIA specifically, we did identify a subpopulation with a relatively high burden of cerebrovascular disease that could benefit from a targeted public health intervention. Given the low cost and the substantial efficiency of this approach in terms of cost per participant reached, and since a major goal of acute management of TIA is urgent evaluation to prevent early recurrent stroke, this subpopulation may present an attractive target for interventions designed to reduce delays in presenting to medical attention for TIA/stroke.

A secondary goal of our study was to assess the performance of a self-reported version of $ABCD^2$ score for TIA. The $ABCD^2$ score was originally developed to assess the risk of stroke after TIA using simple elements available to front-line clinicians, [3] but this score has also been shown to work in part by distinguishing TIA from TIA mimics. [18] Here, we faced the additional challenge from the measurement issues that arise from using self-reported responses from individuals with various levels of health literacy. Accordingly, we found that a modified $ABCD^2$ score by self-report could not reliably rule out a TIA or stroke. Some participants (2 of 12) with the lowest score of 0 had symptoms such as diplopia or amaurosis fugax that are not specifically captured by the score, but would still require urgent evaluation.

With regards to the performance of other self-reported items to predict a cerebrovascular diagnosis, we found a strong association between a higher number of episodes of similar symptoms within the last 12 months and a non-cerebrovascular diagnosis. Having multiple stereotyped episodes of symptoms previously without a resultant stroke may make a given episode less likely to be TIA and may make seizure, migraine or other episodic disorders more likely. [19] The predictive value of this finding will require further validation and confirmation of the dose-response relationship that is suggested by our data.

Since such a high proportion of participants in our study had TIA or stroke, we speculate that all of the individuals that participated in our study may have been well served to seek medical attention regardless of risk score, particularly since the online questionnaire was unable to reliably identify low-risk individuals. Some individual participants indicated that they lacked a primary care provider or medical insurance or otherwise had limited access to medical care, while others indicated that they did not understand that TIA was a medical emergency, or were unable to get an urgent appointment, but had already planned on seeking medical attention at some point. The value of some form of risk stratification at the outset may not be to identify those without worrisome symptoms, but to provide some interactivity and engagement in order to enhance behavior change while participants are deciding on next actions. We suspect that if individuals are given feedback and recommendations that are to some extent individualized and interactive rather than presented as static blanket recommendations, they may be more likely to take action after TIA, though a formal assessment of this possibility would require additional study.

Our methods also highlight opportunities to improve the efficiency of clinical research more generally by quickly and efficiently reaching hundreds of potential participants on a daily basis and by enrolling participants over a large geographic area. Direct-to-participant recruitment portals that incorporate initial eligibility screening by self-report may demonstrate a sufficiently high yield for TIA and stroke diagnoses to serve as a primary recruitment method for some types of clinical research. Furthermore, our study frames the potential role for validated and interactive self-assessment online tools address public health problems more generally. A previous study have demonstrated a relationship between internet search queries and influenza epidemics [20] and another study showed that the frequency of internet search queries for stroke related search terms by state ("stroke signs", "stroke symptoms", "mini stroke", excluding "heat") was associated with stroke prevalence. [21] There remain potential medicolegal issues including whether providing tailored or personalized information constitutes medical advice, and valid concerns about maintaining privacy and confidentiality of health information online. But as disparities in access [22,23,24] and adoption of internet technology across demographic and socio-

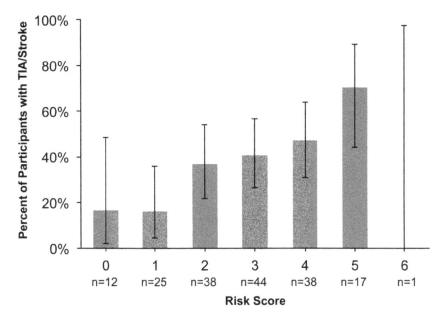

Figure 1. Percent of participants with transient ischemic attack or stroke by self-reported ABCD^2 score. A modified ABCD^2 score was calculated from self-reported components of the score (age $>=60=1$ point; Clinical Features: Speech Disturbance without weakness $=1$ point, Unilateral Weakness $=2$ points; Duration: 10–59 minutes $=1$ point, >60 minutes $=2$ points; Diabetes $=1$ point). The blood pressure item was excluded since this was not likely to be available by self-report, so the range of this risk score was 0 to 6. The grey bars show the proportion observed and the black vertical lines represent the 95% confidence interval around that proportion. The one enrollee with a score of 6 had migraine.

Table 3. Multivariable Predictors of TIA/Stroke Diagnosis Among 175 Users Searching for Information on Transient Ischemic Attack or Mini-Stroke Symptoms Online.

	TIA/Stroke	
	OR (95% CI)	P
Model 1: Components of the ABCD^2 score excluding blood pressure		
Age $>=60$	1.47 (0.76, 2.85)	0.25
Clinical features		
Speech Disturbance	1.09 (0.48, 2.49)	0.84
Unilateral weakness	1.79 (0.80, 3.96)	0.15
Duration of symptoms		
10–59 minutes	2.78 (1.13, 6.81)	0.03
>60 minutes	3.02 (1.32, 6.92)	<0.01
Diabetes	1.53 (0.69, 3.39)	0.30
Model 2: Model 1+ no previous episodes		
Age $>=60$	1.25 (0.61, 2.56)	0.54
Clinical features		
Speech Disturbance	1.10 (0.42, 2.46)	0.98
Unilateral weakness	1.93 (0.81, 4.56)	0.14
Duration of symptoms		
10–59 minutes	3.05 (1.15, 8.07)	0.03
>60 minutes	2.39 (0.98, 5.82)	0.06
Diabetes	2.58 (1.05, 6.37)	0.04
No previous episodes (within 1 year)	5.97 (2.80, 12.7)	<0.01

Components of the ABCD^2 score excluding acute blood pressure are included in Model 1. Model 2 adds the number of previous episodes of similar symptoms in the past year.

demographic strata narrow, [14] internet-based interventions to efficiently target public health problems may become more attractive. Future studies may include questionnaires in the ED regarding internet-based activity prior to presentation in the ED and evaluations of the impact of internet-based tools on the actual the behavior of subjects with possible TIA and ultimately on processes measures of treatment and patient outcomes.

Limitations

Our study should be interpreted in light of a number of limitations. First, about 1% of visitors to the website enrolled in the study and so the participants in this study were highly selected. Although the motivations for enrollment were not captured in our study, many visitors quickly moved from the website within a few seconds, which suggests that they were not finding what they had expected or what they were looking for. We speculate that individuals with symptoms without a straightforward diagnosis despite prior medical evaluations, those with chronic medical conditions, or those with barriers to accessing care might be overrepresented in our study. Second, the authentication of participants and their responses and the difficulty of reaching some participants by telephone limit the generalizability of our results and illustrate a particular challenge for internet-based research. Third, we attempted to mitigate misclassification of TIA and stroke outcomes by formally assessing interrater reliability and masking the neurologists to questionnaire responses, but since follow-up was conducted by telephone and access to additional clinical information such as neuroimaging studies or results of a neurologic exam was limited to self-report the potential for misclassification remains. For the lay-public, the use of the term, "mini-stroke," a much more common search term than "TIA", serves to confuse the distinction between TIA and stroke and the clinical distinction between TIA and minor stroke may be difficult to make even for experienced clinicians. [25,26] Fourth, although the neurologists were masked to responses to the questionnaire, they were free to elicit any information into their final assessments and may have incorporated items that were elicited by the online questionnaire into their assessments.

Conclusion

Individuals seeking information on possible TIA or stroke symptoms online can be efficiently and readily identified, sometimes before they have sought formal medical attention. Although elements of a self-reported $ABCD^2$ score was not able to rule out a cerebrovascular etiology, the burden of true stroke and TIA in this selected subpopulation may be sufficiently high to justify future targeted interventions to encourage urgent medical evaluation.

We thank Christine Wong, MD (California Pacific Medical Center, data collection) and Babak Navi, MD (Weill Cornell Medical College, data collection) for assistance conducting follow-up telephone assessments.

Author Contributions

Conceived and designed the experiments: ASK SCJ. Performed the experiments: ASK SNP JDE SCJ. Analyzed the data: ASK. Wrote the paper: ASK SNP JDE SCJ.

References

1. Johnston SC, Gress DR, Browner WS, Sidney S (2000) Short-term prognosis after emergency department diagnosis of TIA. JAMA 284: 2901–2906.
2. Coull AJ, Lovett JK, Rothwell PM (2004) Population based study of early risk of stroke after transient ischaemic attack or minor stroke: implications for public education and organisation of services. BMJ 328: 326.
3. Johnston SC, Rothwell PM, Nguyen-Huynh MN, Giles MF, Elkins JS, et al. (2007) Validation and refinement of scores to predict very early stroke risk after transient ischaemic attack. Lancet 369: 283–292.
4. Lavallée PC, Meseguer E, Abboud H, Cabrejo L, Olivot J-M, et al. (2007) A transient ischaemic attack clinic with round-the-clock access (SOS-TIA): feasibility and effects. Lancet Neurol 6: 953–960.
5. Rothwell PM, Giles MF, Chandratheva A, Marquardt L, Geraghty O, et al. (2007) Effect of urgent treatment of transient ischaemic attack and minor stroke on early recurrent stroke (EXPRESS study): a prospective population-based sequential comparison. Lancet 370: 1432–1442.
6. Giles MF, Rothwell PM (2007) Risk of stroke early after transient ischaemic attack: a systematic review and meta-analysis. Lancet Neurol 6: 1063–1072.
7. Chandratheva A, Lasserson DS, Geraghty OC, Rothwell PM (2010) Population-based study of behavior immediately after transient ischemic attack and minor stroke in 1000 consecutive patients: lessons for public education. Stroke 41: 1108–1114.
8. Sprigg N, Machili C, Otter ME, Wilson A, Robinson TG (2009) A systematic review of delays in seeking medical attention after transient ischaemic attack. J Neurol Neurosurg Psychiatry 80: 871–875.
9. Johnston SC, Fayad PB, Gorelick PB, Hanley DF, Shwayder P, et al. (2003) Prevalence and knowledge of transient ischemic attack among US adults. Neurology 60: 1429–1434.
10. Mandelzweig L, Goldbourt U, Boyko V, Tanne D (2006) Perceptual, social, and behavioral factors associated with delays in seeking medical care in patients with symptoms of acute stroke. Stroke 37: 1248–1253.
11. Lasserson DS, Chandratheva A, Giles MF, Mant D, Rothwell PM (2008) Influence of general practice opening hours on delay in seeking medical attention after transient ischaemic attack (TIA) and minor stroke: prospective population based study. BMJ 337: a1569.
12. Maestroni A, Mandelli C, Manganaro D, Zecca B, Rossi P, et al. (2008) Factors influencing delay in presentation for acute stroke in an emergency department in Milan, Italy. Emerg Med J 25: 340–345.
13. Giles MF, Flossman E, Rothwell PM (2006) Patient behavior immediately after transient ischemic attack according to clinical characteristics, perception of the event, and predicted risk of stroke. Stroke 37: 1254–1260.
14. Lustria ML, Smith SA, Hinnant CC (2011) Exploring digital divides: an examination of eHealth technology use in health information seeking,
    communication and personal health information management in the USA. Health informatics journal 17: 224–243.
15. Hesse BW, Nelson DE, Kreps GL, Croyle RT, Arora NK, et al. (2005) Trust and sources of health information: the impact of the Internet and its implications for health care providers: findings from the first Health Information National Trends Survey. Archives of internal medicine 165: 2618–2624.
16. Palomeras E, Fossas P, Quintana M, Monteis R, Sebastian M, et al. (2008) Emergency perception and other variables associated with extra-hospital delay in stroke patients in the Maresme region (Spain). Eur J Neurol 15: 329–335.
17. Jones WJ, Williams LS, Meschia JF (2001) Validating the Questionnaire for Verifying Stroke-Free Status (QVSFS) by neurological history and examination. Stroke 32: 2232–2236.
18. Josephson SA, Sidney S, Pham TN, Bernstein AL, Johnston SC (2008) Higher ABCD2 Score Predicts Patients Most Likely to Have True Transient Ischemic Attack. Stroke 39: 3096–3098.
19. Johnston SC, Sidney S, Bernstein AL, Gress DR (2003) A comparison of risk factors for recurrent TIA and stroke in patients diagnosed with TIA. Neurology 60: 280–285.
20. Ginsberg J, Mohebbi MH, Patel RS, Brammer L, Smolinski MS, et al. (2009) Detecting influenza epidemics using search engine query data. Nature 457: 1012–1014.
21. Walcott BP, Nahed BV, Kahle KT, Redjal N, Coumans JV (2011) Determination of geographic variance in stroke prevalence using Internet search engine analytics. Neurosurgical focus 30: E19.
22. Choi N (2011) Relationship between health service use and health information technology use among older adults: analysis of the US National Health Interview Survey. Journal of medical Internet research 13: e33.
23. Wasserman IM, Richmond-Abbott M (2005) Gender and the Internet: Causes of Variation in Access, Level, and Scope of Use*. Social Science Quarterly 86: 252–270.
24. Zach L, Dalrymple PW, Rogers ML, Williver-Farr H (2012) Assessing internet access and use in a medically underserved population: implications for providing enhanced health information services. Health information and libraries journal 29: 61–71.
25. Ferro JM, Falcao I, Rodrigues G, Canhao P, Melo TP, et al. (1996) Diagnosis of transient ischaemic attack by the nonneurologist. A validation study. Stroke 27: 2225–2229.
26. Quinn TJ, Cameron AC, Dawson J, Lees KR, Walters MR (2009) ABCD2 scores and prediction of noncerebrovascular diagnoses in an outpatient population: a case-control study. Stroke 40: 749–753.

9

Non-Focal Neurological Symptoms Associated with Classical Presentations of Transient Ischaemic Attack: Qualitative Analysis of Interviews with Patients

Susan Kirkpatrick[1], Louise Locock[1], Matthew F. Giles[2], Daniel S. Lasserson[3*]

1 Health Experiences Research Group, Department of Primary Care Health Sciences, University of Oxford, Oxford, United Kingdom, **2** Stroke Prevention Unit, Nuffield Department of Clinical Neuroscience, University of Oxford, Oxford, United Kingdom, **3** Department of Primary Care Health Sciences, University of Oxford, Oxford, United Kingdom

Abstract

Background: Improving the recognition of transient ischaemic attack (TIA) at initial healthcare contact is essential as urgent specialist assessment and treatment reduces stroke risk. Accurate TIA detection could be achieved with clinical prediction rules but none have been validated in primary care. An alternative approach using qualitative analysis of patients' experiences of TIA may identify novel features of the TIA phenotype that are not detected routinely, as such techniques have revealed novel early features of other important conditions such as meningococcaemia. We sought to determine whether the patient's experience of TIA would reveal additional deficits that can be tested prospectively in cohort studies to determine their additional diagnostic and prognostic utility at the first healthcare contact.

Methodology and Findings: Qualitative semi-structured interviews with 25 patients who had experienced definite TIA as determined by a stroke specialist; framework analysis to map symptoms and key words or descriptive phrases used against each individual, with close attention to the detail of the language used. All interview transcripts were reviewed by a specialist clinician with experience in TIA/minor stroke. Patients described non-focal symptoms consistent with higher function deficits in spatial perception and awareness of deficit, as well as feelings of disconnection with their immediate surroundings. Of the classical features, weakness and speech disturbance were described in ways that did not meet the readily recognisable phenotype.

Conclusion/Significance: Analysis of patients' narrative accounts reveals a set of overlooked features of the experience of TIA which may provide additional diagnostic utility so that providers of first contact healthcare can recognise TIA more easily. Future research is required in a prospective cohort of patients presenting with transient neurological symptoms to determine how frequent these features are, what they add to diagnostic information and whether they can refine measures to predict stroke risk.

Editor: Jean-Claude Baron, University of Cambridge, United Kingdom

Funding: The research was supported by the National Institute for Health Research (NIHR) Oxford Biomedical Research Centre Programme. The views expressed are those of the authors and not necessarily those of the NHS, the NIHR or the Department of Health. The funders had no role in study design, data collection and analysis, decision to publish, or preparation of the manuscript.

Competing Interests: The authors have declared that no competing interests exist.

* E-mail: daniel.lasserson@phc.ox.ac.uk

Introduction

There is a high risk of stroke within the first few days after transient ischaemic attack (TIA) [1] which can be reduced substantially after urgent specialist assessment and treatment [2,3]. Accurate recognition of TIA at the first healthcare contact is therefore crucial in reducing early stroke risk. Patients with TIA initially seek healthcare from primary care practices and emergency departments [4] and although the relative use of these two sources of first contact healthcare varies by country [5], accurate detection of TIA in both these settings is needed. There are key investigations that stratify stroke risk, such as brain imaging [6], but the diagnosis remains essentially clinical and relies on the report of the episode by the patient with any available witness account.

Detection of TIA therefore relies heavily on the clinical history, which is a largely interrogative process [7]. Nevertheless, there is evidence to suggest that this is a difficult and complex task for primary care physicians – around 50% of referrals to TIA clinics do not have a cerebrovascular diagnosis [8] and vignette studies have demonstrated variation in the ability of primary care physicians to suspect TIA from simple clinical details [9–11].

Improving the recognition of TIA is therefore crucial for stroke prevention and whilst there are simple clinical approaches such as clinical prediction rules, which prompt the clinician to ask certain questions that form components of a scoring system [12], this may be limited for TIA recognition. Although a number of stroke recognition tools exist such as the Recognition of Stroke in the Emergency Room (ROSIER) [13] and the Face, Arm and Speech test (FAST) [14], they are based on the demonstration of physical deficit which is unlikely to be present in TIA, particularly in patients presenting to primary care where there is often significant delay between symptom onset and initial assessment [4]. There is only one report of a recognition tool specifically for TIA which is based on the physical signs elicited from patients with stroke [15], rather than from patients' descriptions of their experience of TIA.

An alternative approach to address the evidence gap of improving recognition of TIA is to use qualitative data to reveal novel or previously unrecognised clinical features that are associated with TIA. Qualitative analysis of interviews with patients can mine the experience of transient neurological events to uncover clinical features that may not be elicited through standard medical history taking. Although qualitative methodologies are not routinely used in diagnostic research, these methods have yielded insights which can aid the diagnostic process, for example interviews with parents of children with meningococcaemia [16] have shown that there are novel clinical features that are not routinely elicited in clinical history taking. Furthermore, these novel features are prognostic and have recently changed national guidance in the UK for suspicion of meningococcaemia in primary care [17].

Quantitative methods are not always appropriate to investigate novel or unrecognised clinical associations due to reliance on questionnaires requiring dichotomous data collection (i.e. feature present or absent) as this will require pre-specified questions. Furthermore, data collection methods which briefly ask for several lines of clinical narrative about the symptoms may also not reveal novel or unrecognised features. A qualitative approach with semi-structured interviews allows patients more time to explore and recount the narratives of their episode of transient neurological deficit and novel or unrecognised clinical features can be sought for in the qualitative analysis of interview transcripts. Whilst definitive prospective studies using quantitative methods will always be required to ascertain diagnostic and prognostic significance of clinical features, the qualitative approach is an initial step to investigate the presence of novel features which can then be tested in subsequent cohort studies.

Therefore we undertook semi-structured qualitative interviews with patients with TIA and their carers to gain additional information about the experience of their event. Patients bring to the consultation their 'embodied knowledge'– internal sensations and observations which may be hidden to the physician, or which may not fit with current diagnostic criteria and are therefore overlooked, even if mentioned by the patient [18].

We restricted the analysis to patients with a diagnosis of definite, rather than possible TIA in order to increase the likelihood that novel or unrecognised descriptors of deficit are not due to inclusion of patients without a cerebrovascular cause for their symptoms.

Methods

Sampling and recruitment

The data is drawn from a wider qualitative interview study in the UK using a maximum variation sampling approach. This is designed to capture the broadest possible range of experiences [19]. Variation was sought across demographic variables and types of TIA experience (e.g. one or several TIAs; different types of presentation; different types of referral route). Participants were recruited from a number of sources including the Oxford Vascular study (OXVASC), primary care practices, TIA clinics, support organisations and community groups, and media advertising. The Primary Care Clinical Studies Group of the UK National Institute for Health Research Stroke Research Network acted as expert advisory group to the study. Participants gave written informed consent to be interviewed, and after checking their interview transcript signed a further form giving permission for their interview to be used for teaching, research, publication and online dissemination on the patient information website www.healthtalkonline.org (see below). Ethics approval for the consent procedure and research methods was granted by Berkshire Research Ethics Committee (reference number 91H050516).

Data collection

37 people (including some family members) were interviewed in 2010 across the UK, usually in the participant's own home. Interviews lasted between one and two hours and were video or audio recorded. They comprised two sections; an unstructured narrative ('tell me your story') followed by semi structured prompting about their experiences of diagnosis, treatment and life after TIA. Anonymised data from the study (video and audio interview extracts) are freely available at http://www.healthtalkonline.org/Nerves_and_brain/transient_ischaemic_attack,

As part of their opening narrative, all participants described what their symptoms were like and what made them think something was wrong. Family members were excluded from this analysis.

Clinical review of transcripts

Because of the range of recruitment sources, the sample included some people with a clinically confirmed diagnosis (notably those recruited through OXVASC), but also others (for example recruited through support groups) where we were reliant on self-report. To overcome this, these interview transcripts were reviewed by a TIA specialist clinician (MG) and participants whose diagnosis was not clinically definite TIA were excluded from the analysis.

Analysis

Two researchers (SK, LL) re-read and discussed sections of the interviews where symptoms were described. Using framework analysis [20] an initial chart was drawn up mapping symptoms and key words used against each individual. Findings were then discussed with authors MG and DL. Analysis focused on both the vivid and nuanced descriptions given of classic TIA symptoms, as well as additional observations made by participants.

Findings

After clinical review of transcripts, we included 19 men (12 aged 50–69 years, 6 aged 70–90 years, 1 over 90 years) and 6 women (1 less than 30 years, 1 aged 30–49 years, 3 aged 50–69 years and 1 over 90 years). All participants were white British. Given the criterion of clinically definite TIA, the data predictably included many conventional descriptions of 'classic' symptoms including motor problems, numbness and speech difficulties. However, clusters of symptoms were reported which included both classic and other symptoms; and some who had two or more TIAs reported different symptoms on each occasion. Below we focus on people's accounts, grouped by mapped symptoms and using pseudonyms, paying particular attention to the nuanced language used.

Spatial perception and coordination

There were many reports of poor spatial awareness and lack of coordination. Julian (who was already booked to see his primary care physician after experiencing transient speech loss the previous day) described what happened when he got in the car:

'As I started to reverse I realised I had no understanding of where the car was in space... not being able to know where I was in a car, where was I in three-dimensional space, that was very frightening.'

Peter experienced a combination of numbness and perception problems:

'When I woke up in the morning, my left hand, it felt a bit odd. It was as if I had been lying on it. A little bit of numbness and tingling in my fingers. And then I realised that I could feel the weight of my arm....I sat up and had a cup of tea and it was already starting to fade away, the symptoms were vanishing. But I did have a problem with holding things....[Normally] you know where your hand is. But in this case I didn't. If I looked at my hand, I could easily pick up my coffee and I could put it down again. But if I wasn't looking at my hand, I really wasn't too sure where it was. I think this is called periception and it had just disintegrated.'

He was so puzzled by the heavy feeling in his arm that he went to weigh his arm on the bathroom scales. At the time this seemed to him a logical response to his puzzlement.

Feelings of disconnection and disorientation

Feeling disoriented and out of touch with reality was commonly reported, and was described in a range of vivid terms. Here Alan's description blends physical symptoms of losing speech and the use of his arm with a sense of distance and disconnectedness.

'I would liken to it to having your head put in a goldfish bowl. Because there was this, I was separated from her [partner]. And I was totally unable to communicate...It came like waves when I was in the ambulance. One minute I was there, and the next minute I wasn't. And it was the same with my arm. I sat in the ambulance and I lost my arm completely, and it just wouldn't function, and it was just like it was somebody else's arm somehow... It's almost like being in a dream. And you can hear a voice from another room'.

Mary described it as 'brain fog'. Gregory remembered 'a dip, a small dizziness' while out walking the dog, before he developed more classic symptoms. June felt 'woozy and funny. I just couldn't put my finger on what was wrong'. Celia likened it to an 'out of body experience'.

Incomplete awareness of deficit

A few people identified either a total or partial lack of awareness of what was happening to them. Chloe's account seems to suggest complete lack of awareness of deficit.

'So then the ambulance men came in, and my colleague was sat next to me and I didn't know what he was doing, but unbeknown to me I was paralysed down my left side but I didn't realise, I had no idea whatsoever. And he was holding me up'

In other cases people reported an uneasy partial awareness, a vague feeling that all was not well, yet not identifying the nature of the deficit. It is intriguing how often these accounts express a double state of knowing/not knowing, sensing/not sensing, being there/not being there.

'I felt absolutely nothing. I had no idea it was happening.....It's being totally unaware - and yet you know there's something.' (Alan)

'I knew something was going on. But I didn't quite know.' (Celia)

'I wasn't totally functioning because I knew everything, but I could sense things, yet not sense things. I felt I was on automatic pilot.' (Richard)

Visual disturbance

Visual disturbance is a known symptom of TIA, but personal accounts reveal interesting ways in which this is experienced. Both Andrew and Julian reported two separate TIAs, with visual symptoms occurring only on the second occasion. Andrew had classic symptoms of speech loss one evening – he wrote 'stroke' on a piece of paper for his wife, but before she could call an ambulance his symptoms disappeared. The next morning he lost part of his field of vision in one eye but had no idea this could be a second TIA until he called his GP. Julian lost his speech briefly and made an appointment for the next day to see his primary care physician. As he got dressed, he noticed

'a strange visual disturbance on the left eye, the left periphery of that vision, a set of flashing chevron multi-coloured lights'.

Among the commonly reported visual disturbances of flashing lights, losing part of the field of vision, blurring, and double vision, a few people reported visual displacement. For Mervyn this was the first indication something was wrong. He said,

'looking at the TV in the bedroom I had like a split vision whereby part of the TV was down there and part was up there. So it was like it was on a sort of fault line.' Shortly after he found himself unable to give his wife 'a straight answer to her questions.'

Kevin experienced something similar in combination with other classic symptoms.

'Suddenly I just couldn't formulate words. Words wouldn't come out of my mouth, my wife asked me a question I just simply couldn't answer...So I stood up in alarm I suppose, feeling a bit leaden but nothing worse than that...I then looked out of the window and it looked as if the window had slipped to the left, moved to the left, strangely, and was fuzzy round the outside.'

Daniel experienced huge difficulty finding words (see below) but also had some visual symptoms which he found it hard to describe.

'When I was looking out to the window it was almost like looking out through - dear me, how can I explain it? A window with patterning on. We did have a longer net curtain than is there now, but it wasn't that. It was like a pattern on it.'

Articulation/word-finding

Some of the most vivid descriptions focus on people's inability to articulate or find words at the time of their TIA.

'I had a normal conversation, turned to speak to the other character, and lost the ability to speak, which was very confusing and quite perturbing. I literally couldn't take the thought from my brain to my mouth and articulate what I wanted to say.' (Julian)

'I tried to respond but...it didn't work, and I wasn't quite sure what I was trying to respond with, because I'd forgotten what speech was.' (Alan)

In Kevin's case, this was combined with a sense of disconnect-edness.

'I couldn't put words together and I couldn't think of the words I needed to say....It wasn't an out of body experience - but I felt detached from what was happening to me. I was consciously trying to think of the words but it was as if I was thinking of the words for another person, rather than being part of me. There was a distance.'

Bernard, a professional writer, remembered becoming unchar-acteristically inarticulate:

'My secretary was here. I was trying to fill in a form but I was also dictating a letter to her and somehow the words started to get really jumbled. I couldn't think what I was doing, but I wasn't aware there was anything wrong except that for some reason I was being stupid. And so I tried to go and fill in a form that I'd already started and I knew I was making mistakes. So I tried to correct them and this made it much worse.... Finally I said to [secretary] in perfectly conventional English, "Oh for God's sake, clear off home. I don't want you to see me in this stupid state."

Daniel's account gives particularly rich insights:

'[Wife] asked me a question and I tried to answer the question. But discovered that the words that I wanted were floating around, well to my mind they were floating around in a very large bubble. And when I tried to catch the words, they squeezed out from between my fingers. And it's so real, it's unbelievable how it's coming back. But the words - I just couldn't hold them. I just couldn't. And I couldn't make any sense of anything….It was a bit like having a drawer with all the words you use in alphabetical order, or in some sort of order that you know where they are and you can just use them, but some clot had been into this drawer and used all my words and put them back in the wrong place … [They] took me to hospital where I was still not really able to say that much, but I did manage to begin to tell people what I felt and what I wanted, but I was still finding that some of these words were still squeezing out from under my fingers. It was like trying to hold a goldfish and it just squeeze away.'

Discussion

Our study of patients' experiences of transient ischaemic attack demonstrates not only great variation in the description of classical features of speech and visual disturbance, but also that there are additional features which are not elicited in standard medical history taking, for example incomplete awareness of deficit and descriptions of disconnection. These novel features arise from the experience of deficit, rather than the physical nature of the deficit itself. Therefore the physical phenotype of stroke that is used as the basis for clinical description of TIA may not capture all of the available diagnostic information that can be revealed by the patient with TIA.

There is very little research about subjective experiences of TIA and existing studies have not addressed methods to improve recognition of TIA at first healthcare contact by widening the currently held phenotype [21–23]. Existing qualitative studies have largely focussed on the albeit important areas of emotions and cognitions following on from the experience of TIA, rather than probing that experience to provide greater information about the nature of TIA itself. Nevertheless, early reports from a community based TIA and stroke cohort study in Oxford (Oxford Community Stroke Project) did suggest that novel symptoms may be associated with visual TIA [24] although these findings have not been followed up in subsequent studies.

The strengths of this study are that rigorous qualitative methods were used to produce a robust analysis and interpretation of the patient experiences and that the methods used to select patients for the sample reduced the risk that non-cerebrovascular disease caused the transient deficits. As such the novel findings are a reflection of a richer clinical phenotype of TIA. However, as with all qualitative studies, the sample is not statistically representative and therefore cannot be used to identify how many people have

particular symptoms or to correlate symptoms with type of TIA or future stroke risk. In particular there were only six women in the sample and there were no patients from ethnic minorities, so there is uncertain generalisation of our findings to a wider population. A further limitation of our study is the lack of a gold standard for TIA diagnosis which has been demonstrated particularly for categories of 'possible TIA' [25], and whilst we restricted our sample to patients with clinically definite TIA, we were unable to exclude the possibility that not all patients had a TIA.

Further research to test the potential additive value of patients' experiences of deficit is needed before our findings could be used to improve the accuracy of diagnosis and prognosis in patients with TIA. Detecting true transient ischaemic attack is complex as there are many presentations with transient neurological symptoms [26] and we do not know if the experiences of the transient deficit caused by cerebrovascular disease is different from the experiences of transient deficit caused by non-cerebrovascular conditions. For example, the associated phenomenon we describe of variable awareness of deficit may be related to ischaemia in cortical structures which mediate anosognosia in completed stroke, and may not be present in non-ischaemic transient neurological symptoms. Furthermore, there is evidence that even with the use of the ABCD2 risk score, generalists do not accurately classify high risk TIA at the first healthcare contact [27] and so determining the prognostic significance of our findings with subsequent cohort studies could be used to improve the recognition of high risk TIA at first healthcare contact. Therefore prospective studies which include a phenotype of experience of deficit described above are needed to determine the impact of our findings on diagnosis of TIA among patients presenting with transient neurological symptoms and of prognosis of TIA in terms of improving the clinical recognition of patients with a high early risk of recurrent stroke.

Prompt recognition of TIA at the first healthcare contact is vital for stroke prevention. Listening to the patient voice has the potential to provide additional diagnostic information which contributes to accurate detection of TIA at initial healthcare contact, but prospective cohort studies of patients presenting with novel neurological features that are appropriately representative in terms of gender and ethnicity are needed to determine diagnostic and prognostic significance.

Acknowledgments

The authors are grateful to Professor Peter Rothwell, Head of the Oxford Vascular Study (OXVASC) for recruitment of patients already enrolled in OXVASC.

Author Contributions

Conceived and designed the experiments: DSL LL MG SK. Performed the experiments: LL SK. Analyzed the data: DSL LL SK MG. Wrote the paper: DSL LL SK MG.

References

1. Coull AJ, Lovett JK, Rothwell PM (2004) Population based study of early risk of stroke after transient ischaemic attack or minor stroke: implications for public education and organisation of services. BMJ 328: 326.

2. Lavallee PC, Meseguer E, Abboud H, Cabrejo L, Olivot JM, et al. (2007) A transient ischaemic attack clinic with round-the-clock access (SOS-TIA): feasibility and effects. Lancet Neurol 6: 953–960.

3. Rothwell PM, Giles MF, Chandratheva A, Marquardt L, Geraghty O, et al. (2007) Effect of urgent treatment of transient ischaemic attack and minor stroke on early recurrent stroke (EXPRESS study): a prospective population-based sequential comparison. Lancet 370: 1432–1442.

4. Lasserson DS, Chandratheva A, Giles MF, Mant D, Rothwell PM (2008) Influence of general practice opening hours on delay in seeking medical attention after transient ischaemic attack (TIA) and minor stroke: prospective population based study. BMJ 337: a1569.

5. Manawadu D, Shuaib A, Collas DM (2010) Emergency department or general practitioner following transient ischaemic attack? A comparison of patient behaviour and speed of assessment in England and Canada. Emerg Med J 27: 364–367.

6. Easton JD, Saver JL, Albers GW, Alberts MJ, Chaturvedi S, et al. (2009) Definition and evaluation of transient ischemic attack: a scientific statement for healthcare professionals from the American Heart Association/American Stroke

Association Stroke Council; Council on Cardiovascular Surgery and Anesthesia; Council on Cardiovascular Radiology and Intervention; Council on Cardiovascular Nursing; and the Interdisciplinary Council on Peripheral Vascular Disease. The American Academy of Neurology affirms the value of this statement as an educational tool for neurologists. Stroke 40: 2276–2293.

7. Koudstaal PJ, van Gijn J, Staal A, Duivenvoorden HJ, Gerritsma JG, et al. (1986) Diagnosis of transient ischemic attacks: improvement of interobserver agreement by a check-list in ordinary language. Stroke 17: 723–728.

8. Murray S, Bashir K, Lees KR, Muir K, MacAlpine C, et al. (2007) Epidemiological aspects of referral to TIA clinics in Glasgow. Scott Med J 52: 4–8.

9. Donders RC, Kappelle LJ, Algra A, van Dijk GW, van Gijn J (1999) How do general practitioners diagnose and manage patients with transient monocular loss of vision of sudden onset? J Neurol 246: 1145–1150.

10. Quik-van Milligen MLT KM, de Melker RA, Touw-Otten FWMM, Koudstaal PJ, van Gijn J (1992) Transient ischemic attacks and the general practitioner: Diagnosis and management. Cerebrovasc Dis 2: 102–106.

11. Tomasik T, Windak A, Margas G, de Melker RA, Jacobs HM (2003) Transient ischaemic attacks: desired diagnosis and management by Polish primary care physicians. Fam Pract 20: 464–468.

12. Moons KG, Altman DG, Vergouwe Y, Royston P (2009) Prognosis and prognostic research: application and impact of prognostic models in clinical practice. BMJ 338: b606.

13. Nor AM, Davis J, Sen B, Shipsey D, Louw SJ, et al. (2005) The Recognition of Stroke in the Emergency Room (ROSIER) scale: development and validation of a stroke recognition instrument. Lancet Neurol 4: 727–734.

14. Harbison J, Hossain O, Jenkinson D, Davis J, Louw SJ, et al. (2003) Diagnostic accuracy of stroke referrals from primary care, emergency room physicians, and ambulance staff using the face arm speech test. Stroke 34: 71–76.

15. Dawson J, Lamb KE, Quinn TJ, Lees KR, Horvers M, et al. (2009) A recognition tool for transient ischaemic attack. QJM 102: 43–49.

16. Thompson MJ, Ninis N, Perera R, Mayon-White R, Phillips C, et al. (2006) Clinical recognition of meningococcal disease in children and adolescents. Lancet 367: 397–403.

17. Visintin C, Mugglestone MA, Fields EJ, Jacklin P, Murphy MS, et al. (2010) Management of bacterial meningitis and meningococcal septicaemia in children and young people: summary of NICE guidance. BMJ 340: c3209.

18. Abel EK, Browner CH (1998) Selective Compliance with Biomedical Authority and the Uses of Experiential Knowledge. In: Lock M, Kaufert P, editors. Pragmatic Women and Body Politics. Cambridge: Cambridge University Press. pp. 310–326.

19. Patton M (1990) Qualitative evaluation and research methods. Beverly Hills, CA: Sage.

20. Ritchie J, Spencer L (1993) Qualitative data analysis for applied policy research. In: Bryman A, Burgess R, editors. Analysing Qualitative Data. London: Routledge. pp. 173–194.

21. Gibson J, Watkins C (2012) People's experiences of the impact of transient ischaemic attack and its consequences: qualitative study. J Adv Nurs 68: 1707–1715.

22. Kamara S, Singh S (2012) What are the patient-held illness beliefs after a transient ischaemic attack, and do they determine secondary prevention activities: an exploratory study in a North London General Practice. Prim Health Care Res Dev 13: 165–174.

23. Spurgeon L, Humphreys G, James G, Sackley C (2012) A Q-Methodology Study of Patients' Subjective Experiences of TIA. Stroke Res Treat 2012: 486261.

24. Dennis MS, Bamford JM, Sandercock PA, Warlow CP (1989) Lone bilateral blindness: a transient ischaemic attack. Lancet 1: 185–188.

25. Castle J, Mlynash M, Lee K, Caulfield AF, Wolford C, et al. (2010) Agreement regarding diagnosis of transient ischemic attack fairly low among stroke-trained neurologists. Stroke 41: 1367–1370.

26. Bots ML, van der Wilk EC, Koudstaal PJ, Hofman A, Grobbee DE (1997) Transient neurological attacks in the general population. Prevalence, risk factors, and clinical relevance. Stroke 28: 768–773.

27. Wong J, Fotherby M, Eveson D (2012) Comparison of ABCD2 scoring between first healthcare-contact and stroke-specialist physicians for transient ischaemic attack in a rapid-access clinic. Age Ageing 41: 115–118.

10

24 Hour ST Segment Analysis in Transient Left Ventricular Apical Ballooning

Frank Bode*, Christof Burgdorf, Heribert Schunkert, Volkhard Kurowski

Medical Department II, University of Luebeck, Luebeck, Germany

Abstract

Objective: The etiologic basis of transient left ventricular apical ballooning, a novel cardiac syndrome, is not clear. Among the proposed pathomechanisms is coronary vasospasm. Long-term ST segment analysis may detect vasospastic episodes but has not been reported.

Methods: 30 consecutive patients with transient left ventricular apical ballooning, left ventricular dysfunction and normal or near-normal coronary arteries were investigated. A 24-hour Holter ECG was obtained after emergency admission. ST segment analysis was performed automatically in 2 leads and confirmed by visual inspection. Criteria for an ischemic event were: 1. ST elevation or 2. horizontal or down-sloping ST segments $\geq$1 min duration and $\geq$100 μV J+80 point deviation corrected for baseline ST-deviation.

Results: Patients presented with ST segment elevation (n = 19) and/or T wave inversion (n = 20) on admission ECG. Ejection fraction was 50$\pm$12%. No transient ST elevations were observed during Holter ECG analysis. In 3 patients, 8 transient episodes of ST depression were recorded. Durations of episodes varied between 75s and 790s (mean 229s). Maximal ST deviation averaged -191 ± 71 μV. Ischemic burden was -1 to -22 mVs (mean -8 mVs). 27 patients showed no ischemic events.

Conclusions: ST segment analysis of 24 h Holter recordings revealed minor ischemic events in only 10% of patients with transient left ventricular apical ballooning. Overall, ST segment changes were not indicative of recurrent coronary spasm playing a major role in the genesis of transient left ventricular apical ballooning.

Editor: Claudio Moretti, S.G.Battista Hospital, Italy

Funding: The authors have no support or funding to report.

Competing Interests: The authors have declared that no competing interests exist.

* E-mail: frank.bode@uk-sh.de

Introduction

The transient left ventricular apical ballooning syndrome, also known as takotsubo cardiomyopathy, is an acute cardiac syndrome that has only recently been generally recognized [1], [2], [3], [4], [5]. The syndrome is characterized by regional contractile dysfunction of the left ventricular apex and/or midmyocardium [6], [7] in the absence of obstructive atherosclerotic coronary disease. Regional wall-motion abnormalities extend beyond a single epicardial vascular distribution. The syndrome most frequently affects postmenopausal women immediately after an episode of acute emotional or physical stress [8], [9]. The clinical presentation is similar to that of patients with acute myocardial infarction. Patients often complain chest pain at rest or dyspnea. New electrocardiographic ST segment elevations or T wave inversions are commonly found during the acute onset of the syndrome [10]. Cardiac enzyme and biomarker levels are elevated. Acute left-sided heart failure, hemodynamic instability and arrhythmias may develop. Left ventricular dysfunction is generally reversible and overall in-hospital prognosis is favorable [8], [11]. The cause of the syndrome is unknown. Endomyocardial biopsy in the acute phase of the syndrome revealed no evidence of myocarditis [3], [12]. Spontaneous or provocable multivessel epicardial spasm was reported in a subset of patients undergoing coronary angiography, suggesting a possible role of coronary spasm in the genesis of the syndrome [1], [8], [13]. Intermittent spontaneous vasospasm can be detected in Holter ECG recordings by ST segment analysis. We evaluated the incidence of transient ischemic episodes suggestive of intermittent coronary vasospasm in the acute phase of left ventricular apical ballooning by ST segment analysis in 24 h Holter recordings.

Methods

After approval by the ethics committee of the University of Luebeck, Germany, 30 consecutive patients with transient left ventricular apical ballooning syndrome were investigated. Patients were admitted to our institution for acute anginal symptoms or dyspnea within 48 hours of symptom onset. All patients presented with 12-lead ECGs suspective of acute myocardial ischemia. ECG changes were classified according to the presence of ST segment elevations $\geq$100 μV and/or T wave inversions. Patients underwent immediate left heart catheterization. They were included after akinesia or hypokinesia had been detected in the apical and/or midventricular region by laevocardiography while coronary angiograms ruled out obstructive coronary artery disease (Fig. 1).

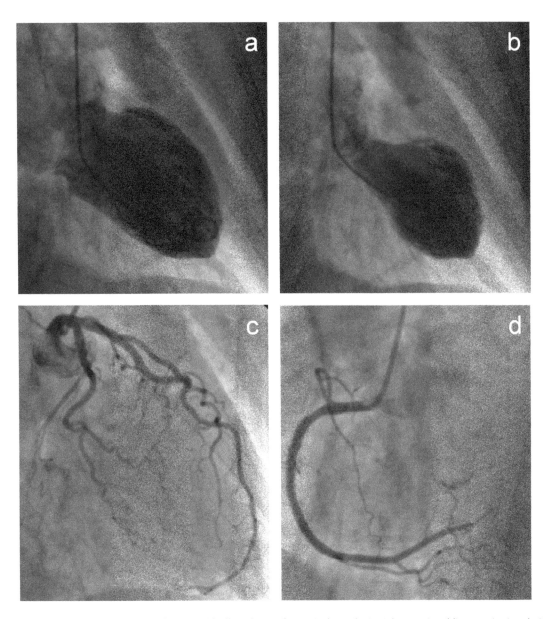

Figure 1. Typical left ventricular apical ballooning. Left ventriculography in right anterior oblique projection during diastole (1a) and systole (1b) demonstrating akinesia of the apical and midventricular segments. Selective coronary angiograms of the left (1c) and right coronary artery (1d) excluding obstructive coronary artery disease.

Cardiac marker levels were determined repetitively on admission, 6, 12 and every 24 hours after admission. Troponin T was measured quantitatively by ELISA test (ES 300 System, Roche Diagnostics) with a cut-off at 0.1 ng/ml for a positive test.

All patients underwent 24 h Holter ECG recording within two days following hospital admission after written informed consent had been obtained. Patients were instructed to protocol any symptoms during acquisition. Two bipolar leads were recorded simultaneously. The recorders used were Reynolds Medical Tracker 3 and the analyzer was a Pathfinder 600 (Reynolds Medical Limited, Hertford, England). Following analog-digital conversion of the tape recordings, the following points from the digitized ECG were used for measurements:

1. PR reference point: The midpoint of the PR segment
2. J point: The end of the QRS complex

3. J+80 measurement point: The point on the ST segment 80 ms after the J point

These points were selected from an average beat superimposition display with adjustable markers. Ischemic episodes were defined as 1. ST elevation or 2. horizontal or down-sloping ST segment depression for at least one minute with at least 100 μV J+80 measurement point deviation compared to J+80 measurement points at baseline. The baseline was defined as the mean value of PR reference points during a 5-minute period within 30 minutes prior to the episode, where baseline conditions were considered to be present based upon a relatively slow heart rate and steady ST segment. Each episode was characterized by slope of ST segment, duration, and ischemic burden (duration multiplied by deviation), and confirmed by visual inspection. Positional changes were excluded.

Variables are presented as mean±SD. Patient data were statistically compared by paired or unpaired t test for continuous variables and by Fishers exact test for parametric variables. P values <0.05 defined statistical significance.

Results

Study Population

All 30 patients were postmenopausal women with a mean age of 71±8 years (range 56–84). Symptom onset was 12±11 hours before hospital admission. An episode of emotional stress preceded clinical presentation in 15 patients. Left ventricular ejection fraction was 50±12% during ventriculography on admission. Coronary angiographies revealed no obstructive coronary artery disease and no macrovascular spasm in any vessel. Initial and maximal troponin T serum levels were 0.72±1.08 ng/ml and 0.90±1.07 ng/ml, respectively (p = 0.002). Initial and maximal creatine kinase levels were 158±93 IU/l and 253±202 IU/l (p = 0.008), creatine kinase MB levels were 24±13 IU/l and 29±16 IU/l (p = 0.005), respectively. Patients underwent hemodynamic monitoring and received heart failure therapy as required. No nitrates or calcium channel blockers known to prevent coronary spasm were applied. Treatment with ß-blockers (n = 23) and angiotensin-converting enzyme inhibitors (n = 24) or angiotensin receptor antagonists (n = 2) was initiated within the first three days. All patients showed symptomatic and hemodynamic improvement during hospitalization for 11±6 days. Echocardiographic reevaluation before discharge showed regression of left ventricular wall motion abnormalities with an improved left ventricular ejection fraction of 61±10% (p<0.001 as compared to ventriculography on admission).

ECG Presentation

12-lead ECGs on admission revealed no left ventricular hypertrophy or left bundle branch block that could have precluded accurate interpretation of ST segment activity. Digoxin and other medications known to affect ST segment morphology were absent. All patients were in sinus rhythm. Patients presented with ST segment elevation of at least 100 μV (n = 19) and/or T wave inversion (n = 20) on admission ECG. Patients displaying ST segment elevations on admission had a more recent symptom onset (8±8 hours) than patients without ST segment elevation (18±13 hours; p = 0.037). ST segment elevation resolved within the first two days, whereas T wave inversion resolved more slowly and often only partially.

Holter ECG Analysis

All 30 Holter recordings were of good quality. No transient ST elevations were observed during Holter ECG analysis. Positional changes mimicking transient ST depression were seen in 5 patients, none of whom had nonpositional ischemic events. In three patients, 8 nonpositional transient episodes of ST depression were recorded (Fig. 2 and 3; Table 1). Durations of episodes varied between 75s and 790s (mean 229s). Maximal ST deviation averaged −191±71 μV. Ischemic burden was −1 to −22 mVs (mean −8 mVs). Heart rate was 74±19 bpm before and 77±19 bpm during episodes (p = 0.718). No patient reported clinical symptoms during automatically detected episodes of ST depression.

Characteristics of Patients with Ischemic Events

The three patients with transient ST segment depression displayed T wave inversion but no ST segment elevation on admission ECG. Maximal cardiac marker levels were lower in those patients than in the remaining study population (maximal troponin T level 0.19±0.13 ng/ml vs. 0.98±1.10 ng/ml; p = 0.015) but not lower than in the other patients without ST segment elevation (0.21±0.16; p = 0.823). Apart from this observation, patients with transient episodes of ST depression showed no specifically different clinical features or history from the 27 patients which showed no ischemic events.

Discussion

The present study investigated for the first time the incidence of transient ischemic episodes in the acute phase of transient left ventricular apical ballooning syndrome by 24 h Holter recordings. ST segment analysis revealed only few, brief ischemic episodes in a minority of patients. Our findings were not indicative of recurrent coronary spasm forming a crucial substrate of this novel cardiac syndrome.

Relevance of Ischemic Episodes

ST segment analysis by Holter monitoring is an established method for detection of intermittent ST deviations indicative of ischemia. A good correlation has been established between ischemic events during exercise tests and ST segment changes during Holter Monitoring [14], [15]. Holter monitoring has facilitated the assessment of silent ischemia in different clinical settings [16], [17]. Due to the transient nature of coronary vasospasm, Holter Monitoring appears to be the proper method for detecting brief spontaneous episodes of resulting ischemia. ST segment analysis by Holter monitoring is indicated for detection of vasospastic angina [18].

The 10% of our patients which displayed transient ischemic events in Holter recordings belonged to a subgroup of patients without ST segment elevation during initial ECG presentation and with a comparatively small release of cardiac markers on admission. Moreover, the brief ischemic events that were detected during Holter recordings caused no symptoms and triggered no further rise in cardiac markers. In contrast, in patients with ST segment elevation on admission reaching high peak plasma levels of cardiac markers, Holter analysis found no transient ischemic events. Thus, electrical and laboratory correlates of myocardial damage were sparse in patients with transient ischemic events. These findings argue against recurrent episodes of ischemia as a relevant pathomechanism driving the syndrome.

Pathology of the Syndrome

Originally reported in the Japanese population [1], [13], the transient left ventricular apical ballooning syndrome has recently been described in European and U.S. patients [19], [20]. Most patients meet the criteria for the diagnosis of myocardial infarction upon presentation, but obstructive epicardial coronary disease is absent. Some features of the syndrome are similar to those seen in myocarditis, but no evidence of myocarditis could be demonstrated in endomyocardial biopsies or viral serology [3], [10], [12]. Regional perfusion abnormalities have been documented by coronary flow measurements and SPECT imaging, which were reversible after the acute phase of the syndrome. Beyond regional perfusion abnormalities, fatty acid and glucose metabolism was found to be impaired in affected regions, indicative of the presence of myocardial "stunning" [21], [22], [23], [24]. Several mechanisms have been proposed to underlie the transient left ventricular apical ballooning syndrome, including multivessel epicardial spasm [10], microvascular coronary spasm [3], [13] and catecholamine-mediated myocardial dysfunction [12], [25].

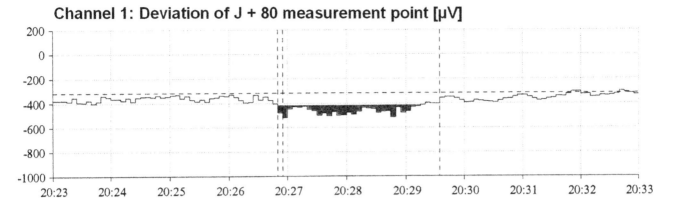

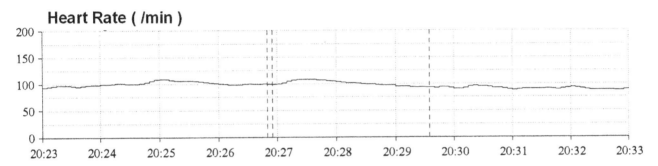

Figure 2. Automatic analysis of ST segment changes during Holter recording. The upper image depicts the deviation of the J +80 measurement point (80 ms after J point) within a 10 minute period (pt. no. 7). At 20 h 26 min 50 s an ischemic episode of 2 min 45s duration was detected. J +80 measurement point deviation >100 µV is marked in black. The lower image depicts the corresponding heart rate (HR).

Proposed Mechanisms

Patients with transient left ventricular apical ballooning syndrome often present in the setting of acute mental or physical stress, associated with **enhanced sympathetic outflow** [5], [12], [26]. It remains unproven whether elevated catecholamine levels represent the causal factor of the syndrome or an

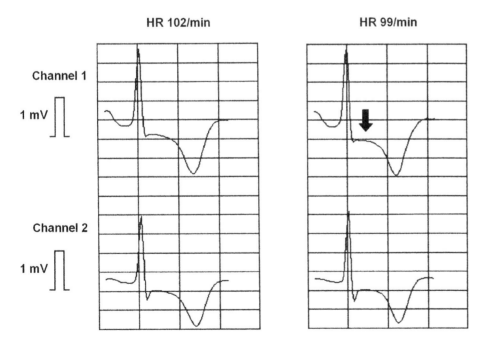

Figure 3. ST segment detail. Recordings show baseline ST depression in both recording channels (left tracing). During an automatically detected ischemic event at 20 h 26 min 59s an additional transient ST depression occurs in channel 1 (arrow, right tracing).

Table 1. Ischemic events.

Patient No.	Event	Time (h:min:s)	Duration (min:s)	Heart Rate before event (bpm)	Heart Rate during event (bpm)	Max. Deviation (μV)	Ischemic Burden (mVs)
1	ST depression	00:54:15	02:10	55	56	−138	−2
1	ST depression	14:02:20	01:15	56	55	−132	−1
1	ST depression	18:11:45	03:40	60	55	−124	−1
7	ST depression	12:15:00	13:10	86	89	−209	−22
7	ST depression	12:55:00	01:30	83	90	−202	−3
7	ST depression	13:57:05	04:05	89	91	−173	−3
7	ST depression	20:26:50	02:45	102	99	−201	−7
16	ST depression	12:46:20	02:00	57	81	−345	−22

epiphenomenon secondary to hemodynamic abnormalities. On one hand, plasma catecholamine levels were higher in transient left ventricular apical ballooning syndrome than in control patients with comparable hemodynamic compromise due to acute myocardial infarction [12]. In a rat model of emotional stress, regional wall motion abnormalities could be reproduced while α- and ß-blocker pretreatment abolished those changes [27]. These findings supported a causal role of sympathetic stimulation. On the other hand, analysis of heart rate variability and turbulence, surrogate markers of autonomic tone, showed that the cardiac sympathetic modulation was not elevated in transient left ventricular apical ballooning syndrome, but sympathovagal balance was rather preserved [28].

Transient epicardial spasm would be required to occur in multiple vessels in order to cause the diffuse wall motion abnormalities located beyond a single epicardial distribution. Spontaneous multivessel spasm has been observed in up to 6% of patients in single centers [13]. A recent meta-analysis of 212 patients reported an overall incidence of only 1.4% [8]. Provocable coronary vasospasm in at least one coronary artery has been found in 10/14 (71%) [13], 10/48 (21%) [2], 2/5 (40%) [1] and 1/7 (14%) [3] of patients. Multivessel spasm could be provoked by ergonovine or acetylcholine in 29% of 84 evaluated patients [8]. Multivessel epicardial spasm might therefore play a role in some patients presenting with the syndrome. Yet, in patients with persistent ST elevations and no evidence of epicardial spasm during coronary angiography (19 of 30 patients in our study population), this genesis is not plausible.

While macrovascular changes are rarely observed, ***microvascular dysfunction*** could be responsible for inducing myocardial ischemia and subsequent myocardial stunning. Microvascular function has been assessed by invasive measurements of coronary flow reserve [29], [30], [31] and TIMI frame count techniques [13], [23], [32]. The vast majority of data supported the hypothesis that abnormal microcirculation contributes to the pathophysiology of the syndrome. Coronary flow reserve was impaired and TIMI myocardial perfusion grade was reduced in most patients. The severity of myocardial injury as measured by peak troponin levels and the presence of ST elevation has been correlated to the impairment of myocardial perfusion [32]. It remains unclear whether microvascular dysfunction is the primary cause of the syndrome or a secondary phenomenon. Abnormal microcirculation might be secondary to the cardiomyopathy and elevated LV filling pressures. But this has been refuted by the assessment of normal microcirculation in patients without the syndrome who showed similar degrees of LV dysfunction and filling pressures [32].

Microvascular coronary spasm might be operative as primary cause of microvascular dysfunction. Nicorandil, a K_{ATP} channel opener that causes vasodilatation of arterioles and large coronary arteries, reduced the extend of ST segment elevation when injected into the coronary arteries, suggesting that microvascular spasm may underly abnormal microcirculation [33]. While the long-term clinical history of each of our patients was devoid of episodes of chest discomfort or variant angina, in particular, and thus revealed no overt disposition for coronary spasms, alterations in vasomotor activity might have been acquired. The predominance of postmenopausal women in patients presenting with the syndrome has suggested that changes in sex hormone activity are involved in its development. Reduced estrogen levels may alter endothelial function and microcirculatory vasomotor activity in response to catecholamines [34], [35], [36], [37]. Estradiol supplementation in ovariectomized female rats attenuated stress-induced wall-motion abnormalities [34].

An increased susceptibility to repetitive coronary spasm was not supported by the results of our study. Few patients showed minor transient ST segment changes with small ischemic burden during the acute phase of the syndrome, while in 90% of patients Holter ECG recording revealed no transient ischemia. Therefore microvascular dysfunction could not be attributed to recurrent coronary spasm in the majority of our patients. Only few patients who have suffered from a first apical ballooning episode experience a repeat episode. This clinical course might further argue against a persistent susceptibility to coronary spasm, thereby supporting our results.

It has to be considered that microcirculatory impairment during the acute phase is not causative to the syndrome but could result from primary myocardial injury. The syndrome might speculatively represent catecholamine-mediated toxicity and metabolic injury rendering the heart to diffuse microvascular dysfunction and myocardial stunning [4], [25], [38]. Opposed to this, Angelini postulated that a catecholamine surge by itself would be insufficient to explain the occurrence of the syndrome [39]. Due to the documentation of provocable diffuse spasm of all coronary distal branches in patients recovering from apical ballooning, his pathophysiologic theory regards the catecholamine surge only as a precipitating factor in labile, endothelially dysfunctional patients. The liability to extreme spasticity is postulated to be transient, varying from a few hours to a few weeks [39]. Our Holter recordings were obtained within 48 h after hospital admission.

Without using provocation tests, we found no relevant indication of recurrent coronary spasms in this early phase after manifestation. An unusual spasticity was not supported by our findings. Thus, only in rare cases a persistent susceptibility to coronary spasm might contribute to the development of transient left ventricular apical ballooning syndrome.

Limitations

Holter ECG recordings were obtained within 48 h after hospital admission. Due to the dynamic nature of transient left ventricular ballooning with acute onset and short-term recovery, the Holter recording might not reflect the initial susceptibility to coronary vasospasm. A spasm preceding the onset of an apical ballooning episode cannot be excluded by any method applied after clinical presentation. We did not use pharmacologic provocation to test the susceptibility to coronary spasms in our patients and to correlate them with the Holter results. Yet, the low incidence of brief spontaneous ischemic episodes during Holter evaluation argues against the usefulness of provocation tests to detect clinically relevant vasospastic instability.

Conclusions

While the pathophysiological roles of multivessel epicardial spasm, microvascular coronary spasm and catecholamine-mediated myocardial dysfunction in transient left ventricular apical ballooning syndrome are still under debate, ST segment analysis during the acute phase of the syndrome provided further evidence against repetitive vasospasm as a relevant contributor to the genesis of the syndrome. Microvascular dysfunction could not be attributed to recurrent vascular spasms in the majority of patients.

Author Contributions

Conceived and designed the experiments: FB CB HS VK. Performed the experiments: FB CB VK. Analyzed the data: FB CB HS VK. Contributed reagents/materials/analysis tools: FB HS. Wrote the paper: FB CB HS VK.

References

1. Dote K, Sato H, Tateishi H, Uchida T, Ishihara M (1991) Myocardial stunning due to simultaneous multivessel coronary spasms: a review of 5 cases. J Cardiol 21: 203–214.
2. Tsuchihashi K, Ueshima K, Uchida T, Oh-mura N, Kimura K, et al. (2001) Transient left ventricular apical ballooning without coronary artery stenosis: a novel heart syndrome mimicking acute myocardial infarction. Angina Pectoris-Myocardial Infarction Investigations in Japan. J Am Coll Cardiol 38: 11–18.
3. Abe Y, Kondo M, Matsuoka R, Araki M, Dohyama K, et al. (2003) Assessment of clinical features in transient left ventricular apical ballooning. J Am Coll Cardiol 41: 737–742.
4. Bybee KA, Kara T, Prasad A, Lerman A, Barsness GW, et al. (2004) Systematic review: transient left ventricular apical ballooning: a syndrome that mimics ST-segment elevation myocardial infarction. Ann Intern Med 141: 858–865.
5. Pilgrim TM, Wyss TR (2008) Takotsubo cardiomyopathy or transient left ventricular apical ballooning syndrome: A systematic review. Int J Cardiol 124: 283–292.
6. Bonnemeier H, Schafer U, Schunkert H (2006) Apical ballooning without apical ballooning. Eur Heart J 27: 2246.
7. Hurst RT, Askew JW, Reuss CS, Lee RW, Sweeney JP, et al. (2006) Transient midventricular ballooning syndrome: a new variant. J Am Coll Cardiol 48: 579–583.
8. Gianni M, Dentali F, Grandi AM, Sumner G, Hiralal R, et al. (2006) Apical ballooning syndrome or takotsubo cardiomyopathy: a systematic review. Eur Heart J 27: 1523–1529.
9. Lee YP, Poh KK, Lee CH, Tan HC, Razak A, et al. (2009) Diverse clinical spectrum of stress-induced cardiomyopathy. Int J Cardiol 133 : 272–275.
10. Kurisu S, Inoue I, Kawagoe T, Ishihara M, Shimatani Y, et al. (2004) Time course of electrocardiographic changes in patients with tako-tsubo syndrome: comparison with acute myocardial infarction with minimal enzymatic release. Circ J 68: 77–81.
11. Bahlmann E, Schneider C, Krause K, Hertting K, Boczor S, et al. (2008) Tako-Tsubo cardiomyopathy characteristics in long-term follow-up. Int J Cardiol 124: 32–39.
12. Wittstein IS, Thiemann DR, Lima JA, Baughman KL, Schulman SP, et al. (2005) Neurohumoral features of myocardial stunning due to sudden emotional stress. N Engl J Med 352: 539–548.
13. Kurisu S, Sato H, Kawagoe T, Ishihara M, Shimatani Y, et al. (2002) Tako-tsubo-like left ventricular dysfunction with ST-segment elevation: a novel cardiac syndrome mimicking acute myocardial infarction. Am Heart J 143: 448–455.
14. Wolf E, Tzivoni D, Stern S (1974) Comparison of exercise tests and 24-hour ambulatory electrocardiographic monitoring in detection of ST-T changes. Br Heart J 36: 90–95.
15. Samniah N, Tzivoni D (1997) Assessment of ischemic changes by ambulatory ECG monitoring. Comparison with 12-lead ECG during exercise testing. J Electrocardiol 30: 197–204.
16. Gill JB, Cairns JA, Roberts RS, Costantini L, Sealy BJ, et al. (1996) Prognostic importance of myocardial ischemia detected by ambulatory monitoring early after acute myocardial infarction. N Engl J Med 334: 65–70.
17. Gottlieb SO, Weisfeldt ML, Ouyang P, Mellits ED, Gerstenblith G. (1986) Silent ischemia as a marker for early unfavorable outcomes in patients with unstable angina. N Engl J Med 314: 1214–1219.
18. Crawford MH, Bernstein SJ, Deedwania PC, DiMarco JP, Ferrick KJ, et al. (1999) ACC/AHA Guidelines for Ambulatory Electrocardiography: Executive Summary and Recommendations. Circulation 100: 886–893.
19. Desmet WJ, Adriaenssens BF, Dens JA. (2003) Apical ballooning of the left ventricle: first series in white patients. Heart 89: 1027–1031.
20. Sharkey SW, Lesser JR, Zenovich AG, Maron MS, Lindberg J, et al. (2005) Acute and reversible cardiomyopathy provoked by stress in women from the United States. Circulation 111: 472–479.
21. Kurisu S, Inoue I, Kawagoe T, Ishihara M, Shimatani Y, et al. (2003) Myocardial perfusion and fatty acid metabolism in patients with tako-tsubo-like left ventricular dysfunction. J Am Coll Cardiol 41: 743–748.
22. Ito K, Sugihara H, Katoh S, Azuma A, Nakagawa M (2003) Assessment of Takotsubo (ampulla) cardiomyopathy using 99mTc-tetrofosmin myocardial SPECT-comparison with acute coronary syndrome. Ann Nucl Med 17: 115–122.
23. Bybee KA, Prasad A, Barsness GW, Lerman A, Jaffe AS, et al. (2004) Clinical characteristics and thrombolysis in myocardial infarction frame counts in women with transient left ventricular apical ballooning syndrome. Am J Cardiol 94: 343–346.
24. Kurowski V, Kaiser A, von Hof K, Killermann DP, Mayer B, et al. (2007) Apical and Midventricular Transient Left Ventricular Dysfunction Syndrome (Tako-Tsubo Cardiomyopathy): Frequency, Mechanisms and Prognosis. Chest 132: 809–816.
25. Mann DL, Kent RL, Parsons B, Cooper Gt. (1992) Adrenergic effects on the biology of the adult mammalian cardiocyte. Circulation 85: 790–804.
26. Takizawa M, Kobayakawa N, Uozumi H, Yonemura S, Kodama T, et al. (2007) A case of transient left ventricular ballooning with pheochromocytoma, supporting pathogenetic role of catecholamines in stress-induced cardiomyopathy or takotsubo cardiomyopathy. Int J Cardiol 114: e15–17.
27. Ueyama T, Kasamatsu K, Hano T, Yamamoto K, Tsuruo Y, et al. (2002) Emotional stress induces transient left ventricular hypocontraction in the rat via activation of cardiac adrenoceptors: a possible animal model of 'tako-tsubo' cardiomyopathy. Circ J 66: 712–713.
28. Ortak J, Kurowski V, Wiegand UK, Bode F, Weitz G, et al. (2005) Cardiac autonomic activity in patients with transient left ventricular apical ballooning. J Am Coll Cardiol 46: 1959–1961.
29. Ako J, Takenaka K, Uno K, Nakamura F, Shoji T, et al. (2001) Reversible left ventricular systolic dysfunction-reversibility of coronary microvascular abnormality. Jpn Heart J 42: 355–363.
30. Yanagi S, Nagae K, Yoshida K, Matsumura Y, Nagashima E, et al. (2002) Evaluation of coronary flow reserve using Doppler guide wire in patients with ampulla cardiomyopathy: three case reports. J Cardiol 39: 305–312.
31. Kume T, Akasaka T, Kawamoto T, Yoshitani H, Watanabe N, et al. (2005) Assessment of coronary microcirculation in patients with takotsubo-like left ventricular dysfunction. Circ J 69: 934–939.
32. Elesber AA, Prasad A, Bybee KA, Valeti U, Motiei A, et al. (2006) Transient cardiac apical ballooning syndrome: prevalence and clinical implications of right ventricular involvement. J Am Coll Cardiol 47: 1082–1083.
33. Ito K, Sugihara H, Kawasaki T, Yuba T, Doue T, et al. (2001) Assessment of ampulla (Takotsubo) cardiomyopathy with coronary angiography, two-dimensional echocardiography and 99mTc-tetrofosmin myocardial single photon emission computed tomography. Ann Nucl Med 15: 351–355.
34. Ueyama T, Hano T, Kasamatsu K, Yamamoto K, Tsuruo Y, et al. (2003) Estrogen attenuates the emotional stress-induced cardiac responses in the animal model of Tako-tsubo (Ampulla) cardiomyopathy. J Cardiovasc Pharmacol 42: S117–119.
35. Celermajer DS, Sorensen KE, Spiegelhalter DJ, Georgakopoulos D, Robinson J, et al. (1994) Aging is associated with endothelial dysfunction in healthy men years before the age-related decline in women. J Am Coll Cardiol 24: 471–476.
36. Sader MA, Celermajer DS (2002) Endothelial function, vascular reactivity and gender differences in the cardiovascular system. Cardiovasc Res 53: 597–604.

37. Taddei S, Virdis A, Ghiadoni L, Mattei P, Sudano I, et al. (1996) Menopause is associated with endothelial dysfunction in women. Hypertension 28: 576–582.

38. White M, Wiechmann RJ, Roden RL, Hagan MB, Wollmering MM, et al. (1995) Cardiac beta-adrenergic neuroeffector systems in acute myocardial dysfunction related to brain injury. Evidence for catecholamine-mediated myocardial damage. Circulation 92: 2183–2189.

39. Angelini P (2008) Transient left ventricular apical ballooning: A unifying pathophysiologic theory at the edge of Prinzmetal angina. Catheter Cardiovasc Interv 71: 342–352.

11

Direct Stimulation of Adult Neural Stem/Progenitor Cells *In Vitro* and Neurogenesis *In Vivo* by Salvianolic Acid B

Pengwei Zhuang[1], **Yanjun Zhang**[1]*, **Guangzhi Cui**[1], **Yuhong Bian**[2], **Mixia Zhang**[1], **Jinbao Zhang**[1], **Yang Liu**[1], **Xinpeng Yang**[1], **Adejobi Oluwaniyi Isaiah**[1], **Yingxue Lin**[1], **Yongbo Jiang**[1]

1 Tianjin State Key Laboratory of Modern Chinese Medicine, Key Laboratory of Traditional Chinese Medicine Pharmacology, Chinese Materia Medica College, Tianjin University of Traditional Chinese Medicine, Tianjin, China, **2** Chinese Medical College, Tianjin University of Traditional Chinese Medicine, Tianjin, China

Abstract

Background: Small molecules have been shown to modulate the neurogenesis processes. In search for new therapeutic drugs, the herbs used in traditional medicines for neurogenesis are promising candidates.

Methodology and Principal Findings: We selected a total of 45 natural compounds from Traditional Chinese herbal medicines which are extensively used in China to treat stroke clinically, and tested their proliferation-inducing activities on neural stem/progenitor cells (NSPCs). The screening results showed that salvianolic acid B (Sal B) displayed marked effects on the induction of proliferation of NSPCs. We further demonstrated that Sal B promoted NSPCs proliferation in dose- and time-dependent manners. To explore the molecular mechanism, PI3K/Akt, MEK/ERK and Notch signaling pathways were investigated. Cell proliferation assay demonstrated that Ly294002 (PI3K/Akt inhibitor), but neither U0126 (ERK inhibitor) nor DAPT (Notch inhibitor) inhibited the Sal B-induced proliferation of cells. Western Blotting results showed that stimulation of NSPCs with Sal B enhanced the phosphorylation of Akt, and Ly294002 abolished this effect, confirming the role of Akt in Sal B mediated proliferation of NSPCs. Rats exposed to transient cerebral ischemia were treated for 4 weeks with Sal B from the 7th day after stroke. BrdU incorporation assay results showed that exposure Sal B could maintain the proliferation of NSPCs after cerebral ischemia. Morris water maze test showed that delayed post-ischemic treatment with Sal B improved cognitive impairment after stroke in rats.

Significance: Sal B could maintain the NSPCs self-renew and promote proliferation, which was mediated by PI3K/Akt signal pathway. And delayed post-ischemic treatment with Sal B improved cognitive impairment after stroke in rats. These findings suggested that Sal B may act as a potential drug in treatment of brain injury or neurodegenerative diseases.

Editor: Josef Priller, Charité-Universitätsmedizin Berlin, Germany

Funding: This work was supported by the National Natural Science Foundation of China (nos. 30873395 and 30472177), National Basic Research Program of China (no. 2011CB505302), National Science & Technology Major Project "Key New Drug Creation and Manufacturing Program" (2012ZX09101202) and the Program for Changjiang Scholars and Innovative Research Team in University (no. IRT0973). The funders had no role in study design, data collection and analysis, decision to publish, or preparation of the manuscript.

Competing Interests: The authors have declared that no competing interest exist.

* E-mail: zyjsunye@163.com

Introduction

Ischemic brain damage is one of the most dangerous ailments that lead to learning and memory disability, physical dysfunction and even death. Up to now, no effective treatment has been reported [1]. Neurons as terminally differentiated cells cannot regenerate after injury in traditional view. However, appropriate exercise training can facilitate some neurological function recovery after stroke in clinical practice [2,3], with the evidence that neurogenesis occurs in the adult brain. Neural stem/precursor cells (NSPCs) had been found and confirmed in adult brain in past decades that it can differentiate into neurons or glial cells as a result of neurogenesis [4–7], NSPCs can be stimulated in several pathological conditions, such as neurological diseases, cerebral ischemic in adult brain, and many reports showed that they are an excellent candidate for developing therapeutic strategies to repair the injured CNS [8,9]. Although the NSPCs would be stimulated to proliferation and differentiation during the brain injury, often

this response is not sufficient to overcome the damage. It is essential to study the signalling mechanisms that are activated by small molecular materials in the NSPCs to enhance their response pharmacologically. NSPCs proliferation and neurogensis involves a series of intracellular signaling pathways [10,11]. Among these pathways, the activation of Notch, mitogen-activated protein kinases (MAPKs) and phosphatidylinositol-3-kinase (PI3K)/Akt pathways are known to play major roles in cell growth and survival responses [12–14]. Numerous studies have shown that small molecular materials such as growth factors [15], retinoic acid [16] and Traditional Chinese Medicine (TCM) active constituent [17,18] can regulate the biological characteristics of neural stem cell and promote neurogenesis. Therefore, regulation of neurogenesis by NSPCs is anticipated as a noble therapeutic strategy for brain damage.

Herbs have been used for treating diseases for centuries, and a lot of natural compounds that with neural beneficial from medicinal plants had been discovered [19]. Treatment of stroke by TCM has a wealth of clinical experience and theoretical basis, and a large number of effective clinical prescriptions have been accumulated. In recent years a large number of studies have shown that TCM prescription and its active ingredient can improve cerebral ischemic injury in experimental animal [20,21]. Ginsenoside Rb1 and Rg1, for example, improved spatial learning and increase hippocampal synaptophysin level in mice [22]. Curcumin had been demonstrated to stimulate developmental and adult hippocampal neurogenesis, and a biological activity that may enhance neural plasticity and repair [23]. A recent report has shown that NeuroAid (MLC601 and MLC901), a Traditional Chinese Medicine is used in China for patients after stroke, reduced the increase in escape latency and in swim distance induced by ischemia [24]. With an extensive clinical experience, there are ample opportunities to discover natural compounds that effectively promote the proliferation of NSPCs and neurogenesis from TCM.

Sal B was discovered in an *in vitro* screening assay for searching the NSPCs proliferation-inducing natural molecules. It is one of the major ingredients in the water-soluble extracts of *S. miltiorrhiza Bunge* which has been reported to reduce cerebrovascular disease [25–27]. As a well-known Chinese herbal medicine, Danshen (*Salvia miltiorrhiza*) has been widely used in traditional Chinese medicinal preparation for the treatment of ischemic disease, and the medicinal properties of this plant have been extensively studied [28,29]. Several studies have demonstrated the effect of salvianolic acids on preventing brain injury [27,30]. Importantly, Sal B was reported to be capable of improving the recovery of motor function after cerebral ischemia in rats [31,32]. However, research on the mechanism of Sal B in treatment of stroke, and the molecular mechanisms responsible for the reported beneficial

cerebrovascular effects of Sal B are fairly rare. Meanwhile, the effect of delayed treatment with Sal B after ischemic stroke is still unclear. Therefore, the effect of chronic Sal B treatment beginning seven days after ischemic stroke on neurological deficits and pathophysiology after the transient cerebral ischemic model in rats were studied in our research.

Considering the significance of neurogenesis-related brain recovery, the present study was undertaken to examine the promotive effects of Sal B on NSPCs proliferation and neurogenesis. We provide evidence that Sal B increasing the proliferation of NSPCs in vitro and in vivo. These actions are at least in part mediated by altering the PI3K/Akt signaling pathway. Additionally, delayed post-ischemic administration of Sal B had beneficial effects on the recovery of cognitive function. The stimulative effects of Sal B on NSPCs self-renew and neurogenesis might be associated with a favorable outcome for stroke and other neurological disease.

Results

Salvianolic acid B induced the proliferation of cultured NSPCs *in vitro*

Forty-five herbal compounds, which are extensively used clinically for treating stroke in China, were screened in an *in vitro* proliferation assay to identify compounds that could induce proliferation of NSPCs. As shown in Fig. 1, among these natural compounds screened, berberine and Sal B displayed marked activity promoting NSPCs proliferation. In the following study, the proliferative effect of berberine and Sal B were systematically investigated but the action of berberine was proved to be an

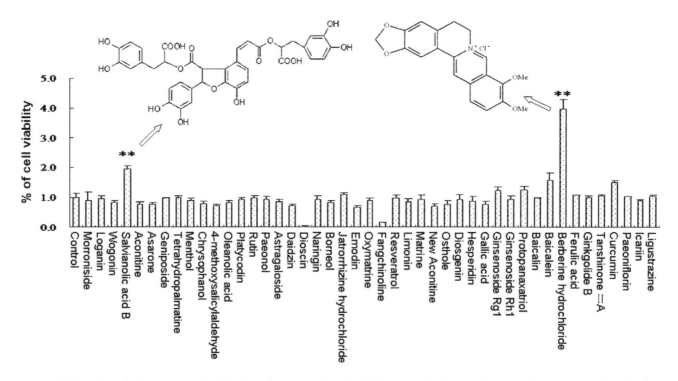

Figure 1. Screening for NSPCs proliferation-inducing natural materials. The proliferation-inducing activities on NSPCs of a total of 45 natural compounds, which were from medicinal materials extensively used in China to treat stroke clinically, were tested using a MTS assay, and the results are expressed in fold change relative to the corresponding controls. The proliferation-inducing effect of the most potent compound, Sal B (A) and berberine (B), were indicated by the arrow and its structure is shown in the inset. Data represent the mean ± S.D. from three independent experiments. **Significant difference from the control group at *P*<0.01.

illusion by BrdU incorporation assay (See Figure S1 in the Supporting Information).

To study the proliferation-inducing effect of Sal B in detail, we investigated effects of Sal B on the viability of NSPCs *in vitro* using the MTS assay, NSPCs were treated with Sal B at different concentrations and for different durations. We investigated Sal B at 5, 10, 20, 30, 40, 50 µM dose exposure for 24 hours, and at 20 µM dose incubated for 24, 48, 72 hours on promoting NSPCs proliferation. The results showed that the viability of NSPCs significantly increased as the dose ($P<0.01$, $F_{(6, 35)} = 103.06$) and time increases ($P<0.01$, Fig. 2A–B). The number and size of neurospheres were increased by addition of 20 µM of Sal B (Figure 2C–D). These results suggested that Sal B significantly increased the viability of NSPCs in dose- and time- dependent manners.

The MTS assay is a good indicator of cell viability. However, it does not give explicit information on cell proliferation. To provide further evidence that Sal B promotes NSPCs proliferation, a BrdU-incorporation assay was performed. BrdU incorporated cells were detected by immunocytochemistry with anti-BrdU antibody. As shown in Fig. 3, Sal B significantly increased BrdU-labeled cells compared with untreated control ($P<0.01$, $F_{(3, 40)} = 6.63$, Fig. 3).

Effect of Salvianolic acid B on self-renew genes of NSPCs

To confirm the effects of Sal B on maintaining the self-renew cell fate of NSPCs, we further investigated whether treatment of the NSPCs with Sal B could influence their self-renew potential. We studied the effect of Sal B on cell fate specification using RT-PCR method. NSPCs were treated with Sal B (5, 10, 20 µM) for 3 days in proliferation condition, and then the total RNA was extracted. The effect of Sal B on mRNA expression of the self-renew genes, Nestin and Notch-1, was evaluated. The results showed that Sal B up-regulated the expression of Nestin ($P<0.01$, $F_{(5, 24)} = 6.92$) and Notch-1 ($P<0.01$, $F_{(5, 24)} = 6.10$) mRNA of NSPCs (Fig. 4). These observations suggested that Sal B can maintain self-renewal of NSPCs.

NSPCs proliferation mediated by Akt activation

To investigate the molecular mechanism of Sal B on promoting proliferation of NSPCs, we checked the PI3K/Akt, MEK/ERK and Notch signaling pathways, which were closely related to the proliferation and differentiation of NSPCs [12–14]. The Akt pathway inhibitor Ly294002, ERK pathway inhibitor U0126, and Notch pathway inhibitor DAPT were used. NSPCs were maintained in the presence or absence of Sal B (20 µg/mL), Ly294002 (20 µM), U0126 (10 µM) and DAPT (10 µM) for 2 days. The proliferative response of Sal B/inhibitors was studied using the cell proliferation assay.

MTS results showed that Sal B (20 µg/mL) increased the cell survival (Control 0.17 ± 0.01 *vs* Sal 0.30 ± 0.01, n = 5, $P<0.01$). Inhibition of Akt activity by Ly294002 significantly reduced the number of NSPCs, the effects of Sal B on promoting NSPCs proliferation were abolished by the PI3K inhibitor Ly294002, Notch and ERK1/2 had no significant effect on the Sal B -mediated cell survival ($P<0.01$, $F(7, 40) = 158.48$, Fig. 5). These results suggested that PI3K/Akt pathway is involved in Sal B-induced proliferation of NSPCs.

We further investigated the phosphorylation of Akt in Sal B-treated cultures. NSPCs were stimulated with Sal B (20 µM) for 15, 30, 60, 120 min and the phosphorylation of Akt was detected using phospho-specific antibodies. Western blotting results showed that Sal B could increase the level of Akt phosphorylation at all of the time tested compared with control (Fig. 6A). The effect of Ly294002 on the blocking of Akt phosphorylation induced by Sal B was investigated by treated NSCPs with Ly294002 (20 µM) and/or Sal B for 30 min. As a result, Ly294002 (PI-3K inhibitor) abolished the phosphorylation of Akt induced by Sal B (Fig. 6B). These results suggested that PI3K/Akt signaling was involved in Sal B mediated proliferation of NSPCs.

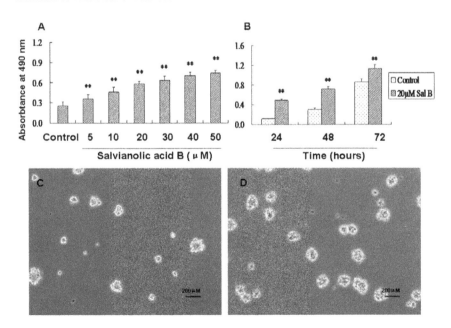

Figure 2. The promotive effect of salvianolic acid B on NSPCs proliferation. (A) Sal B dose-dependently promoted NSPCs proliferation. (B) Sal B time-dependently promoted NSPCs proliferation. Data represent mean ± S.D. from three independent experiments. **Significant difference from the control group at $P<0.01$. (C–D) Representative microphotographs of formed neurospheres in the absence (C) or presence (D) of Sal B (20 µM). Sal B increased the size of formed neurospheres. Scale bars: 200 µm.

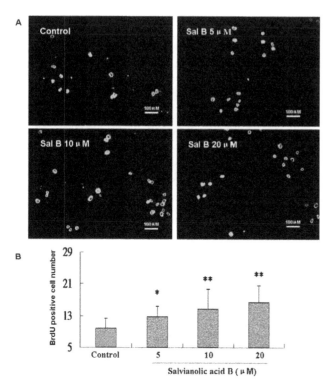

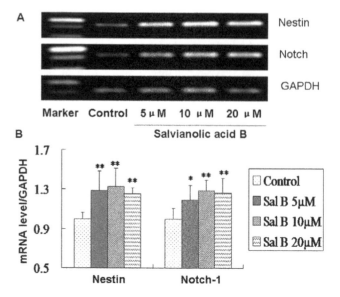

Figure 4. Salvianolic acid B up-regulated the self-renew genes of NSPCs. (A) The mRNA levels of NSPCs self-renew markers were analyzed by RT-PCR. (B) The expression levels were semi-quantified by densitometric measurements, normalized with GAPDH internal control, compared with control, and expressed as means ± S.D from three independent experiments. *Significant difference from the control group at $P<0.05$. **Significant difference from the control group at $P<0.01$.

Figure 3. The effect of Salvianolic acid B on BrdU-incorporation in cultured NSPCs. Dissociated NSPCs were cultured on poly-L-lysine-coated 12-well chamber slides with or without Sal B for 12 h and were subsequently incubated with BrdU (10 µg/ml) for other 12 h. After treatment, cells were fixed, immunostained with anti BrdU antibody. (A) Visualization of BrdU-positive cells by the Immunofluorescence staining assay on NSPCs. Scale bar: 100 µm. (B) BrdU-positive cells were counted in 10 randomly selected fields from three different chambers. Data represent the mean ± S.D. from three independent experiments. *Significant difference from the control group at $P<0.05$. **Significant difference from the control group at $P<0.01$.

Salvianolic acid B protected the learning and memory functions

Since cerebral ischemia can cause prolonged spatial memory disturbance in rats [33], we performed Morris water-maze test to examine the hippocampus involvement and Sal B effect on in learning and memory. Each animal was tested twice a day for 5 consecutive days on their escape latency to the hidden platform. Fig. 8A showed the escape latencies of the three groups of animals during acquisition training (5 days). In all the groups, escape latencies became shorter across training sessions ($F_{(2,30)} = 31.54$, $P<0.01$, Repeated measures ANCOVA). The decreased escape

Salvianolic acid B increased the number of BrdU-positive cells *in vivo*

In the following study, the effect of Sal B on recovery of brain functions after transient cerebral ischemia was evaluated. Firstly, we investigated whether Sal B (50 mg/kg) exposure *in vivo* would affect NSPCs behavior. Since BrdU is incorporated into dividing and proliferating cells, BrdU labeling has been widely used in many investigations concerning neurogenesis. BrdU (50 mg/kg IP) was administered to the rats in sham, vehicle, and ischemia groups once every 2 hours over a period of 8 hours at the 21th day after injection to label the proliferating cells after ischemia. The next day the rats were perfused with 0.01 M PBS (pH 7.2), then with 4% paraformaldehyde (PFA) in PBS. The dividing cells labeled with BrdU were visualized using BrdU immunohistochemistry. BrdU labeled neurons were found in all groups in the dentate gyrus of the hippocampus (Fig. 7). A few BrdU-positive cells were observed in the SGZ of hippocampal dentate gyrus in the control, and BrdU immunoreactivity did not significantly differ between vehicle and sham-operated animals in 21 days. We observed a significant 2.5-fold increase in the numbers of BrdU positive cells in the SGZ of hippocampal dentate gyrus in Sal B treated group (50 mg/kg) (n = 4, $p<0.01$), which is consistent with our *in vitro* findings that Sal B enhanced NSPCs proliferation.

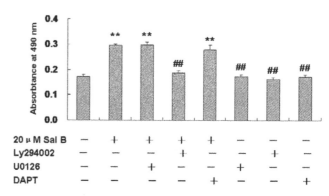

Figure 5. Salvianolic acid B promoted NSPCs proliferation in a PI3K/Akt -independent pathway. NSPCs were cultured in the proliferation medium containing Sal B (20 µM) in the presence and absence of the PI3K inhibitor Ly294002 (20 µM), MEK inhibitor U0126 (10 µM) or Notch inhibitor DAPT (10 µM) for 2 days. Cell survival was assessed by MTS assay. Data represent the mean ± S.D. from three independent experiments. **$P<0.01$ as compared with control,##$P<0.01$ as compared with Sal B-treated cells.

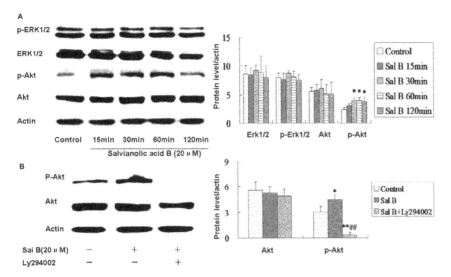

Figure 6. Salvianolic acid B activated PI3K/Akt in NSPCs. Cell lysates from NSPCs treated or untreated with Sal B (20 μM) were subjected to Western blot analysis with antibodies against both total and phosphorylated forms of ERK1/2, and Akt. Actin was used as loading control. (A) Sal B increased the phosphorylation of Akt. Akt phosphorylation in Sal B-treated runners (15 min, 30 min, 60 min, 120 min) were significantly greater than control runners. Histograms represent the change in the phosphorylation of Akt normalized to anti-actin antibodies (n = 4). **Significant difference from the control group at $P<0.01$. (B) PI3K/Akt inhibitors Ly294002 regulated the Sal B-mediated phosphorylation of Akt. Ly294002 abolished the phosphorylation of Akt induced by Sal B. Histograms represent the change in the phosphorylation of Akt normalized to anti-actin antibodies (n = 4). *$P<0.05$ as compared with control, **$P<0.01$ as compared with control, ##$P<0.01$ as compared with Sal B-treated cells. No change in total Akt was observed.

latency during the learning process in the three groups clearly reflected memory for the escape platform place. Repeated measures ANCOVA revealed no interaction between training days and groups ($F_{(2,30)} = 0.90$, $P>0.05$). However, differences were observed between the three groups ($F_{(2,30)} = 9.96$, $P<0.01$, Repeated measures ANCOVA), sham-operated animals memorized the position of the hidden platform very quickly, reaching it in a shorter latency during the training. In contrast, the untreated ischemic animals showed a severe deficiency compared to the control. Although they were gradually trained and showed better

performance, their escape latencies were still much longer than those of the control animals. And there are signifitient difference between sham and model of the escape latency in the day 4 (Sham 32.76 ± 18.54 vs Model 54.55 ± 26.05, n = 10, $P<0.05$) and day 5 (Sham 16.38 ± 6.56 vs Model 48.89 ± 27.39, n = 10, $P<0.01$). Administration of Sal B (50 mg/kg) significantly ameliorated such deficiencies.

After 5 days of studying the acquisition of place learning, rats had learned the escape platform position. To determine the degree of memory, on the sixth day the animal was placed in the pool for

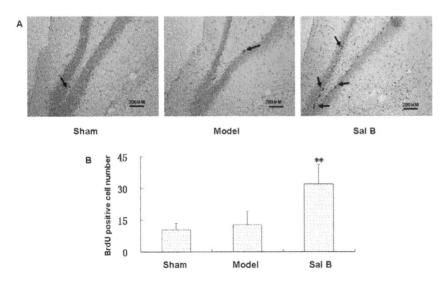

Figure 7. Salvianolic acid B increased the number of BrdU-positive cells *in vivo*. (A) Representative photomicrographs showing BrdU-positive cells in the hippocampus of sham, ischemia and ischemia+Sal B (50 mg/kg)-treated rats. BrdU-labeled cells were indicated by arrows. Scale bar: 200 μm. (B) Quantification of BrdU-positive cells in the hippocampus. Each column represents the represent the mean ± S.D. (n = 10). **Significant difference from the sham group at $P<0.01$.

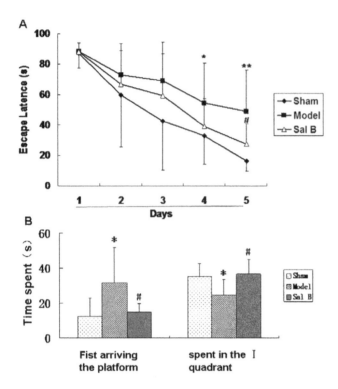

Figure 8. Delayed post-ischemic treatment with salvianolic acid B improved cognitive impairment in Morris water maze task. (A) Place learning with multiple trials. There was a decrease in escape latencies with training in all three groups. (B) In the transfer task, the escape latencies (mean ± S.D.) are compared among sham-operated, untreated ischemic, and Sal B treated groups (n = 8). And the animals from the Sal B-treated group spent more time in the quadrant that contained the escape platform during the place learning than untreated group. *$P < 0.05$ as compared with sham group, #$P < 0.05$ as compared with model group.

90 s without the escape platform and the time the animal spent to arrive the position and in the quadrant which had the escape platform during the training experiment was recorded. Time spent data were shown in Fig. 8. In relation to the transfer of this task, animals in untreated group remained for a similar total period of time in the four quadrants. Animals from sham and Sal B (50 mg/kg) groups spent longer in the quadrant which had contained the escape platform during the initial place learning than in the remaining quadrants. These results showed that Sal B could improve the learning and memory ability of cerebral ischemic animals.

Discussion

NSPCs proliferation is important to produce of neurogenesis. Compounds that can promote neural stem cell proliferation are seen to support neurogenesis. In the present study, we selected a total of 45 natural compounds from medicinal materials which are extensively used in China to treat stroke clinically, and tested their proliferation-inducing activities on NSPCs using a MTS assay. The screening results showed that several natural compounds such as berberine and Sal B displayed marked effects on the proliferation of NSPCs. In the further research, we found that although berberine could increase the value of MTS assay, it reduced the BrdU incorporation. The action of berberine was proved to be an illusion since BrdU incorporation was considered as an important sign of cell proliferation. Additionally, morpho-

logically berberine could cause cell swelling and decrease the cell number (see Figure S1 in the Supporting Information). Therefore berberine was cytotoxic to neural stem cell and could not promote proliferation.

To explore whether Sal B could promote the NSPCs proliferation, we next systemic examined the promotive effects of Sal B on NSPCs proliferation. Cortical NSPCs were isolated at embryonic day 13.5, the cells were plated in non-adherent conditions, evaluation with MTS assays demonstrated that Sal B induced NSPCs proliferation in a dose- and time-dependent manner. On the molecular level, DNA synthesis of NSPCs in Sal B-treated cultures was determined by BrdU incorporation assay. Immunostaining results showed that the BrdU positive cells were up regulated by Sal B treatment. Consistent with the MTS assay, the BrdU incorporation studies established that metabolic activity of cells was enhanced with the presence of Sal B when compared with the control. These observations suggested that Sal B indeed promoted the proliferation of the NSPCs. Next we conducted a RT-PCR analysis with NSPCs self-renew marker, Nestin and Notch-1. The results showed that the nestin and Notch-1 mRNA expression was up-regulated significantly by Sal B treatment. The results were consisted with the promotion of NSPCs proliferation induced by Sal B. In summary, these observations suggest that Sal B could maintain the NSPCs self-renew and promote proliferation.

Several intricate cell signaling cascades are crucial for determining whether NSPCs proliferation or differentiation. Notch, MEK/ERK and PI3K/Akt pathways are the most frequently ones that associated with regulation of cell growth, survival, and differentiation [34]. We sought to determine which signaling pathway was activated by which Sal B facilitated the NSPCs self-renew. If these signal pathways play important proliferation roles in NSPCs, inhibition of PI3K/Akt should reduce Sal B-induced proliferation. MTS results showed that the absorbance value could be increased by Sal B, and PI3K/Akt specific inhibitor Ly294002 but not Notch specific inhibitor DAPT and MEK/ERK specific inhibitor U0126 could block this effect. The results suggested that PI3K/Akt signal pathway was involved in the Sal B-induced proliferation of NSPCs.

To gain further insight into the mechanisms by which Sal B modulates PI3K/Akt signalling and by which PI3K/Akt mediates Sal B induced self-renew, we evaluated the role of the PI3K/Akt pathway. Akt is a serine/threonine kinase, which can be activated by phosphorylation and subsequently enhance cell survival by activates multiple downstream targets [35,36]. We demonstrated that exposure to Sal B induced the activation of Akt. If PI3K/Akt signal pathway plays an important profileation role, inhibition of PI3K/Akt should reduce Sal B-induced phosphorylation of Akt. Consistent with our hypothesis, the results showed that Sal B-induced activation of Akt was completely inhibited by the PI3K/Akt-inhibitor, Ly294002. In short, these findings supported the hypothesis that PI3K/Akt signal pathway was the signal mediator in Sal B-stimulated NSPCs proliferation.

In order to examine the effects of Sal B on proliferation of NSPCs in vivo, transient cerebral ischemic rats and BrdU labeling were employed. New neurons can be generated in the hippocampal of adult rats after transient ischemia of the forebrain [37–39]. Many researchers had reported that cerebral ischemic could transient stimulated neurogenesis in the adult hippocampus. As far as we know, Liu et al. [40] first demonstrated increased neurogenesis in the gerbils hippocampus after transient global ischemia, the BrdU incorporation peaks 11 days after ischemia and that incorporation subsides to control levels by 3 weeks after ischemia. Similar results were described after transient global ischemia in mice [41] and rats [42]. But most of the cells were not fully mature during the 2- to 5-week period after ischemia and could not form a functional link [42]. Therefore, in our view, the behavior performance could not be better at that time. In accordance with previous reports, the NSPCs responded to the injury by proliferation in this study. Cerebral ischemic made the NSPCs proliferation after 7 days (See Figure S2 in the Supporting Information), but the proliferation ability of the rats in the vehicle group declined quickly 28 days after cerebral ischemic. However, Sal B (25 mg/kg) treatment significantly increased the number of BrdU-positive cells in the dentate gyrus 21 days after injection, suggested that Sal B exposure could maintain the ability of the NSPCs proliferation *in vivo*.

Since Sal B promote NSPCs proliferation *in vitro* and *in vivo*, we next sought to correlate the regeneration of new neurons and recovery of brain functions. The present study demonstrated that delayed post-ischemic treatment (7 days after ischemic stroke) with Sal B (25 mg/kg) improved cognitive impairment after stroke in rats. Since NSPCs proliferation in hippocampus was important site for spatial learning and memory [43,44], we speculated that the enhancement of functional recovery by Sal B might be dependent on its action on NSPCs proliferation. But more extensive experiments were still necessary to demonstrate that Sal B could cross over the blood–brain barrier and act on NSPCs. Further study will be carried out to clarify this point. Although our present study showed that Sal B promoted the adult hippocampus neurogenesis and improved the cognitive functions in cerebral ischemia rats, there is no direct evidence to show that Sal B could pass through the blood-brain barrier [45], and the exact mechanism(s) by which Sal B acts on adult neurogenesis remain unclear. More advanced research is needed in the future to further clarify the pathways and mechanisms of Sal B in promoting adult neurogenesis including using appropriate tool drugs to block certain pathways to confirm NSPCs proliferation by Sal B on contributing to the cognitive improvement.

In conclusion, the results of this work clearly demonstrated that Sal B was capable of promoting proliferation of NSPCs and improving the learning and memory ability of cerebral ischemic rats. Additionally, we confirmed that Sal B promoteed NSPCs self-renew and neurogensis were at least in part mediated by the PI3K/Akt signaling pathway. These findings suggested that Sal B may act as a potential drug in treatment brain injury or neurodegenerative disease.

Materials and Methods

Reagents

Salvianolic acid B (Sal B, purity >99%) was purchased from the Chinese National Institute for the Control of Pharmaceutical and Biological Products (Beijing, China), When used, it was freshly prepared in phosphate buffer solution (PBS); B27 (without retinoic acid) was purchased from Invitrogen (Carlsbad, CA, USA); Recombinant human fibroblast growth factor 2 (FGF-2) was from Millipore (Temecula, CA); Antibodies for ERK1/2, phospho-ERK1/2, Akt, phosphor-Akt (Ser-473) were obtained from Cell Signaling Technology (Beverly, MA). Antibody for β-actin was purchased from senta; 1,4-diamino-2,3-dicyano-1,4-bis(2-amino-phenylthio)-butadiene (U0126) and 2-(4-morpholinyl)-8-phenyl-4H-1-benzopyran-4-one (Ly294002) was from CalBiochem (San Diego, CA). U0126 and Ly294002 were solubilized in dimethyl-sulphoxide.

Cell culture

Primary neurospheres were isolated from the cerebral cortex of 13.5-day-embryonic Wistar rats, according to the method described by Davis et al [46]. Briefly, the cerebral cortex was carefully isolated from adjacent tissues, and collected in cold serum-free medium consisting of DMEM/F-12 (1:1; Invitrogen, Carlsbad, CA, USA). The tissue was digested at 37°C for 10 min by acctuase (Millipore, Temecula, CA), and mechanically disrupted into single cells by filtering through a nylon mesh of 70 μm. The dissociated cells were then plated at a concentration of 2×10^5 cells/ml in T75 culture flasks for 20 ml, and cultured in neurosphere proliferation media consisting of Dulbecco's Modified Eagle's Medium (DMEM): F12 supplemented with 2% (v/v) B27 supplement (Invitrogen, Carlsbad, CA, USA), 20 ng/ml epidermal growth factor (EGF; PEPROTECH, Rocky Hill, NJ, USA), and 20 ng/ml fibroblast growth factor 2 (FGF2). After 6 days in culture, the proliferating cells formed the neurospheres, which were suspended in the medium. Subsequently, the neurospheres were passaged by treatment with accutase about 5 min at 37°C until they were gently dissociated, and then subcultured as single cells in a new T75 culture flask at a density of 20,000 cells/ml in the fresh culture medium. The procedure of subculture was repeated again to achieve the purified cortical NSPCs and proliferating neurospheres. The 3–5 passages of NSPCs were used for the following experiments.

MTS assay

For *in vitro* cell proliferation assay, A Cell Titer 96 AQ$_{neous}$ One Solution Cell Proliferation Assay (Promega, Charbonnières-les-Bains, France) was used. NSPCs were plated at 30, 000 cells/well in a 96-well plate in the presence and absence of Sal B (0.5, 1, 5, 10, 20 μM), U0126 (10 μg/ml), DAPT (10 μg/ml) and Ly294002 (20 μg/ml) in a 96-well plate. Cell proliferation was assessed at day 2 of cell culture. According to the manufacturer's recommendations, 40 μl MTS solution was then added into each of the wells. Then cells were incubated for 2 h at 37°C in the humidified 5% CO_2 atmosphere incubator, and results were obtained at a wavelength of 490 nm using a microplate reader (FlexStation 3, Molecular Devices, USA). The same volume of medium without cells was used as blank. Results were expressed in Optical Density (OD).

In vitro BrdU-incorporation assay

For *in vitro* BrdU-incorporation assay, cultured NSPCs were incubated with or without Sal B for 24 h, the cells were labeled with BrdU (10 μg/ml) during the last 12 h of incubation, then the cells were plated onto poly-L-lysine coated slides for 2 h, fixed in 4% paraformaldehyde, washed with phosphate-buffered saline (PBS) and incubated in 2 N HCl at 37°C for 10 min. After washing with PBS, the cells were incubated with mouse anti-BrdU antibody (1:100, senta) at 4°C for 24 h in PBS. After washing in PBS, they were then incubated at room temperature for 1 h in PBS containing FITC conjugated anti-mouse IgG secondary antibody (1:200, senta). BrdU-positive cells were evaluated using a fluorescent microscope (Leica, German). BrdU positive cells were counted in 10 randomly selected fields from three different chambers.

RT-PCR analysis

Cells were harvested and total RNA was isolated from treated or untreated NSPCs with TRIzol (Roche), the first strand cDNA was synthesized from 0.4 μg of total RNA using Reverse Transcriptase (Takala) and Random primer as described in the manufacture's instructions. After synthesis, 5 μl of cDNA was used in PCR reaction with gene-specific primers, The sequences of the PCR primer pairs (5′ to 3′) that were used for each gene are as follows: rat nestin, 5′- TTCCCTTCCCCCTTGCCTAATACC-3′ (forward) and 5′- TGGGCTGAGCTGTTTTCTACTTTT-3′ (reverse); Notch-1, 5′- ATGGCCTCCAACGATACTCCT-3′ (forward) and 5′- ACATGTACCCCCATAGTGGCA-3′ (reverse). Products were analyzed on 1.5% agarose gel and visualized by ethidium bromide staining. The relative amount of each transcript was normalized to the level of β-actin.

Western blot analysis

Protein extracts were prepared and subjected to Western blot analysis. Cells were harvested and lysed with RIPA lysis buffer. The protein concentrations of the lysates were determined with a Bradford protein assay kit (Bio-Rad) according to the manufacturer's instructions. An equal amount of protein was fractionated by SDS-polyacrylamide gel electrophoresis (PAGE) and transferred onto polyvinylidine difluoride membranes. After blocking with 5% skim milk in TBS-T, the membrane was probed with primary antibodies (goat anti-actin 1:1000, Santa Cruz; rabbit anti-ERK1/2 1:500, rabbit anti-phospho-ERK1/2 1:300, rabbit anti-Akt 1:500 or rabbit anti-phospho-Akt (Ser-473) 1:300, Cell Signaling Technology) in a blocking solution of non-fat milk (5%). Secondary horseradish peroxidase-conjugated rabbit anti-goat 1:2000, goat anti-rabbit 1:2000 (Santa Cruz) antibody in non-fat milk blocking solution (5%) was then applied. The immunoreactivity was visualized with ECL Western blotting detection reagents (Millipore).

Induction of the transient global ischemia

Adult (8–10 week-old) male Wistar rats weighing 200–250 g were subjected to transient forebrain ischemia by a method combining those described previously [47,48]. The rats were housed singly in temperature-controlled conditions with a 12 hr light/dark cycle (lights on: 8:00 AM) following surgery. They had access to food and water ad libitum. Experimental procedures were conducted in accordance with recommendations of the Animal Ethics Committee of Tianjin University of Traditional Chinese Medicine (TCM-2009-034-E01). In brief, twelve hours before the induction of ischemia, rats were anesthetized with sodium pentobarbital, the bilateral carotid arteries were exposed to facilitate the occluding on the following day, and then the vertebral arteries were irreversibly occluded by electrocoagulation. The next day, ischemia was induced by bilaterally occluding carotid arteries with aneurysm clips, and carotid arteries were clamped for 6 min exactly. Rats lost their righting reflex during ischemic, the clips were removed to restore cerebral blood flow. The rats that remain their righting reflex in 1 min after occluding of the both carotid arteries were considered to be failure of ischemia and eliminated. Sham-operated rats were anesthetized, the carotid arteries were isolated, but they were not clamped.

Drug adminstration

The study was carried out on rats divided into three groups (n = 13). (i) Sham group+vehicle (Sham), (ii) Ischemic group+vehicle (Model) and (iii) Ischemic group+Sal B (Sal B). Seven days after cerebral ischemia, Sal B (50 mg/kg) was dissolved in distilled water, and injected i.p. once daily for 4 weeks, and three mice in each group were used for histological analysis at day 21 after innjection. All controls received an amount of vehicle equivalent to drug treatment conditions.

In vivo proliferation assay

For *in vivo* proliferation analysis of Sal B, that had not been behaviorally tested were evaluated for BrdU labeling. BrdU (50 mg/kg; Sigma) was injected i.p. once every 2 hours over a period of 8 hours at the 21th day after injection to label the proliferating cells. Twenty-four hours after the last BrdU injection, rars were anesthetized with ether and perfused with PBS, followed by a cold 4% paraformaldehyde solution. Brains were collected and post-fixed overnight in a 4% paraformaldehyde solution at 4°C. Coronal sections (20 μm thickness) were obtained throughout the hippocampus. For analysis concerning BrdU immunohistochemistry, sections were incubated in 50% formamide/2×saline sodium citrate (SSC) for 2 h at 65°C, followed by a rinse with PBS. Sections were then incubated in 2 N HCl for 30 min at 37°C to denature double-stranded DNA, and rinsed in 0.1 M borate buffer (pH 8.5). After blocking for 2 h with 1% BSA in PBS, sections were incubated overnight at 4°C with mouse anti-BrdU monoclonal antibody (1:100; senta). Followed by rinsing in PBS, sections were incubated for 2 h at RT with biotinylated goat anti-mouse IgG (1:200; senta), and incubated for 2 h at RT with the ABC kit. BrdU positive cells were visualized by incubating sections with Vector DAB.

Morris water maze task

The learning and memory ability was examined using the Morris water-maze [49]. A cylindrical tank 1.5 m in diameter was filled with water (22±1°C), and a transparent platform 10 cm in diameter was placed at a constant position in the center of one of the four quadrants within the tank. The platform was set 2 cm below the water level where the rats could not see it directly. Rats were allowed to swim freely for 1 min to become habituated to the apparatus. From the next day, in the hidden platform trials, acquisition trials were carried out 2 times per day for 5 days. In each trial, rats were placed into the water at a fixed starting position, and the time taken to escape onto the hidden platform and the swimming path length were measured. Rats were given 90 s to find the hidden platform during each acquisition trial. If it failed to locate the platform within 90 s, it was guided there. The rat was allowed to stay on the platform for 20 s. Performance was tested 24 h after the final training day in a probe trial during which the platform was removed, the rat was placed in the start and its behavior was monitored for 90 s.

Statistical analysis

SPSS11.5 for Windows (SPSS Inc.) was used to analyze the data. Data are expressed as the mean ± S.D. and analyzed by ANOVA followed by the post-hoc Least Significant Difference (LSD) test. Differences were considered statistically significant if P values were less than 0.05. To analyze water-maze place-navigation performance, the average escape latency of 5 trials per day per animal was calculated and evaluated by repeated-measures ANCOVA.

Supporting Information

Figure S1 Berberine failed to promote the NSPCs proliferation. (A) Berberine increased the value of MTT assay. (B) Berberine reduced the BrdU incorporation. **Significant difference from the control group at $P<0.01$. (C) Morphologically berberine caused cell swelling and decreased the cell number. Scale bar: 200 μm.

Figure S2 Regeneration of Hippocampal NSPCs Following Ischemia. BrdU positive cells in the granule cell layer in the intact (A) and ischemic (B, DAI7) animals. The inset shows an enlarged display of a typical BrdU positive cell. Scale bar: 200 μm.

Acknowledgments

We would like to thank Dr. Hui Wang and Prof. Yan Zhu for their helpful discussion and critical reading of our manuscript. We would also like to thank Mr. Huaien Bu for technical assistant of the Statistical analysis.

Author Contributions

Conceived and designed the experiments: YJZ PWZ. Performed the experiments: PWZ GZC MXZ XPY YL JBZ AOI. Analyzed the data: YJZ PWZ YHB. Contributed reagents/materials/analysis tools: JBZ YXL YBJ. Wrote the paper: YJZ PWZ AOI.

References

1. Doyle KP, Simon RP, Stenzel-Poore MP (2008) Mechanisms of ischemic brain damage. Neuropharmacology 55: 310–318.
2. Duncan P, Studenski S, Richards L, Gollub S, Lai SM, et al. (2003) Randomized clinical trial of therapeutic exercise in subacute stroke. Stroke 34: 2173–2180.
3. Kwakkel G, van Peppen R, Wagenaar RC, Wood Dauphinee S, Richards C, et al. (2004) Effects of augmented exercise therapy time after stroke: a meta-analysis. Stroke 35: 2529–2539.
4. Reynolds BA, Weiss S (1992) Generation of neurons and astrocytes from isolated cells of the adult mammalian central nervous system. Science 255: 1707–1710.
5. Weiss S, Reynolds BA, Vescovi AL, Morshead C, Craig CG, et al. (1996) Is there a neural stem cell in the mammalian forebrain? Trends Neurosci 19: 387–393.
6. Reynolds BA, Weiss S (1996) Clonal and population analyses demonstrate that an EGF-responsive mammalian embryonic CNS precursor is a stem cell. Dev Biol 175: 1–13.
7. McKay R (1997) Stem cells in the central nervous system. Science 276: 66–71.
8. Ming GL, Song H (2011) Adult neurogenesis in the mammalian brain: significant answers and significant questions. Neuron 70: 687–702.
9. Lie DC, Song H, Colamarino SA, Ming GL, Gage FH (2004) Neurogenesis in the adult brain: new strategies for central nervous system diseases. Annu Rev Pharmacol Toxicol 44: 399–421.
10. Johnson MA, Ables JL, Eisch AJ (2009) Cell-intrinsic signals that regulate adult neurogenesis in vivo: insights from inducible approaches. BMB Rep 42: 245–259.
11. Khodosevich K, Monyer H (2010) Signaling involved in neurite outgrowth of postnatally born subventricular zone neurons in vitro. BMC Neurosci 11: 18.
12. Imayoshi I, Sakamoto M, Yamaguchi M, Mori K, Kageyama R (2010) Essential roles of Notch signaling in maintenance of neural stem cells in developing and adult brains. J Neurosci 30: 3489–3498.
13. Choi YS, Cho HY, Hoyt KR, Naegele JR, Obrietan K (2008) IGF-1 receptor-mediated ERK/MAPK signaling couples status epilepticus to progenitor cell proliferation in the subgranular layer of the dentate gyrus. Glia 56: 791–800.
14. Bruel-Jungerman E, Veyrac A, Dufour F, Horwood J, Laroche S, et al. (2009) Inhibition of PI3K-Akt signaling blocks exercise-mediated enhancement of adult neurogenesis and synaptic plasticity in the dentate gyrus. PLoS One 4: e7901.
15. Leker RR, Lasri V, Chernoguz D (2009) Growth factors improve neurogenesis and outcome after focal cerebral ischemia. J Neural Transm 116: 1397–1402.
16. Jacobs S, Lie DC, DeCicco KL, Shi Y, DeLuca LM, et al. (2006) Retinoic acid is required early during adult neurogenesis in the dentate gyrus. Proc Natl Acad Sci U S A 103: 3902–3907.
17. Yabe T, Hirahara H, Harada N, Ito N, Nagai T, et al. (2010) Ferulic acid induces neural progenitor cell proliferation in vitro and in vivo. Neuroscience 165: 515–524.
18. Heurteaux C, Gandin C, Borsotto M, Widmann C, Brau F, et al. (2010) Neuroprotective and neuroproliferative activities of NeuroAid (MLC601, MLC901), a Chinese medicine, in vitro and in vivo. Neuropharmacology 58: 987–1001.
19. Kim H (2005) Neuroprotective herbs for stroke therapy in traditional eastern medicine. Neurol Res 27: 287–301.
20. Feigin VL (2007) Herbal medicine in stroke: does it have a future? Stroke 38: 1734–1736.
21. Wu B, Liu M, Liu H, Li W, Tan S, et al. (2007) Meta-analysis of traditional Chinese patent medicine for ischemic stroke. Stroke 38: 1973–1979.
22. Mook-Jung I, Hong HS, Boo JH, Lee KH, Yun SH, et al. (2001) Ginsenoside Rb1 and Rg1 improve spatial learning and increase hippocampal synaptophysin level in mice. J Neurosci Res 63: 509–515.
23. Kim SJ, Son TG, Park HR, Park M, Kim MS, et al. (2008) Curcumin stimulates proliferation of embryonic neural progenitor cells and neurogenesis in the adult hippocampus. J Biol Chem 283: 14497–14505.
24. Quintard H, Borsotto M, Veyssiere J, Gandin C, Labbal F, et al. (2011) MLC901, a traditional Chinese medicine protects the brain against global ischemia. Neuropharmacology 61: 622–631.
25. Kim DH, Park SJ, Kim JM, Jeon SJ, Kim DH, et al. (2011) Cognitive dysfunctions induced by a cholinergic blockade and Aβ(25–35) peptide are attenuated by salvianolic acid B. Neuropharmacology 61: 1432–1440.
26. Tang MK, Ren DC, Zhang JT, Du GH (2002) Effect of salvianolic acids from Radix Salviae miltiorrhizae on regional cerebral blood flow and platelet aggregation in rats. Phytomedicine 9: 405–409.
27. Chen T, Liu W, Chao X, Zhang L, Qu Y, et al. (2011) Salvianolic acid B attenuates brain damage and inflammation after traumatic brain injury in mice. Brain Res Bull 84: 163–168.
28. Zhou L, Zuo Z, Chow MS (2005) Danshen: an overview of its chemistry, pharmacology, pharmacokinetics, and clinical use. J Clin Pharmacol 45: 1345–1359.
29. Ji XY, Tan BK, Zhu YZ (2000) Salvia miltiorrhiza and ischemic diseases. Acta Pharmacol Sin 21: 1089–1094.
30. Jiang M, Wang XY, Zhou WY, Li J, Wang J, et al. (2011) Cerebral protection of salvianolic acid A by the inhibition of granulocyte adherence. Am J Chin Med 39: 111–120.
31. Tang M, Feng W, Zhang Y, Zhong J, Zhang J (2006) Salvianolic acid B improves motor function after cerebral ischemia in rats. Behav Pharmacol 17: 493–498.
32. Du GH, Qiu Y, Zhang JT (2000) Salvianolic acid B protects the memory functions against transient cerebral ischemia in mice. J Asian Nat Prod Res 2: 145–152.
33. Yonemori F, Yamada H, Yamaguchi T, Uemura A, Tamura A (1996) Spatial memory disturbance after focal cerebral ischemia in rats. J Cereb Blood Flow Metab 16: 973–980.
34. Shioda N, Han F, Fukunaga K (2009) Role of Akt and ERK signaling in the neurogenesis following brain ischemia. Int Rev Neurobiol 85: 375–387.
35. Chan CB, Liu X, Pradoldej S, Hao C, An J, et al. (2011) Phosphoinositide 3-kinase enhancer regulates neuronal dendritogenesis and survival in neocortex. J Neurosci 31: 8083–8092.
36. Le Belle JE, Orozco NM, Paucar AA, Saxe JP, Mottahedeh J, et al. (2011) Proliferative neural stem cells have high endogenous ROS levels that regulate self-renewal and neurogenesis in a PI3K/Akt-dependant manner. Cell Stem Cell 8: 59–71.
37. Nakatomi H, Kuriu T, Okabe S, Yamamoto S, Hatano O, et al. (2002) Regeneration of hippocampal pyramidal neurons after ischemic brain injury by recruitment of endogenous neural progenitors. Cell 110: 429–441.
38. Wang C, Zhang M, Sun C, Cai Y, You Y, et al. (2011) Sustained increase in adult neurogenesis in the rat hippocampal dentate gyrus after transient brain ischemia. Neurosci Lett 488: 70–75.
39. Yagita Y, Kitagawa K, Ohtsuki T, Takasawa Ki, Miyata T, et al. (2001) Neurogenesis by progenitor cells in the ischemic adult rat hippocampus. Stroke 32: 1890–1896.
40. Liu J, Solway K, Messing RO, Sharp FR (1998) Increased neurogenesis in the dentate gyrus after transient global ischemia in gerbils. J Neurosci 18: 7768–7778.
41. Takagi T, Nozaki K, Takahashi J, Yodoi J, Ishikawa M, et al. (1999) Proliferation of neuronal precursor cells in the dentate gyrus is accelerated after transient forebrain ischemia in mice. Brain Res 831: 283–287.
42. Kee NJ, Preston E, Wojtowicz JM (2001) Enhanced neurogenesis after transient global ischemia in the dentate gyrus of the rat. Exp Brain Res 136(3): 313–20.
43. Canales JJ (2010) Comparative neuroscience of stimulant-induced memory dysfunction: role for neurogenesis in the adult hippocampus. Behav Pharmacol 21: 379–393.
44. Banta Lavenex P, Lavenex P (2009) Spatial memory and the monkey hippocampus: not all space is created equal. Hippocampus 19: 8–19.
45. Xu M, Fu G, Qiao X, Wu WY, Guo H, et al. (2007) HPLC method for comparative study on tissue distribution in rat after oral administration of salvianolic acid B and phenolic acids from Salvia miltiorrhiza. Biomed Chromatogr 21(10): 1052–63.
46. Davis AA, Temple S (1994) A self-renewing multipotential stem cell in embryonic rat cerebral cortex. Nature 372: 263–266.
47. Nitatori T, Sato N, Waguri S, Karasawa Y, Araki H, et al. (1995) Delayed neuronal death in the CA1 pyramidal cell layer of the gerbil hippocampus following transient ischemia is apoptosis. J Neurosci 15: 1001–1011.
48. Pulsinelli WA, Brierley JB, Plum F (1982) Temporal profile of neuronal damage in a model of transient forebrain ischemia. Ann Neurol 11: 491–498.
49. Morris R (1984) Developments of a water-maze procedure for studying spatial learning in the rat. J Neurosci Methods 11: 47–60.

12

Acute, Delayed and Chronic Remote Ischemic Conditioning Is Associated with Downregulation of mTOR and Enhanced Autophagy Signaling

Sagar Rohailla⁹, Nadia Clarizia⁹, Michel Sourour, Wesam Sourour, Nitai Gelber, Can Wei, Jing Li, Andrew N. Redington*

Division of Cardiology, Labatt Family Heart Center, Hospital for Sick Children, University of Toronto, Ontario, Canada

Abstract

Background: Remote ischemic conditioning (RIC), induced by brief periods of limb ischemia has been shown to decrease acute myocardial injury and chronic responses after acute coronary syndromes. While several signaling pathways have been implicated, our understanding of the cardioprotection and its underlying mediators and mechanisms remains incomplete. In this study we examine the effect of RIC on pro-autophagy signaling as a possible mechanism of benefit.

Methods and Results: We examined the role of autophagy in the acute/first window (15 minutes after RIC), delayed/second window (24 hours after RIC) and chronic (24 hours after 9 days of repeated RIC) phases of cardioprotection. C57BL/6 mice (N = 69) were allocated to each treatment phase and further stratified to receive RIC, induced by four cycles of 5 minutes of limb ischemia followed by 5 minutes of reperfusion, or control treatment consisting solely of handling without transient ischemia. The groups included, group 1 (1W control), group 2 (1W RIC), group 3 (2W control), group 4 (2W RIC), group 5 (3W control) and group 6 (3W RIC). Hearts were isolated for assessment of cardiac function and infarct size after global ischemia using a Langendorff preparation. Infarct size was reduced in all three phases of cardioprotection, in association with improvements in post-ischemic left ventricular end diastolic pressure (LVEDP) and developed pressure (LVDP) ($P<0.05$). The pattern of autophagy signaling varied; 1W RIC increased AMPK levels and decreased the activation of mammalian target of rapamycin (mTOR), whereas chronic RIC was associated with persistent mTOR suppression and increased levels of autophagosome proteins, LC3II/I and Atg5.

Conclusions: Cardioprotection following transient ischemia exists in both the acute and delayed/chronic phases of conditioning. RIC induces pro-autophagy signaling but the pattern of responses varies depending on the phase, with the most complete portfolio of responses observed when RIC is administered chronically.

Editor: John Calvert, Emory University, United States of America

Funding: The authors have no support or funding to report.

Competing Interests: The authors have declared that no competing interests exist.

* Email: andrew.redington@sickkids.ca

⑨ These authors contributed equally to this work.

Introduction

The additional injury incurred as a result of reperfusion after prolonged coronary ischemia currently limits clinical strategies against myocardial ischemia-reperfusion (IR) injury. Despite a greater understanding of the mechanisms underlying IR injury, interventions aimed at improving post-ischemic cardiac function have been suboptimal [1]. A promising strategy involves exposing remote tissues to brief periods of sub-lethal ischemia, which protects the myocardium against damage during and after a subsequent prolonged ischemic insult, a phenomenon termed remote ischemic conditioning (RIC) [2]. Induced by brief periods of limb ischemia and reperfusion using a blood pressure cuff or tourniquet, RIC has been rapidly translated from animal models to proof-of-principle clinical trials in acute IR syndromes [3–5].

RIC induced by limb ischemia is a neuro-humoral stimulus resulting in the release of circulating cytoprotective factors which induce protection against IR injury in distant organs. The mechanisms underlying RIC-induced cytoprotection have recently been reviewed in detail ([2]), but key components of cardioprotection involve stimulation of g-protein coupled receptors on the cell-surface, induction of a intracellular kinase signaling, opening of potassium-ATP (K^+_{ATP}) channels and preventing the formation of the mitochondrial transition pore (mPTP). The cardioprotection afforded by RIC is usually described as biphasic. There is an early/acute cytoprotective phase, termed the first window (1W) of protection, which essentially recapitulates the changes in intracellular kinase signaling pathways previously described for local ischemic conditioning (IC) [6–9]. Approximately twenty-four hours after the original stimulus, a 'second window' (2W) of protection emerges, that likely relates to transcriptional changes induced within the cell [10]. While the effects of the delayed response may be less robust, there is emerging clinical [11,12] and experimental [13,14] evidence that RIC, repeated over time (chronic RIC-3W), may have additional disease-modifying effects. For example, chronic RIC administered for 28 consecutive days in rats was associated with a reduction in post-myocardial infarction (MI) left ventricular remodeling and improved survival at 12 weeks [14].

The exact mechanisms underlying these responses remain to be delineated precisely, however there is emerging evidence for a key role of autophagy signaling in the adaptive and maladaptive responses to IR injury [15]. Indeed, several studies have highlighted a protective role of autophagy in myocardial IR injury. In one study, inhibition of mammalian target of rapamycin (mTOR), a known negative regulator of autophagy, led to a decrease in infarct size in mice [16]. A separate study using microarray analysis of mice that underwent chronic local IC, through repetitive coronary occlusion, revealed upregulation of genes associated with autophagy and the unfolded protein response [17,18]. The possible role of RIC in autophagy modulation remains unknown. We therefore studied in-vivo myocardial signaling and assessed cardioprotection in a mouse Langendorff isolated heart model, to examine autophagy responses in the acute, delayed and chronic phases of cardioprotection afforded by RIC.

Materials and Methods

All animal protocols were approved by the Animal Care and Use Committee of the Hospital for Sick Children in Toronto and conformed to the *Guide for the Care and Use of Laboratory Animals* published by the National Institutes of Health (NIH publication No. 85-23, revised 1996).

Induction of remote ischemic conditioning (RIC)

RIC was induced by four cycles of 5 minutes of limb ischemia (by tourniquet tightened at the inguinal level) followed by 5 minutes of reperfusion as previously described [6]. Distal limb pallor was observed during occlusion, followed rapidly by brisk reactive hyperemia during reperfusion.

Experimental design

C57/BL6 male mice (8–10 weeks old, N = 69) were habituated to handling by experimenters for ten minutes a day two days prior to induction of RIC. Control animals were treated identically with the tourniquet applied around the leg but not tightened and were handled for the same duration as RIC.

Myocardial autophagy signaling

Mice were divided in to three treatment categories based on conditioning modality which include: acute/first window (1W), delayed/second window (2W) and chronic/third window (3W). Within each category, mice were further stratified to receive RIC according to the protocol described or control treatment consisting solely of handling without applying transient ischemia to the limb. The groups include, group 1 (1W control), group 2 (1W RIC), group 3 (2W control), group 4 (2W RIC), group 5 (3W control) and group 6 (3W RIC).

At the end of each experiment, mice were anesthetized with pentobarbital (60 mg/kg via an intra-peritoneal injection) and their hearts were isolated for further study of protein expression using western blot analysis or cardiac function using a Langendorff isolated heart model of global ischemia. To assess the first window

of RIC, mice were sacrificed fifteen minutes after the end of the RIC or handling. Mice in the second window groups underwent a similar protocol but were sacrificed 24 hours after handling or RIC. To assess the chronic effects of repeated RIC, mice underwent 9 days of repeated limb ischemia or handling and were sacrificed twenty-four hours after the last day of treatment. (See figure 1 for experimental protocol).

Immunoblotting

Following RIC or control treatment, mouse hearts were excised and cut transversely to separate the atrium and ventricle. Ventricular tissue was then used for western blot experiments. Stored heart tissue was homogenized using lysis buffer (1% NP40, 150 mM NaCl, 1 mM EGTA, 1 mM EDTA, 2.5 mM $Na_4O_7P_2$, 1 mM β-glycerolphosphate, 1 mM Na_3VO_4 and a cocktail of protease inhibitors (Roche)). The homogenate was centrifuged at 10,000×g at 4°C for 30 min to obtain cytosolic protein. An equal amount of protein (30 μg protein) from each sample was separated by 10% SDS–polyacrylamide gels and transferred onto nitrocellulose membranes (Bio-Rad). Membranes were incubated with Atg5 (catalog #8540 – Cell Signaling Tech.), phosphor-mTOR (Ser2481) (catalog #2974 – Cell Signaling Tech.), beclin-1 (catalog #3495 – Cell Signaling Tech.), p62 (catalog #5114 – Cell Signaling Tech.), LC3I/II (NB100-2331 – Novus Biologicals), phospho-AMPK (Thr 172) (catalog #2531 – Cell Signaling Tech.), cathepsin L (catalog #AF1515 – R&D Systems) or GAPDH (catalog #G8795 - Sigma-Aldrich Inc.) overnight at 4°C. The membranes were then washed and subsequently incubated with peroxidase-conjugated secondary antibody (Santa Cruz, CA) and detected with the ECL plus Detection Kit (Amersham, Piscataway, NJ). Immunoblots were scanned using an Odyssey LI-COR and quantified using Image Studio (Ver 2.1).

Assessment of cardioprotection in mouse Langendorff preparation using global ischemia/reperfusion injury

Mice from each study group were assessed for cardiac function following global ischemia-reperfusion injury. After completion of experimental intervention, mice received heparin (200 IU, i.p. Sigma) and were anesthetized with pentobarbital (60 mg/kg, i.p. Ceva Sante animale) and then intubated and ventilated. Hearts were rapidly excised by bilateral thoracotomy, placed in ice-cold buffer and the aorta cannulated with a 20-gauge metal cannula. Isolated hearts were mounted on the Langendorff perfusion apparatus (Radnoti Technologies Inc., Monrovia, CA, USA), and perfused under non-recirculating conditions at a constant pressure of 80 mmHg with 37°C Krebs–Henseleit buffer (KHB) (consisting of the following in mmol/L: NaCl 120.0, $NaHCO_3$ 25.0, KCl 4.7, $MgSO_4$ 1.2, KH_2PO_4 1.2, $CaCl_2$ 2.5, EDTA 0.5 and glucose 15). The left atrial appendage was removed, and a balloon, made with saran wrap and PE60 polyethylene tubing, was inserted into left ventricular (LV) through the mitral valve and was connected to a pressure transducer. The balloon was inflated with water to adjust left ventricular end-diastolic pressure (LVEDP) to 7–10 mmHg at the beginning of the experiment and the volume kept constant for the duration of the study. After a 20 min stabilization period, subjected to 30 min of no-flow global ischemia followed by 60 min of reperfusion. Hemodynamic measurements, including heart rate (HR), peak left ventricular pressure (LVP), maximum rate of contraction (+dP/dtmax), maximum rate of relaxation (−dP/dtmin), and LVEDP will be recorded on a data acquisition system (PowerLab, ADInstruments) throughout the procedure. The LV developed pressure (LVDP) was calculated as the difference between the systolic and end-diastolic LV pressures.

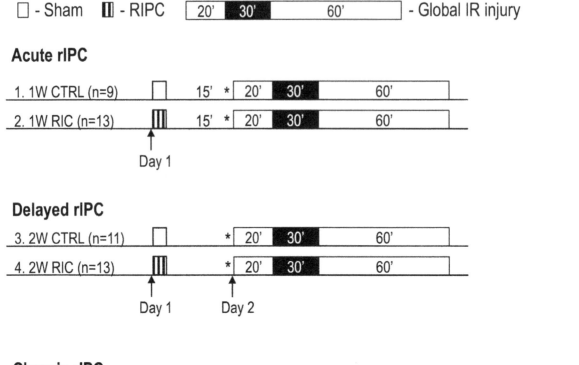

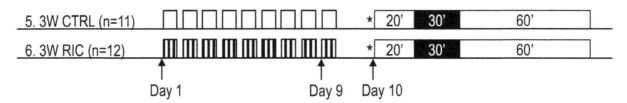

Figure 1. Schematic summary of RIC treatment groups and experimental protocol. Control groups 1, 3 and 5 were left untreated and underwent handling alone without RIC. Treatment groups 2, 4, and 6 underwent RIC via four cycles of 5 min of femoral artery occlusion, followed by 5 min of reperfusion. Following the treatment protocol, mouse hearts were removed (denoted by *), mounted on a isovolumic Langendorff perfusion apparatus, and subjected to 20 min of equilibration, 30 min of no-flow global ischemia and 60 min of reperfusion. The infarcted area was visualized using TTC following global ischemia in each group.

Measurement of infarct size

After reperfusion the hearts were weighed and frozen at $-80°C$. The frozen heart was transversely cut into six 1-mm thick slices using a Mouse Heart Slicer Matrix (Zivic Instruments) which were stained with 1.25% 2,3,5-triphenyltetrazolium chloride (TTC) in 200 mM Tris/HCL solution (pH 7.4) for 15 min in a 37°C water bath. After staining, heart slices were fixed for 2–4 hours in 10% neutral buffered formaldehyde. Both sides of each slice was then photographed at 1200 DPI resolution using a computer scanner (CanoScan 4400F). Images were processed with Adobe Photoshop CS2 software to measure infarct size and left-ventricle area using automated planimetry. Viable myocardium stains red due to the reaction of tetrazolium salts with NADH and dehydrogenase enzymes while infarcted tissue, that does not possess enzymes, appears pale. Infarct sizes of each slice were expressed as the percentage of the total left ventricle area.

Statistical Analysis

The analysis method for array data is discussed previously. For all other comparisons, statistical significance was determined using one-way ANOVA, followed by post hoc testing (Newman–Keuls)

where appropriate. Values of $P \leq 0.05$ were considered statistically significant. Data are shown as mean ± S.E. (standard error).

Results

Chronic RIC reduces infarct size following global ischemia

Myocardial infarct size was assessed by TTC staining (figure 2). As previously shown in other studies we observed a significant ($P < 0.05$) reduction in 1W RIC treated mice (32.9±2.6%). compared with 1W controls (45.1±3.4%) We also observed protection against infarction after delayed and chronic preconditioning. Both 2W RIC (30.6±5.1%) and 3W RIC (31.3±3.4%) treated mice had significantly ($P < 0.05$) reduced infarct sizes compared to their respective control groups, 2W control (58.6±5.0%) and 3W control (48.8±4.8%).

Chronic RIC protects post-ischemic left ventricular function

We also examined the effects of acute and chronic RIC on left ventricular function using an isolated Langendorff heart model of global ischemia. As previously shown, acute 1W RIC ameliorates

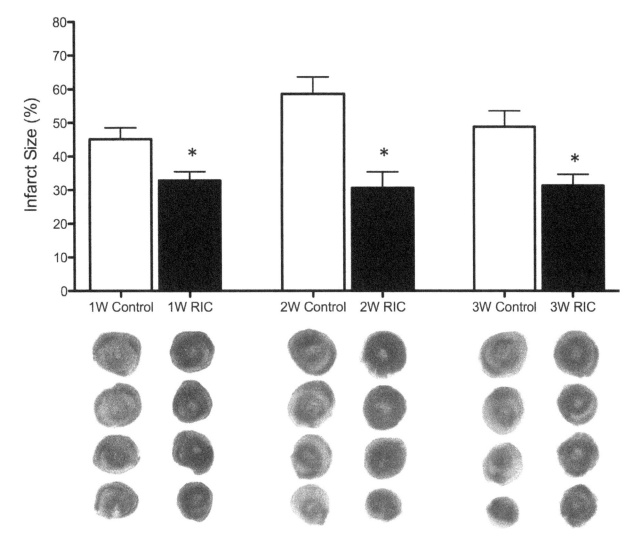

Figure 2. RIC reduces heart infarct size in the acute, delayed and chronic phases of conditioning. (A) Infarct size expressed as percentage of left ventricle area for each of the treatment groups. Values are means ± S.E.M. An (*) denotes a statistically significant difference compared to controls (P<0.05). (B) Representative cross-sections of mouse hearts from each of the treatment groups after I/R and staining with TTC to visualize the infarcted area.

the effects of ischemia-reperfusion injury on the heart with improvements in LVDP and LVEDP. Measured as a percentage of baseline function, we found that after 60 minutes of reperfusion, there was a significantly (P<0.05) greater level of recovery in developed pressure (figure 3A) in 1W RIC mice compared to controls (98.0±4.9% vs. 67.9±4.7%). Consistent with previous reports we also observed marked differences in diastolic recovery after RIC during the first window of treatment (figure 3B), as 1W RIC mice had a significantly (P<0.001) attenuated increase in diastolic pressure (LVEDP) compared to 1W controls (11.9±1.1 mmHg vs. 34.9±5.7 mmHg) after 60 minutes of reperfusion.

Interestingly we showed for the first time that delayed and chronic RIC delivered daily for nine days produces similar cardioprotective benefits as acute 1W RIC (figure 4 and 5 A, B). LVDP was significantly greater (P<0.05) in both 2W and 3W RIC mice compared to the untreated controls (2W RIC – 87.5±5.5% vs. 63.2±8.2% and 3W RIC - 93.6±4.1% vs. 62. 3±6.0%) after global ischemia and 60 minutes of reperfusion. Furthermore, we also observed a significant attenuation of post-infarct diastolic

pressures after delayed and chronic preconditioning compared to controls (2W – 154±2.6 mmHg vs. 38.4±5.4 mmHg and 3W RIC - 16. 9±2.8 mmHg vs. 40.1±5.6 mmHg) at the end of reperfusion.

RIC enhances autophagy-signaling pathways

A main objective of the study was to examine the effects of acute, delayed and chronic RIC on components of cellular autophagy signaling pathways, including AMPK, mTOR, beclin-1, Atg5, LC3II/I, cathepsin L and p62. Using western blot analysis, we assessed the protein expression of each signaling component in each modality of preconditioning.

Acute conditioning induced a significant (P<0.05) increase in p-AMPK levels – a positive regulator of autophagy activated during energy depletion - (1.9±0.1 – fold increase compared to control) and a concomitant significant decrease in the phosphorylated and activated form of its downstream target molecule, mTOR – a Ser/Thr kinase and negative regulator of autophagy (0.5±0.1 – fold decrease compared to control) (figure 6A, B). In addition we observed nearly a three-fold increase (P<0.05) in microtubule

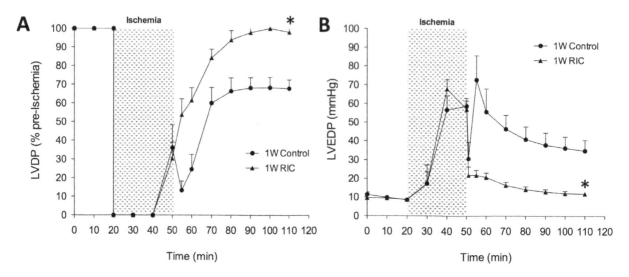

Figure 3. Acute, first window RIC improves post-ischemic cardiac performance in isolated perfused hearts. Representative LVDP (A) and LVEDP (B) tracings are shown from 1W control and RIC groups. Left ventricular developed pressure (LVDP) is expressed as a percentage of pre-ischemic baseline values and left ventricular end diastolic pressure (LVEDP) is expressed in mm Hg. Values are expressed as means ± S.E.M. An (*) denotes a statistically significant difference (P<0.05) compared to control groups after 60 minutes of reperfusion.

associated protein light chain 3, LC3II/I ratio in 1W RIC mice – a critical component of autophagosome membrane formation (2.7±0.4 – fold increase compared to controls). There were no significant differences observed in the other components of autophagy between 1W RIC and control groups.

During delayed preconditioning the acute activation of AMPK is lost with a significant decrease (P<0.05) in its phosphorylated protein expression compared to 2W control mice (0.4±0.2 – fold decrease compared to controls). Interestingly, the inhibition of mTOR is sustained during delayed preconditioning (0.6±0.1 – fold decrease compared to control) (P<0.05) (figure 7A, B). However, we found that autophagy signaling may not be a predominant feature of delayed/second window preconditioning. This is highlighted with a significant (P<0.05) decrease in the expression of beclin-1, a cellular complex important for initiating

autophagy (P<0.05) in 2W RIC mice (0.6±0.1 – fold decrease compared to controls). Other proteins involved in autophagy showed no significant differences between 2W RIC and control groups.

Similar to both acute and delayed preconditioning, we found that phosphorylated-mTOR expression remains decreased in 3W mice (0.7±0.1 – fold decrease compared to control, P = 0.055). This inhibition is likely achieved through a non-AMPK mechanism, as AMPK kinase levels trended towards decreased activation (0.6±0.1 – fold decrease compared to controls). However, unlike delayed preconditioning, it appears that the autophagy machinery is reactivated following chronic stimulation. We observed increases in the levels proteins associated with autophagy signaling, including LC3II/I (1.4±0.2 – fold increase compared to control) (P = 0.0587), Atg5 – an important autophagy-related protein

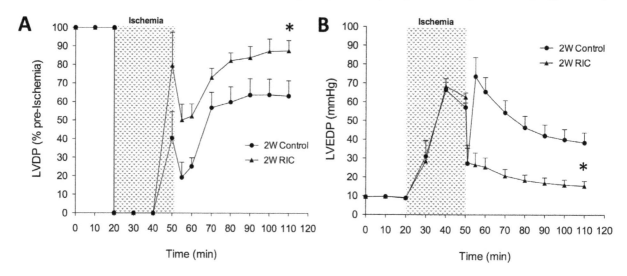

Figure 4. Delayed, second window RIC improves post-ischemic cardiac performance in isolated perfused hearts. Representative LVDP (A) and LVEDP (B) tracings are shown from 2W control and RIC groups. Left ventricular developed pressure (LVDP) is expressed as a percentage of pre-ischemic baseline values and left ventricular end diastolic pressure (LVEDP) is expressed in mm Hg. Values are expressed as means ± S.E.M. An (*) denotes a statistically significant difference (P<0.05) compared to control groups after 60 minutes of reperfusion.

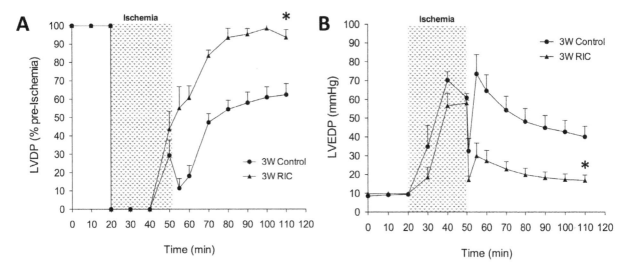

Figure 5. Chronic, third window RIC improves post-ischemic cardiac performance in isolated perfused hearts. Representative LVDP (A) and LVEDP (B) tracings are shown from 3W control and RIC groups. Left ventricular developed pressure (LVDP) is expressed as a percentage of pre-ischemic baseline values and left ventricular end diastolic pressure (LVEDP) is expressed in mm Hg. Values are expressed as means ± S.E.M. An (*) denotes a statistically significant difference (P<0.05) compared to control groups after 60 minutes of reperfusion.

$(1.6\pm0.2$ – fold increase compared to control) (P<0.05) and cathepsin L, $(2.2\pm0.3$ – fold increase compared to control) (P< 0.05) in 3W RIC. P62, a sensor of proteotoxicity consumed by the active autophagosome, was unchanged during each preconditioning modality (figure 8A, B).

Kinase responses in second window and chronic RIC

We have previously reported that RIC acutely induces a portfolio of protective intracellular kinase signaling (e.g. PKCε, Akt, Erk), similar to that seen in local IC. The role of kinase signaling in delayed RIC responses appears much less significant. We found no significant differences in the expression of phosphorylated-Akt and phosphorylated-Erk in 2W RIC mice. Chronic preconditioning was associated with a small but significant (P<0.05) increase in the expression of p-Akt $(1.8\pm0.3$ – fold increase compared to control), but there was no significant change in p-Erk expression. (figure 9A, B).

Discussion

To our knowledge, this is the first study to examine the effects of acute, delayed and chronic RIC on autophagy signaling in the myocardium. Our data show that repeated RIC leads to downregulation of mTOR and subsequent upregulation of pro-autophagy proteins, and is associated with levels of cardioprotection similar to that seen with the acute stimulus.

Delayed and chronic RIC reduce infarction and improve cardiac functional recovery

The acute phase of cardioprotection induced by either local or remote ischemic preconditioning is associated with a well-established portfolio of intracellular kinase responses, which function to prevent mitochondrial-induced cell death. The delayed and chronic mechanisms of preconditioning similarly promote cell survival but have been suggested to do so primarily through changes in gene transcription and *de novo* protein synthesis that modify both the local and systemic responses (e.g. inflammation) to IR injury. The delayed response to RIC, while documented to be present in several organs, has been relatively sparsely studied in

experimental and clinical studies of cardioprotection [19–22]. However, in a clinical trial of children undergoing cardiac surgery, delayed RIC was shown to reduce biomarkers of cardiac injury, and modify the inflammatory response [23]. A very recent experimental study in a rat model found that delayed RIC provided additional cardioprotection over and above that seen with acute sevoflurane-induced cardioprotection, via enhanced HO-1 expression via Nrf2 translocation [24]. There are no prior data examining the myocardial effects of repeated RIC, delivered for daily for 10 days (as in our present studies of 'chronic' cardioprotection), although we have previously demonstrated that such a regime induces sustained reduction in human neutrophil adhesiveness and phagocytotic activity, which may themselves play a role in modulating responses to IR injury [25]. For this reason, we chose to study the cardioprotective effect of this regime in an ex-vivo Langendorff model of IR injury, to avoid potential confounding effects. Consequently, we showed that delayed and chronic RIC preserve post-ischemic cardiac function to a similar degree as acute RIC, with improvements in both post-ischemic LVDP and LVEDP, but that the underlying patterns of kinase and autophagy signaling differs.

The role of autophagy signaling in cardioprotection against IR injury

Autophagy has been identified as a pro-survival strategy utilized by cardiomyocytes during IR injury to prevent protein aggregation and cell death. Ischemia-reperfusion injury results in a battery of biochemical, metabolic and structural changes in the heart. At the onset of ischemia, oxidative phosphorylation is arrested resulting in an abrupt decline in ATP levels and eventually a breakdown of cell homeostasis [1]. The ensuing change in ion distribution across the cell and the accumulation of reactive oxygen species (ROS) damages the cells protein machinery [26]. Restoration of flow during reperfusion exacerbates these response and leads to cell dysfunction and eventual death. Activation of autophagy can help to mitigate the damage of IR injury and support cell function through the clearing damaged protein aggregates, removal of damaged ROS-producing mitochondria and through the recycling of macromolecules for use in cell repair.

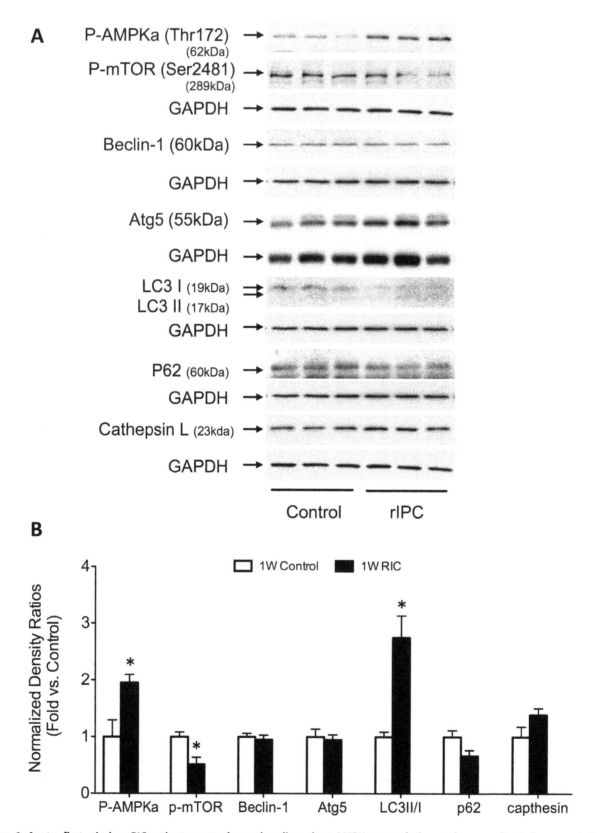

Figure 6. Acute, first window RIC activates autophagy signaling via p-AMPK upregulation and concomitant downregulation of mTOR. (A) Western blots for autophagy related signaling proteins. (B) Quantification of the protein fold change in 1W RIC compared to 1W controls. Values are means ± S.E.M. n = 6–8 per group. An (*) denotes a statistically significant difference (P<0.05) compared to control. (P-: phospho-).

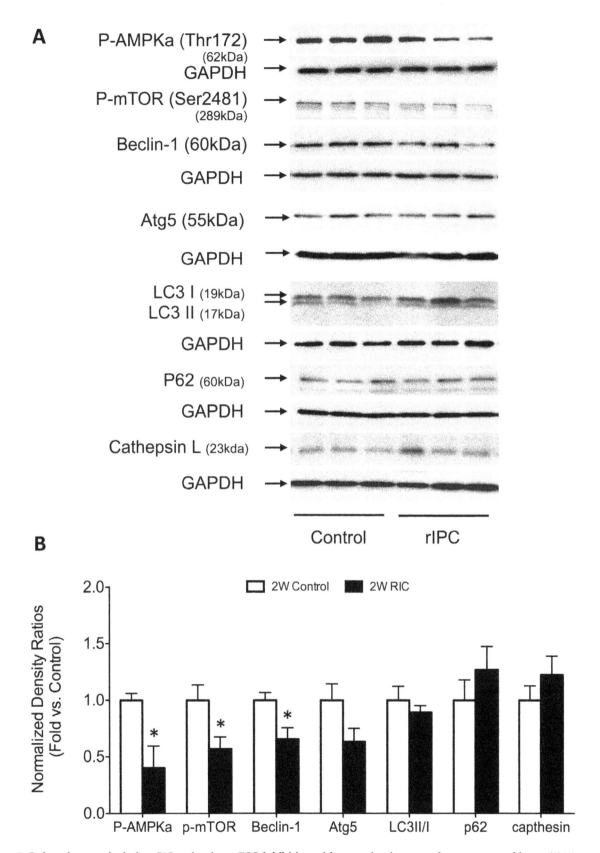

Figure 7. Delayed, second window RIC maintains mTOR inhibition without activating autophagosome machinery. (A) Western blots for autophagy related signaling proteins. (B) Quantification of the protein fold change in 2W RIC compared to 2W controls. Values are means ± S.E.M. n = 6–8 per group. An (*) denotes a statistically significant difference (P<0.05) compared to control. (P-: phospho-).

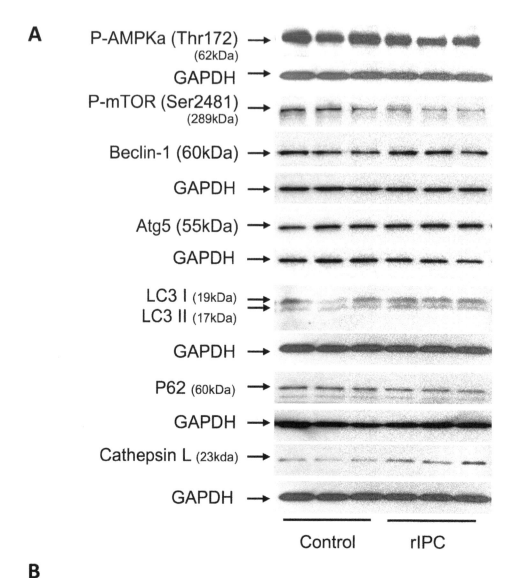

A

P-AMPKa (Thr172) →
(62kDa)

GAPDH →

P-mTOR (Ser2481) →
(289kDa)

Beclin-1 (60kDa) →

GAPDH →

Atg5 (55kDa) →

GAPDH →

LC3 I (19kDa) →
LC3 II (17kDa) →

GAPDH →

P62 (60kDa) →

GAPDH →

Cathepsin L (23kda) →

GAPDH →

Control   rIPC

B

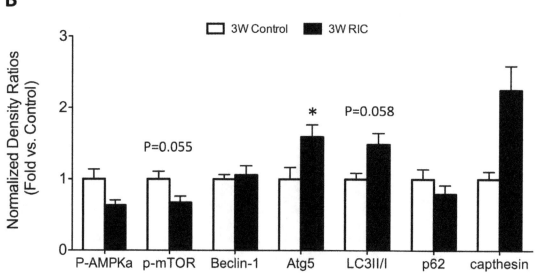

Figure 8. Chronic, third window RIC increases the expression of autophagosome proteins, LC3I/II and Atg5. (A) Western blots for autophagy related signaling proteins. (B) Quantification of the protein fold change in 3W RIC compared to 3W controls. Values are means ± S.E.M. n = 6–8 per group. An (*) denotes a statistically significant difference (P<0.05) compared to control. (P-: phospho-).

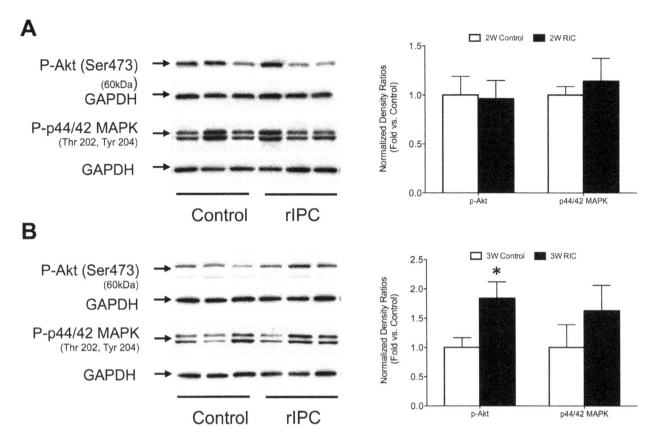

Figure 9. Chronic RIC activates kinase signaling in mouse myocardium. Western blots for phospho-Akt and phospho-Erk (p44/42 MAPK) in 2W(A) and 3W (B) RIC and control groups. Quantification of the protein fold change is shown in the graph to the right of blots. Values are means ± S.E.M. n = 6–8 per group. An (*) denotes a statistically significant difference (P<0.05) compared to control. (P-: phospho-).

Several studies have highlighted the benefits of autophagy during the acute and chronic phases of ischemic injury. For instance, it was found that treatment with autophagosome-lysosomal fusion inhibitor, bafilomycin A1, significantly aggravated post-infarction adverse remodeling in a mouse model of in-vivo IR injury [27]. In the same study it was found that treatment with rapamycin, an inhibitor of mTOR and a pro-autophagic stimulant was associated with improved functional and histological outcomes during the sub-acute and chronic post-infarct phases [27].

It has been suggested that cardioprotective strategies, such as ischemic preconditioning, can enhance autophagy to protect the myocardium from the deleterious effects of IR injury and its associated long-term sequalae [15,28]. While this concept has already been demonstrated in investigations of local IPC, the present study is the first to show that RIC can also augment autophagy as part of its cardioprotective repertoire. Preconditioning may activate the autophagic machinery through one of two mechanisms, which may be differentially activated during the early and delayed/chronic phases. These include (1) PKC- or rising AMP- induced AMPK activation and subsequent mTOR inhibition or (2) Beclin-1 class III PI3K complex formation.

RIC and autophagy

In the present study we show that factors involved in initiating autophagy and subsequent assembly of the autophagosome are induced as early as the first window of remote preconditioning. Within 1 hour of the RIC stimulus, there was a significant rise in the level of phosphorylated-AMPK, inhibition of the downstream regulator mTOR, and increases in LC3II/I, key regulators

involved in autophagosome assembly. Increased AMPK during local ischemia has previously been implicated as an important mechanism in cytosolic ATP maintenance [29]. It is ubiquitously expressed in metabolically active tissues, such as skeletal and cardiac muscle, functioning as an intracellular fuel sensor that is activated upon depletion of energy stores [30]. During IR injury, intracellular stores of ATP are rapidly utilized and are not replenished with decreasing glucose supply. Depleting ATP levels give rise to increasing cytoplasmic adenosine monophosphate (AMP), an end product of ATP utilization and a potent signal for AMPK [31].

It is interesting that remote ischemia induces a similar response in AMPK signaling, even though the myocardium itself is not rendered ischemic. However, activation of AMPK has been previously implicated in the cardioprotective effects of IPC through a PKC-induced AMPK up-regulation of glucose transporters at the cell membrane [32]. In addition to enhancing mechanisms that maintain ATP production, AMPK serves as a master regulator of the autophagy pathway through deactivation of mTOR, itself a negative regulator of autophagy [28]. Interestingly, while we showed in the present study that RIC makes use of AMPK in the early phases of protection, its up-regulation does not appear to be a feature of the delayed and chronic phases. This observation fits with our current understanding of the later phases of RIC. Acute RIC is mediated primarily through activation of the reperfusion injury salvage kinases (RISK), which include the PI3k-Akt-PKC-Erk signaling cascade [33]. Therefore it is possible that the acute kinase response involving PKC leads to AMPK activation through a non-ATP depleting mechanism.

While initiation of autophagic mechanisms occurs during the acute phase of preconditioning, there is prior evidence suggesting it is primarily a phenomenon of long-term cardioprotection. Indeed, autophagy has previously implicated as a factor of local cardioprotection in the chronically preconditioned myocardium. A study by Yan et al. examining the effects of repetitive coronary stenosis in pigs found a marked increase in autophagic protein expression (cathepsin B and D, Beclin 1 and LC3-II) after six episodes of stenosis delivered 12 hourly over 3 days, compared to just one [34]. Further studies by the same group confirmed local conditioning to lead to up-regulation of autophagy with increases in the transcription of autophagy-related proteins [17,18].

In the present study, we showed that the early significant increase in kinase signaling is substantially lost after ten days of repeated limb ischemia, and there is up-regulation of the expression of LC3-II and cathepsin L (a lysosomal cysteine protease involved in autophagy signaling). Additionally, we found a significant increase in autophagic machinery protein Atg5, a rate-limiting protein involved in autophagosome formation, in chronically preconditioned mice. LC3-II and Atg5 are both critical for the final maturation of the autophagosome [35] and their increase after repeated transient ischemia provides further support that autophagy may be a treatment paradigm of long term conditioning. In a human study examining the effects of RIC in patients undergoing coronary artery bypass grafting (CABG), it was found that only LC3II/I was elevated at reperfusion, although other markers of autophagy signaling (Atg5) were unaffected [36]. These findings are consistent with those generated in this study in which we found that not all the autophagosomal components are fully formed during the acute phase of preconditioning. That said, the mechanisms underlying how chronic RIC augments the autophagic machinery remain unclear. It is possible that activation occurs through a beclin-1 mediated process similar to local IPC. However, our results show only a slight increase in beclin-1 expression after chronic RIC. Interestingly we showed that mTOR inhibition is sustained during both the delayed and chronic phases of RIC, the latter without a concomitant increase in AMPK, suggesting that other signaling pathways involved with the preconditioning phenotype may be operating to limit its function. Our data therefore provide proof-of-principle upon which future investigations should be based.

Another measure of autophagic flux in addition to LC3-II and Atg5 is the level of p62 within the cell. As previously discussed, p62 is an adaptor protein that binds to ubiquinated protein products destined for consumption by the autophagsome machinery. As such, accumulation of p62 can be used as a marker of proteotoxicty buildup within the cell and a decrease in the function of autophagic clearance mechanisms [26]. Conversely, low levels of p62 imply active intracellular phagocytsosis. However, given that RIC is a non-lethal stimulus, there is likely no build up of protein aggregates, which may provide some explanation for the low levels of p62 seen during each phase of conditioning examined in this study.

While the underlying mechanisms remain to be elucidated in future studies, there are important implications of our data regarding chronic autophagy signaling. For example, inhibition of mTOR signaling has been shown to be beneficial for remodeling of the post-infarcted myocardium. In a study by Buss et al., it was shown that 28 days of mTOR inhibition using everolimus following experimental myocardial infarction was associated with improvements in LV function and end-diastolic diameters [37]. This was also associated with reduced infarction and an increase in

cellular autophagy mechanisms in the injury zone. The authors concluded that inhibition of mTOR-mediated protein synthesis was critical for preventing pathological LV hypertrophy. The long-term activation of autophagy with mTOR inhibition and its effects on minimizing adverse LV remodeling is consistent with a previous study conducted by our group in which we showed similar benefits with chronic RIC for 28 days after MI in a rat model [14]. While autophagy wasn't directly examined in that study, our current the findings showing chronically conditioned myocardium induces upregulation of autophagy may provide a mechanistic explanation.

Another interesting finding generated from this study involves a potential interaction between autophagy related proteins and elements of the RISK pathway. We observed that chronic RIC recapitulated elements of the RISK pathway that are active components in the acute phases of protection. Specifically, we found an increase in the levels of Akt after nine days of remote conditioning. This finding suggests the growing hypothesis that chronic RIC utilizes multiple signaling mechanisms to generate the cardioprotective phenotype [18]. Indeed, recently Martinez-Lopez et al. has shown that the cell proliferation regulator, extracellular signal regulated kinase (ERK), which is an important component of the RISK pathway of preconditioning, localizes with autophagy proteins (ATG) [38]. Furthermore, their study shows that deletion of Atg5 results in decreased ERK activity. Our results suggest that a similar interaction may exist with, the serine threonine kinase, Akt. The interactions between RISK signaling and autophagy proteins and their relation to the cardioprotective effects of preconditioning warrant further study to better understand the mechanisms various mechanisms at work in the chronically conditioned heart.

There are some limitations to the current study. Firstly, it important to note that while the current findings are the first to examine the existence of autophagy signaling in the cardioprotection of RIC, we did not examine the functional significance of each signal. We have generated a unique set of preliminary observations, which implicate autophagy in the cellular mechanisms of preconditioning for future studies. These may involve investigating the effects of upregulation or inhibition of autophagy on the cardioprotection granted by RIC. Secondly, the findings generated in this study are cardiac specific and may not apply in other organs (e.g. brain, liver kidney), particularly with respect to mTOR activation. For example, a study examining the effects of RIC on the hippocampus after bilateral carotid artery occlusion found that an increase in mTOR activation was associated with neural cell protection [39]. Furthermore, inhibiting mTOR with rapamycin treatment blocked the effects of RIC. These incongruent findings have also been shown in studies of cardioprotection after RIC. In a study of local ischemic preconditioning it was found that mTOR is activated through the actions of Erk-P70S6K. It appears that preconditioning can operate via two available RISK pathways, the PI3K-Akt or the Erk-P70S6k-mTOR pathway [16]. Interestingly both pathways exhibit cross talk in that increased activation of one pathway leads to inhibition of other RISK signaling cascades. In the present study, it appears that RIC predominantly activates a PI3K-Akt pathway, which, in addition to AMPK activation, leads to an overall decrease in mTOR activation, permitting the initiation of autophagy.

In conclusion, we showed for the first time that a similar level of cardioprotection following transient ischemia exists in both the acute and delayed phases of preconditioning. Furthermore, chronically preconditioned mice exhibit cardioprotection against both tissue damage and ventricular dysfunction after ischemia-reperfusion injury similar to that observed with an isolated stimulus. In addition to traditional kinase signaling pathways (e.g. RISK), we identified a potential role for autophagy in the cellular mechanism of preconditioning, which may have broader implications in the protection against post-infarction left-ventricular remodeling and dysfunction.

References

1. Yellon DM, Hausenloy DJ (2007) Myocardial Reperfusion Injury. N Engl J Med 357: 1121–1135. doi:10.1056/NEJMra071667.
2. Hausenloy DJ, Yellon DM (2008) Remote ischaemic preconditioning: underlying mechanisms and clinical application. Cardiovascular Research 79: 377–386. doi:10.1093/cvr/cvn114.
3. Venugopal V, Hausenloy DJ, Ludman A, Di Salvo C, Kolvekar S, et al. (2009) Remote ischaemic preconditioning reduces myocardial injury in patients undergoing cardiac surgery with cold-blood cardioplegia: a randomised controlled trial. Heart 95: 1567–1571. doi:10.1136/hrt.2008.155770.
4. Jenkins DP, Pugsley WB, Alkhulaifi AM, Kemp M, Hooper J, et al. (1997) Ischaemic preconditioning reduces troponin T release in patients undergoing coronary artery bypass surgery. Heart 77: 314–318. doi:10.1136/hrt.77.4.314.
5. Thielmann M, Kottenberg E, Boengler K, Raffelsieper C, Neuhaeuser M, et al. (2010) Remote ischemic preconditioning reduces myocardial injury after coronary artery bypass surgery with crystalloid cardioplegic arrest. Basic Res Cardiol 105: 657–664. doi:10.1007/s00395-010-0104-5.
6. Li J, Xuan W, Yan R, Tropak MB, Jean St Michel E, et al. (2011) Remote preconditioning provides potent cardioprotection via PI3K/Akt activation and is associated with nuclear accumulation of β-catenin. Clin Sci 120: 451–462. doi:10.1042/CS20100466.
7. Hassouna A, Hassouna A, Matata BM, Galiñanes M (2004) PKC- is upstream and PKC- is downstream of mitoKATP channels in the signal transduction pathway of ischemic preconditioning of human myocardium. AJP: Cell Physiology 287: C1418–C1425. doi:10.1152/ajpcell.00144.2004.
8. Hausenloy DJ (2004) Ischemic preconditioning protects by activating prosurvival kinases at reperfusion. AJP: Heart and Circulatory Physiology 288: H971–H976. doi:10.1152/ajpheart.00374.2004.
9. Reid EA (2005) In vivo adenosine receptor preconditioning reduces myocardial infarct size via subcellular ERK signaling. AJP: Heart and Circulatory Physiology 288: H2253–H2259. doi:10.1152/ajpheart.01009.2004.
10. Bolli R (2000) The Late Phase of Preconditioning. Circulation Research 87: 972–983. doi:10.1161/01.RES.87.11.972.
11. Meng R, Asmaro K, Meng L, Liu Y, Ma C, et al. (2012) Upper limb ischemic preconditioning prevents recurrent stroke in intracranial arterial stenosis. Neurology 79: 1853–1861. doi:10.1212/WNL.0b013e318271f76a.
12. Hougaard KD, Hjort N, Zeidler D, Sorensen L, Norgaard A, et al. (2013) Remote Ischemic Perconditioning as an Adjunct Therapy to Thrombolysis in Patients With Acute Ischemic Stroke: A Randomized Trial. Stroke 45: 159–167. doi:10.1161/STROKEAHA.113.001346.
13. Hahn CD, Manlhiot C, Schmidt MR, Nielsen TT, Redington AN (2011) Remote Ischemic Per-Conditioning: A Novel Therapy for Acute Stroke? Stroke 42: 2960–2962. doi:10.1161/STROKEAHA.111.622340.
14. Wei M, Xin P, Li S, Tao J, Li Y, et al. (2011) Repeated Remote Ischemic Postconditioning Protects Against Adverse Left Ventricular Remodeling and Improves Survival in a Rat Model of Myocardial Infarction. Circulation Research 108: 1220–1225. doi:10.1161/CIRCRESAHA.110.236190.
15. Yan W-J, Dong H-L, Xiong L-Z (2013) The protective roles of autophagy in ischemic preconditioning. Acta Pharmacol Sin 34: 636–643. doi:10.1038/aps.2013.18.
16. Khan S, Salloum F, Das A, Xi L, Vetrovec GW, et al. (2006) Rapamycin confers preconditioning-like protection against ischemia–reperfusion injury in isolated mouse heart and cardiomyocytes. Journal of Molecular and Cellular Cardiology 41: 256–264. doi:10.1016/j.yjmcc.2006.04.014.
17. Shen YT, Depre C, Yan L, Park JY, Tian B, et al. (2008) Repetitive Ischemia by Coronary Stenosis Induces a Novel Window of Ischemic Preconditioning. Circulation 118: 1961–1969. doi:10.1161/CIRCULATIONAHA.108.788240.
18. Depre C, Park JY, Shen YT, Zhao X, Qiu H, et al. (2010) Molecular mechanisms mediating preconditioning following chronic ischemia differ from those in classical second window. AJP: Heart and Circulatory Physiology 299: H752–H762. doi:10.1152/ajpheart.00147.2010.
19. Joo JD, Kim M, D'Agati VD, Lee HT (2006) Ischemic Preconditioning Provides Both Acute and Delayed Protection against Renal Ischemia and Reperfusion Injury in Mice. Journal of the American Society of Nephrology 17: 3115–3123. doi:10.1681/ASN.2006050424.
20. Romanque P, Díaz A, Tapia G, Uribe-Echevarría S, Videla LA, et al. (2010) Delayed Ischemic Preconditioning Protects Against Liver Ischemia–Reperfusion Injury In Vivo. Transplantation Proceedings 42: 1569–1575. doi:10.1016/j.transproceed.2009.11.052.
21. Dirnagl U, Becker K, Meisel A (2009) Preconditioning and tolerance against cerebral ischaemia: from experimental strategies to clinical use. The Lancet Neurology 8: 398–412. doi:10.1016/S1474-4422(09)70054-7.
22. Loukogeorgakis SP, Panagiotidou AT, Broadhead MW, Donald A, Deanfield JE, et al. (2005) Remote Ischemic Preconditioning Provides Early and Late Protection Against Endothelial Ischemia-Reperfusion Injury in Humans. Journal of the American College of Cardiology 46: 450–456. doi:10.1016/j.jacc.2005.04.044.
23. Wenwu Z, Debing Z, Renwei C, Jian L, Guangxian Y, et al. (2009) Limb Ischemic Preconditioning Reduces Heart and Lung Injury After an Open Heart Operation in Infants. Pediatr Cardiol 31: 22–29. doi:10.1007/s00246-009-9536-9.
24. Zhou C, Li H, Yao Y, Li L (2014) Delayed Remote Ischemic Preconditioning Produces an Additive Cardioprotection to Sevoflurane Postconditioning Through an Enhanced Heme Oxygenase 1 Level Partly Via Nuclear Factor Erythroid 2-Related Factor 2 Nuclear Translocation. Journal of Cardiovascular Pharmacology and Therapeutics. doi:10.1177/1074248414524479.
25. Shimizu M, Saxena P, Konstantinov IE, Cherepanov V, Cheung MMH, et al. (2010) Remote Ischemic Preconditioning Decreases Adhesion and Selectively Modifies Functional Responses of Human Neutrophils. Journal of Surgical Research 158: 155–161. doi:10.1016/j.jss.2008.08.010.
26. Gottlieb RA, Mentzer RM (2012) Autophagy: an affair of the heart. Heart Fail Rev 18: 575–584. doi:10.1007/s10741-012-9367-2.
27. Kanamori H, Takemura G, Goto K, Maruyama R, Tsujimoto A, et al. (2011) The role of autophagy emerging in postinfarction cardiac remodelling. Cardiovascular Research 91: 330–339. doi:10.1093/cvr/cvr073.
28. Przyklenk K, Reddy Undyala VV, Wider J, Sala-Mercado JA, Gottlieb RA, et al. (2011) Acute induction of autophagy as a novel strategy for cardioprotection: Getting to the heart of the matter. autophagy 7: 432–433. doi:10.4161/auto.7.4.14395.
29. Matsui Y, Takagi H, Qu X, Abdellatif M, Sakoda H, et al. (2007) Distinct Roles of Autophagy in the Heart During Ischemia and Reperfusion: Roles of AMP-Activated Protein Kinase and Beclin 1 in Mediating Autophagy. Circulation Research 100: 914–922. doi:10.1161/01.RES.0000261924.76669.36.
30. Hardie DG (2006) AMPK: A Key Sensor of Fuel and Energy Status in Skeletal Muscle. Physiology 21: 48–60. doi:10.1152/physiol.00044.2005.
31. Gustafsson AB, Gottlieb RA (2009) Autophagy in Ischemic Heart Disease. Circulation Research 104: 150–158. doi:10.1161/CIRCRESAHA.108.187427.
32. Nishino Y (2004) Ischemic preconditioning activates AMPK in a PKC-dependent manner and induces GLUT4 up-regulation in the late phase of cardioprotection. Cardiovascular Research 61: 610–619. doi:10.1016/j.cardiores.2003.10.022.
33. Hausenloy DJ, Lecour S, Yellon DM (2011) Reperfusion Injury Salvage Kinase and Survivor Activating Factor Enhancement Prosurvival Signaling Pathways in Ischemic Postconditioning: Two Sides of the Same Coin. Antioxidants & Redox Signaling 14: 893–907. doi:10.1089/ars.2010.3360.
34. Yan L, Vatner DE, Kim SJ, Ge H, Masurekar M, et al. (2005) Autophagy in chronically ischemic myocardium. Proceedings of the National Academy of Sciences 102: 13807–13812. doi:10.1073/pnas.0506843102.
35. Choi AMK, Ryter SW, Levine B (2013) Autophagy in Human Health and Disease. N Engl J Med 368: 651–662. doi:10.1056/NEJMra1205406.
36. Gedik N, Thielmann M, Kottenberg E, Peters J, Jakob H, et al. (2014) No Evidence for Activated Autophagy in Left Ventricular Myocardium at Early Reperfusion with Protection by Remote Ischemic Preconditioning in Patients Undergoing Coronary Artery Bypass Grafting. PLoS ONE 9: e96567. doi:10.1371/journal.pone.0096567.
37. Buss SJ, Muenz S, Riffel JH, Malekar P, Hagenmueller M, et al. (2009) Beneficial Effects of Mammalian Target of Rapamycin Inhibition on Left Ventricular Remodeling After Myocardial Infarction. Journal of the American College of Cardiology 54: 2435–2446. doi:10.1016/j.jacc.2009.08.031.
38. Martinez-Lopez N, Athonvarangkul D, Mishall P, Sahu S, Singh R (2013) Autophagy proteins regulate ERK phosphorylation. Nature Communications 4. doi:10.1038/ncomms3799.
39. Zare Mehrjerdi F, Aboutaleb N, Habibey R, Ajami M, Soleimani M, et al. (2013) Increased phosphorylation of mTOR is involved in remote ischemic preconditioning of hippocampus in mice. Brain Research 1526: 94–101. doi:10.1016/j.brainres.2013.06.018.

Author Contributions

Conceived and designed the experiments: SR NC MS JL AR. Performed the experiments: SR NC CW MS WS JL NG. Analyzed the data: SR JL AR NG. Contributed to the writing of the manuscript: SR NC.

13

Protection of Ischemic Postconditioning against Neuronal Apoptosis Induced by Transient Focal Ischemia Is Associated with Attenuation of NF-κB/p65 Activation

Jianmin Liang[1,3], **Yongxin Luan**[2], **Bin Lu**[2], **Hongbo Zhang**[1], **Yi-nan Luo**[2,3], **Pengfei Ge**[2,3]*

1 Department of Pediatrics, First hospital of Jilin University, Changchun, China, **2** Department of Neurosurgery, First hospital of Jilin University, Changchun, China, **3** Neuroscience Research Center, First hospital of Jilin University, Changchun, China

Abstract

Background and Purpose: Accumulating evidences have demonstrated that nuclear factor κB/p65 plays a protective role in the protection of ischemic preconditioning and detrimental role in lethal ischemia-induced programmed cell death including apoptosis and autophagic death. However, its role in the protection of ischemic postconditioning is still unclear.

Methods: Rat MCAO model was used to produce transient focal ischemia. The procedure of ischemic postconditioning consisted of three cycles of 30 seconds reperfusion/reocclusion of MCA. The volume of cerebral infarction was measured by TTC staining and neuronal apoptosis was detected by TUNEL staining. Western blotting was used to analyze the changes in protein levels of Caspase-3, NF-κB/p65, phosphor- NF-κB/p65, IκBα, phosphor- IκBα, Noxa, Bim and Bax between rats treated with and without ischemic postconditioning. Laser scanning confocal microscopy was used to examine the distribution of NF-κB/p65 and Noxa.

Results: Ischemic postconditioning made transient focal ischemia-induced infarct volume decrease obviously from $38.6\% \pm 5.8\%$ to $23.5\% \pm 4.3\%$, and apoptosis rate reduce significantly from $46.5\% \pm 6.2$ to $29.6\% \pm 5.3\%$ at reperfusion 24 h following 2 h focal cerebral ischemia. Western blotting analysis showed that ischemic postconditioning suppressed markedly the reduction of NF-κB/p65 in cytoplasm, but elevated its content in nucleus either at reperfusion 6 h or 24 h. Moreover, the decrease of IκBα and the increase of phosphorylated IκBα and phosphorylated NF-κB/p65 at indicated reperfusion time were reversed by ischemic postconditioning. Correspondingly, proapoptotic proteins Caspase-3, cleaved Caspase-3, Noxa, Bim and Bax were all mitigated significantly by ischemic postconditioning. Confocal microscopy revealed that ischemic postconditioning not only attenuated ischemia-induced translocation of NF-κB/p65 from neuronal cytoplasm to nucleus, but also inhibited the abnormal expression of proapoptotic protein Noxa within neurons.

Conclusions: We demonstrated in this study that the protection of ischemic postconditioning on neuronal apoptosis caused by transient focal ischemia is associated with attenuation of the activation of NF-κB/p65 in neurons.

Editor: Thiruma V. Arumugam, National University of Singapore, Singapore

Funding: This work was supported by National Nature and Science Foundation (30973110) and (81171234), the Outstanding Youth Grant (20080139) from the Science and Technology Department of Jilin Province. The funders had no role in study design, data collection and analysis, decision to publish, or preparation of the manuscript.

Competing Interests: The authors have declared that no competing interests exist.

* E-mail: pengfeige@gmail.com

Introduction

Ischemic stroke due to lack of cerebral blood supply is one of the most common causes leading to death or disability in adults worldwide [1]. Either animal study or clinical finding has revealed that reperfusion following ischemia results in brain damage [2,3]. Since it was found that the activation of nuclear factor κB (NF-κB) induced by transient ischemia is prior to DNA fragmentation [4], accumulating evidences have demonstrated that NF-κB plays an important role in regulating transient ischemia-induced neuronal death [5,6]. NF-κB is a nuclear transcription factor comprising five different proteins including p50, RelA/p65, c-Rel, RelB and p52, of which RelA/p65 and p50 have been proved to be responsible for the detrimental effect of NF-κB on neuronal injury

in cerebral ischemia [7]. Schneider et al found that transient ischemia-induced brain damage and neuronal death reduced in NF-κB/p50 deficient mice when compared with that in wild type mice [8]. By contrast, inhibition of NF-κB/65 is found to underlie the protective mechanism of many compounds against brain damage caused by transient ischemia [9,10]. In resting cells, NF-κB is normally sequestered in the cytoplasm by binding to its inhibitory IκB proteins. Under stress conditions such as ischemia and hypoxia, IκB is phosphorylated by its kinase (IKK), which leads to its degradation and disruption of the NF-κB/IκB complex. The activated NF-κB translocates subsequently to nucleus and binds to the κB promoter region of target genes [7]. Within neurons, NF-κB activation up-regulates the expression of pro-apoptotic factors such as Noxa and Bim [11]. By contrast, the activated NF-κB in glial cells could induce the production of neuro-toxic cytokines such as IL-1β, TNF-α and IL-6, which makes secondary injury to neurons [12]. Therefore, regulating the activation of NF-κB has become the target to prevent neuronal injury caused by transient cerebral ischemia.

Ischemic postconditioning, as a procedure consisting of series of rapid intermittent interruptions of blood flow in the early phase of reperfusion, is effective in protecting cerebral damage caused by ischemia/reperfusion [13]. Both animal studies and clinical investigation showed that ischemic postconditioning has protective effects on transient ischemia-induced injury. Wang et al and Ren et al reported respectively that ischemic postconditioning protected rat cerebral injury caused by either transient global or focal ischemia [14,15]. Loukogeorgakis et al observed that ischemic postconditioning attenuated endothelial injury secondary to transient ischemia in human brachial artery [16]. Because ROS (reactive oxygen species) is an important trigger of the activation of NF-κB [17] and the protective effect of ischemic postconditioning on ischemic brain injury is correlated with inhibition of oxidative stress [18,19], we hypothesize that the neuro-protection produced by ischemic postconditioning on transient ischemia-induced brain damage and neuronal apoptosis might be via regulating the activation of NF-κB. Therefore, in this study, we used rat model of transient focal ischemia to investigate the effect of ischemic postconditioning on the activation of NF-κB.

Materials and Methods

Animals

Adult male Wistar rats (weighing 280–300 g; 7 to 8 weeks of age) supplied by Experimental Animal Center, Jilin University, Changchun, China, were housed in a temperature-controlled room (22–25°C) on a 12-h light/dark cycle with free access to food and water. All animal procedures were approved by the ethical committee for animal experiments, Jilin University. All possible measures were taken to reduce animal suffering and numbers of animals in this study.

Surgical procedure

Brain ischemia was produced by using the middle cerebral artery occlusion (MCAO) model in rats as described before [18]. Following overnight fast of the rats, anesthesia was induced with intra-peritoneal administration of chloral hydrate (300 mg/kg). A rectal probe was inserted and core temperature was maintained at $37 \pm 0.5°C$ with a heating pad and lamp. A surgical incision was made to expose the right common carotid artery (CCA), internal carotid artery, and external carotid artery. The external carotid artery was ligated proximal to the origin of any branches, such as the occipital artery. The proximal CCA then was ligated and temporarily closed proximal to the carotid bifurcation by a microvascular clip. A small incision was made in the CCA. The occlusion filament was inserted into the internal carotid artery through the CCA 19 to 21 mm distal from the bifurcation to occlude the origin of the MCA. The filament was prepared of monofilament fishing line and covered with a distal cylinder of silicon rubber (diameter 0.31 to 0.32 mm). After the MCAO was performed, animals were allowed to awaken and resume spontaneous breathing. Two hours after induction of ischemia, the filament was withdrawn. After surgery, animals were then placed into a cage to recover from anesthesia at room temperature and were allowed food and drink.

Ischemic postconditioning protocol

At the start of the study, the rats were assigned randomly into a sham-operated group, an ischemia group and an ischemic postconditioning group. The rats in the ischemia group and ischemic postconditioning group were subjected to 2 h of focal cerebral ischemia as described above. The rats in ischemia group were subjected to 2 h of ischemia only, without any further interruption of reperfusion. Ischemic postconditioning rats were subjected to three cycles of 30 seconds/30 seconds reperfusion/reocclusion after 2 h of ischemia. In sham group, rats were subjected to the same procedures except for occlusion of the MCA.

Evaluation of neurological functional score

Neurological functional scores were evaluated at 24 hours post reperfusion by randomly choosing six rats from each group by staffs blinded to these groups. The test consists of two aspects of neurological function as has been previously described [20]: (1) the postural reflex test to examine upper body posture while the animal is suspended by the tail; (2) the forelimb placing test to examine sensorimotor integration in forelimb placing responses to visual, tactile, and proprioceptive stimuli. Neurological function was graded on a scale of 0 to 12 (normal score, 0; maximal score, 12).

Measurement of infarct size

At 24 h after reperfusion, seven rats from each group were chosen randomly by staffs who were blinded to these rats, killed by an overdose of pentobarbital i.p. and their brains were rapidly removed. Infarct sizes were measured by staining with 2, 3, 5-triphenyl-2H-tetrazolium chloride (TTC; Sigma-Aldrich, St. Louis, MO, USA). Brains were cut into 2-mm-thick coronal sections in a cutting block and 6 slices were stained with 1% TTC solution for 30 min at 37°C followed by overnight immersion in 4% paraformaldehyde. The percentage of brain infarct was measured by normalizing to the entire brain tissue from the animals, as described previously [18].

Brain tissue fixation

After rat was anesthetized, the thorax was opened and the heart was disclosed. Herpin (0.1 mL, 300 IU/kg) was injected into the left ventricle before the catheter was inserted into the main artery via left atrium. Then, PBS was perfused into the vascular system at 4°C for 3 min, and PBS with 4% paraformaldehyde was perfused at 4°C for another 3 min. Subsequently, the brain tissue was taken out and put into PBS fixation solution containing 4% paraformaldehyde at 4°C. Twelve hours later, 20- μm and 50- μm coronal brain slices were cut by vibrotome and the brain slices in similarity were selected for TUNEL staining and immunohistochemistry labeling.

TUNEL staining

TUNEL staining was performed at reperfusion 24 h by using In Situ Cell Death Detection Kit (Roche, Mannheim, Germany) according to the manufacturer's protocol. Brain slices were post-fixed 5 min in ethanol acetic acid (2:1) and rinsed. Then, the sections were incubated in proteinase K (20 μg/ml) for 15 min, followed by 10 min quenching in 3% hydrogen peroxide at room temperature. After three 10 min washes in PBS, the slices were incubated with TUNEL reaction mixture for 1 h at 37°C. Sections were washed in PBS three times for 10 min each and color development was performed in the dark with DAB (3,3′-diaminobenzidine). Hematoxylin was used for counter-staining, and the slices were finally mounted onto gelatin-coated slides and dried in dark room. TUNEL-positive apoptotic cells exhibited brown nuclear or cytoplasmic staining. In three fields of 0.04 mm^2 at the dorsal, ventral, and middle border of the infarct region at the level of the anterior commissure, TUNEL-positive cells were counted by a blinded pathologist and expressed as percent of total cell count.

Immunohistochemical analysis

The 50- μm brain slices were put into 24 wells plate with 500 μL citrate buffer (pH 6.0) and incubated in a 100°C water bath for 10 min. After cooling down, the slices were washed with the TBS solution containing 0.2% TX-100 for 10 min and blocked in the TBS solution containing 3% BSA and 0.2% TX-100 for 1 h at room temperature. Then they were incubated with mixtures of primary antibodies at 4°C overnight. For NF-κB/p65 staining, the primary antibody mixture included 1:300 polyclonal NF-κB/p65(Cell signaling Technology, Danvers, MA, USA) and 1:600 monoclonal anti-NeuN (Abcam, Cambridge, MA, USA) antibodies. For Noxa staining, the primary antibody mixture contained 1:200 polyclonal Noxa (Santa Cruz Biotechnology) and 1:600 monoclonal anti-NeuN (Abcam, Cambridge, MA, USA). After washed up with TBS solution containing 0.1%TX-100 for three times (10 min each) at room temperature, the antibody-labeled brain slices were incubated with 1% BSA containing 1:500 Alexa Fluor 594 Donkey Anti-mouse IgG(Cell signaling Technology, Danvers, MA, USA)for 1 h at room temperature. After the brain slices were washed with TBS solution containing 0.1% TX-100 for three times (10 min), they were incubated with 1:800 Alexa Fluor 488 Donkey Anti-rabbit IgG(Cell signaling Technology, Danvers, MA, USA). Again, the brain slices were washed with TBS solution containing 0.1% TX-100 for three times (10 min each), and then were mounted on slides and dried in dark room. Mounting medium was added on the slides prior to be covered with coverslips for observing by a laser scanning confocal microscope.

Western blotting analysis

At reperfusion 6 h and 24 h, the brain tissues were isolated from ischemic penumbra cortices and homogenized in ice cold buffer (1.5 mmol/L Tris base-HCl pH 7.6, 1 mmol/L DTT, 0.25 mol/L sucrose, 1 mmol/L MgCl$_2$, 1.25 μg/mL pepstatin A, 10 μg/mL leupeptin, 2.5 μg/mL approptonin, 0.5 mmol/L PMSF, 2.5 mmol/L EDTA, 1 mmol/L EGTA, 0.1 mol/L Na$_3$VO$_4$, 50 mmol/L NaF, and 2 mmol/L sodium pyrophosphate). The homogenates were centrifuged (1000×g for 20 min at 4°C) and the protein concentration of the supernatants (containing cytoplasm) and pellets (containing nucleus) was measured. Western blot analysis was conducted with 10% sodium dodecyl sulfate-polyacrylamide gel electrophoresis (SDS-PAGE). Four samples (from four different rats) in every experimental group were used for statistical analysis. After electrophoresis, proteins were transferred onto PVDF membranes. The membranes were probed with the following primary antibodies: 1:800 anti-Noxa (Santa Cruz Biotechnology, Santa Cruz, CA, USA); 1:1000 anti-Caspase-3 (Abcam, Cambridge, MA,USA); 1:1000 anti-NF-κB/p65, 1:1000 anti-p-NF-κB/p65(Ser536), 1:1000 anti-Bim, 1:1000 anti-Bax, 1:1000 anti-IκBα, 1:1000 anti-p-IκBα, 1:1000 anti-Lamin B1 and 1:1000 anti-β-actin (Cell signaling Technology, Danvers, MA). Horseradish peroxidase-conjugated goat anti-rabbit secondary antibody was obtained from Cell Signaling Technology (Danvers, MA, USA). After being incubated with horseradish peroxidase-conjugated goat anti-rabbit IgG (1: 2000), blots were washed and immunoreactive proteins were visualized on a Kodak X-omat LS film (Eastman Kodak Company, New Haven, CT, USA) with an enhanced chemiluminescence. Densitometry was performed with Kodak ID image analyses software (Eastman Kodak Company).

Statistical analysis

All data are expressed as mean ± SD and were analysed by SPSS statistical software, version 17.0 (SPSS Inc., Chicago, IL, USA) for Windows. One-way analysis of variance (ANOVA) was used for statistical comparisons between the different groups. $P <$ 0.05 was considered to be statistically significant.

Results

Ischemic postconditioning reduced cerebral infarction and neuronal apoptosis

In order to confirm the protection of the ischemic postconditioning procedure used in this study, we compared the infarct volume between ischemia group and ischemic postconditioning group. As shown in figure 1, the infarct volume at reperfusion 24 h was 38.7%±5.8% in ischemia group. By contrast, administration of ischemic postconditioning made the infarct volume decrease significantly to 23.6%±4.4% ($p < 0.01$, versus ischemia group). This result indicated that 3 cycles of 30 seconds reperfusion/ reocclusion is an effective ischemic postconditioning procedure to prevent brain injury. Moreover, neurological scores showed that ischemic postconditioning significantly mitigated the damaged neurological dysfunction caused by ischemia and reperfusion.

Because previous reports showed that transient ischemia leaded to brain damage via apoptotic pathway [5], we compared the differences in the apoptosis rate at reperfusion 24 h between ischemia group and ischemic postconditioning group. As figure 2 showed, the apoptosis rate 4.6%±1.5% in the sham group was increased to 46.5%±6.2% by 2 h focal ischemia and 24 h reperfusion. However, ischemic postconditioning suppressed the elevated apoptosis rate to 29.6%±5.3% ($p < 0.01$, versus ischemia group). For further examining the inhibitory effect of ischemic postconditioning on apoptosis, western blotting analysis was used to investigate the expressional changes in Caspase-3. It was found that ischemia/reperfusion induced cleavage of Caspase-3 was attenuated by administration of ischemic postconditioning (Figure 2 F and G). This result suggested the neuro-protection of ischemic postconditioning against ischemic brain damage is via inhibition of apoptosis.

Ischemic postconditioning inhibited the translocation of NF-κBp/65 in neurons.

When NF-κB/p65 is activated, it would translocate from cytoplasm to nucleus to induce apoptosis [11] and its transcriptional activity is also regulated by its phosphorylation by serine/threonine kinases[21]. Thus, we isolated cytoplasm fraction and nucleus fraction by using differential centrifugation and analyzed the protein level of NF-κB/p65 in each fraction by western blotting. As shown in figure 3 A and B, when compared with sham group, the protein level of NF-κB/p65 reduced in cytoplasm but increased correspondingly in nucleus either at reperfusion 6 h or 24 h. Moreover, its content in nucleus increased with the extension of reperfusion time from 6 h to 24 h. However, in the ischemic postconditioning group, the elevation of NF-κB/p65 in nucleus and its reduction in cytoplasm were both reversed significantly when compared with those in ischemia group at each indicated reperfusion time. Additionally, ischemic postconditioning significantly mitigated the phosphorylated level of NF-κB/p65 in both cytoplasm and nucleus induced by ischemia/reperfusion at either reperfusion 6 h or 24 h, indicating the transcriptional activity of NF-κB p65 was inhibited by ischemic postconditioning.

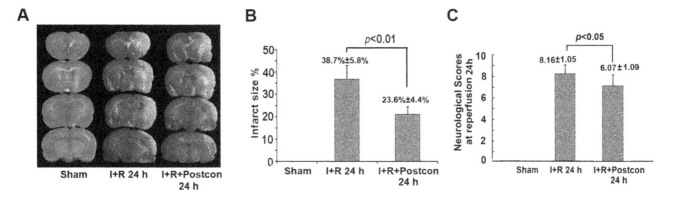

Figure 1. Measurement of cerebral infarction and evaluation of neurological function. A, representative images of TTC staining; B, statistics of infarct size. C, statistics of neurological scores.

In order to clarify whether ischemic postconditioning inhibited the translocation of neuronal NF-κB/p65 within neurons, we used laser scanning confocal microscopy in combination with neuron-specific probe NeuN to observe the distribution of NF-κB/p65. As shown in figure 3 C, the figures of nuclei were round and NF-κB/p65 was located in cytoplasm in sham group. At reperfusion 24 h following 2 h focal ischemia, nuclei shrank in some neurons and NF-κB/p65 distributed mainly in nuclei. By contrast, these changes in nuclei figures and distribution of NF-κB/p65 caused by ischemia and reperfusion were partly reversed by ischemic

postconditioning. Therefore, our results indicated that ischemic postconditioning attenuated ischemia/reperfusion-induced translocation of NF-κB from cytosol to nucleus within cortex neurons.

Ischemic postconditioning suppressed phosphorylation of IκBα

Despite there are several forms of IκB protein that have been identified, IκBα represents the predominant form in brain [22]. Thus, we examined the effects of ischemic postconditioning on the phosphorylation of IκB by using western blotting analysis. As

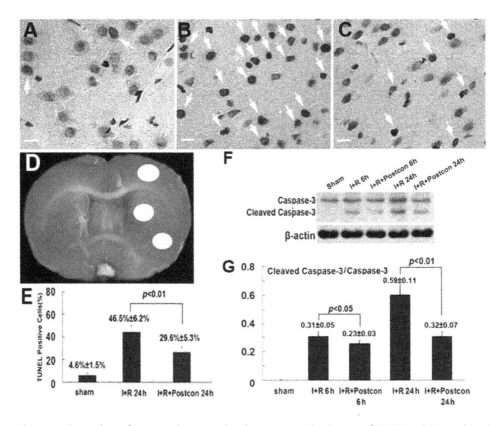

Figure 2. Detection of neuronal apoptosis. The representative images of TUNEL staining under microscope (x40) showed apoptotic cells exhibited brown nuclear or cytoplasmic staining (A, sham group; B, ischemia group; C, ischemic postconditioning group). D, brain region used for counting apoptotic neurons (White region). E, statistics of TUNEL positive cells. F, Western blotting of Caspase-3; G, statistics of the ratio of Cleaved Caspase-3 to Caspase-3. Scale bar: 20 μm.

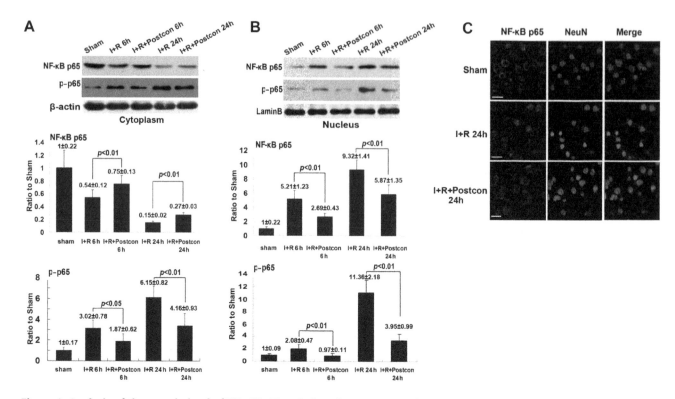

Figure 3. Analysis of the protein level of NF-κB/p65 and phosphor- NF-κB/p65 in cytoplasm and nucleus and observation of the distribution of NF-κB/p65 within neurons. A, representative western blotting image and statistics of NF-κB/p65 and phosphor- NF-κB/p65 in cytoplasm. B, representative western blotting image and statistics of NF-κB/p65 and phosphor- NF-κB/p65 in nucleus. C, representative confocal images of NF-κB/p65. This result showed that ischemic postconditioning reversed abnormal higher level of NF-κB/p65 and phosphor- NF-κB/p65, and the translocation of NF-κB/p65 from cytoplasm to nucleus caused by transient ischemia. Scale bar: 30 μm

shown in figure 4, compared with sham group, the level of phosphorylated IκBα increased significantly at reperfusion 6 h and 24 h, while the IκBα reduced markedly at each time point in ischemia group. Moreover, the reduction of IκBα was concomitant with the elevation of its phosphorylation when reperfusion time was extended from 6 h to 24 h. However, ischemic postconditioning suppressed markedly the phosphorylation of IκBα and maintained IκBα level in cytoplasm either at reperfusion 6 h or 24 h. This result indicated that the inhibitory effect of ischemic postconditioning on the activation of NF-κB/p65 is correlated with suppression of the phosphorylation of IκBα.

Ischemic postconditioning suppressed the expression of proapoptotic proteins mediated by NF-κB

The expressional level of proapoptotic proteins Noxa, Bim and Bax demonstrated to be regulated by activated NF-κB/p65 [7,23] were investigated. As shown in figure 5 and figure 6, when compared with sham group, the expressional levels of proapoptotic proteins Noxa, Bim and Bax were all up-regulated markedly at both reperfusion 6 h and 24 h. Their expression at reperfusion 24 h was higher than those at reperfusion 6 h, respectively. However, the increased expressional levels of these three proapoptotic proteins were all suppressed at each indicated time by ischemic postconditioning. These results were consistent with the changes in NF-κB level in the rats treated with ischemic postconditioning, indicating that inhibition of the abnormal

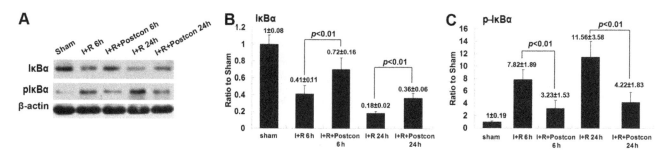

Figure 4. Analysis of the phosphorylation of IκBα. A representative image of western blotting; B, statistics of the protein level of IκBα; C, statistics of the protein level of phosphorylated IκBα. This result showed that ischemic postconditioning inhibited transient ischemia-induced phosphorylation of IκBα.

expression of these pro-apoptotic proteins was due to suppression of NF-κB activation by ischemic postconditioning. Further, we selected Noxa as a representative protein to investigate whether ischemic postconditioning mitigates its abnormal expression within neurons. As shown in figure 5, transient ischemia-induced elevation in the expression of Noxa was located in the cells labelled with neuron-specific probe NeuN. Obviously, administration of ischemic postconditioning mitigated the expression of Noxa within neurons. Thus, these results suggests mitigation of the expression of proapoptotic proteins Noxa, Bim and Bax is associated with the inhibitory effect of ischemic postconditioning on activation of NF-κB/p65.

Discussion

In the present study, we demonstrated that ischemic post-conditioning protected brain damage caused by transient focal ischemia through attenuating apoptotic neurons. Its inhibition of neuronal apoptosis was associated with suppressing ischemia/reperfusion-induced activation of NF-κB/p65 by mitigating over-phosphorylation of IκBα. Correspondingly, the expressional level of proapoptotic proteins Noxa, Bim and Bax mediated by NF-κB/p65 was reduced by ischemic postconditioning.

It has been found that NF-κB/p65 could be activated under various noxious stresses to mature brain, which include transient ischemia, subarachnoid hemorrhage, neurotrauma and epilepsy [5,24–26]. Accumulating evidences suggest that activated NF-κB/p65 plays an important role in modulating cellular programmed death such as apoptosis and autophagy-like death. Nakai et al proved that activated NF-κB/p65 contributed to epilepsy-induced neuronal apoptosis in rat striatum [26]. Zeng et al reported that ischemia-induced activation of NF-κB/p65 aggravated myocardial injury through the activation of Beclin 1-mediated autophagy [27]. In the case of transient ischemia, it is found that activation of NF-κB/p65 is associated closely with neuronal damage [4,5], and inhibition of the activation of NF-κB/p65 produces protection against neuronal apoptosis. Xu et al proved that inhibition of NF-

κB/p65 signaling pathway by matrine contributed to its protective effect on neurons against cerebral focal ischemia [28]. Similarly, the protection of hypothermia and electrical acupuncture on brain damage was proved as well to be via modulating the activation of NF-κB/p65 [29,30].Consistent with these reports, we not only demonstrated that transient ischemia induced activation of NF-κB/p65, but also found that ischemic postconditioning protects neuronal apoptosis caused by cerebral ischemia and reperfusion via inhibiting of NF-κB/p65 activation.

It was reported that NF-κB/p65 could be activated in both neurons and glial cells by transient ischemia, but their roles in ischemic brain damage is different. Zhang et al demonstrated by using transgenic mouse that ischemic damage is due to the activation of neuronal NF-κB/p65, not the glial NF-κB/p65 [5]. However, it is thought that transient ischemia-induced activation of NF-κB/p65 via toll like receptor 4 or 2 in glial cells would exert secondary injury to neurons by producing neuro-toxic cytokins such as TNFα and IL-1β [12]. In the present study, we demonstrated by using double immuno-fluorescence staining that ischemic postconditioning protects neuronal apoptosis via suppression of neuronal proapoptotic proteins. Although we did not investigate the effect of ischemic postconditioning on the activation of glial NF-κB, other researchers reported that ischemic post-conditioning could inhibit the production of toxic cytokines TNFα and IL-1β induced by ischemia [31]. We thus speculate that the transient ischemia-induced activation of glial NF-κB/p65 might be inhibited by ischemic postconditioning.

Activated NF-κB/p65 promotes apoptosis in neurons via upregulating the expression of its downstream proapoptotic proteins, such as nitric oxide synthase II [32], Bax[23], Noxa and Bim[7]. Noxa and Bim are Bcl-2 family members, but only contain BH3 (Bcl-2 homology domain 3)-only domain. They both could activate Bax to release cytochrome c and other death signals from mitochondria, and prevent Bax from being blocked by anti-apoptotic Bcl-2 and Bcl-XL [33]. Noxa and Bim have been demonstrated to be associated with ischemic injury, because previous reports showed that the expression of Bim and Noxa were

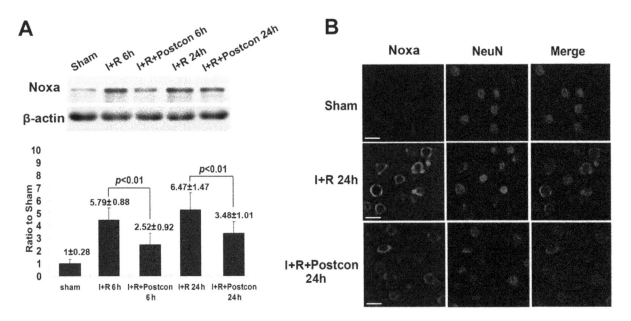

Figure 5. Analysis of the expressional level of Noxa and its changes within neurons. A, representative western blotting image of Noxa and statistical analysis; B, representative confocal images. This result showed that the up-regulated expression of Noxa in neurons was suppressed by ischemic postconditioning. Scale bar: 30 μm

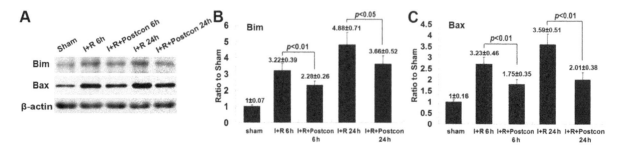

Figure 6. Analysis of the expressional level of Bim and Bax. A, representative western blotting images of Bim, Bax and cleaved caspase-3. B, statistics of the protein level of Bim; C, statistics of the protein level of Bax. This result showed that ischemic postconditioning mitigated the up-regulated expression of Bim and Bax.

rup-regulated at the ischemic heart and brain [34,11]. By contrast, suppression of the expression of Noxa by antisense oligonucleotides rescued hypoxia-induced cell death and decreased infarct volumes caused by focal cerebral ischemia [35]. In this study, we proved that ischemic postconditioning reduced the abnormal protein level of proapoptotic Noxa, Bim and Bax, which might underlie the inhibitive mechanism of ischemic postconditioning on neuronal apoptosis.

Despite it was reported that phosphorylation of NF-κB/p65 on Serine 536 defines an IκBα-independent NF-κB pathway[36], the activation of NF-κB/p65 is mainly regulated by its natural interior inhibitor IκB. Xu et al demonstrated by using recombinant adenoviral expression of dominant negative IκBα that over-expression of IκB rescued neuronal injury caused by cerebral ischemia [37]. The reduction of IκB during the course of cerebral ischemia and reperfusion is mainly due to its degradation by proteasome after it is phosphorylated by IκB kinase (IKK) [7]. However, it was found that NF-κB/p65 phosphorylation coincides with promotion of IκBα degradation [38]. In the present study, we demonstrated that ischemic postconditioning inhibited the ischemia/reperfusion-induced higher level of phosphorylated NF-κB/p65 in both cytoplasm and nucleus, which was consistent with the finding that ischemic postconditioning reversed the decreased level of IκBα caused by cerebral ischemia/reperfusion (figure 4).

Evidence showed that oxidative stress is an upstream event promoting IκB phosphorylation [10,39]. Moreover, Shen et al reported antioxidant attenuated reperfusion injury after global brain ischemia via inhibiting NF-κB activity by mitigating the phosphorylation of IκB [40]. Similarly, Fischer et al proved that anti-oxidative treatment suppressed activation of NF-κB during myocardial ischemia-reperfusion in heart. [41]. On the basis of prior findings that ischemic postconditioning could attenuate the overproduction of ROS caused by transient focal ischemia and reverse the damaged activity in endogenous antioxidant enzyme [18,42], we think that the inhibitory effect of ischemic post-conditioning on the phosphorylation of IκB is also associated with its inhibition of oxidative stress.

The role of NF-κB/p65 during the course of cerebral ischemia and reperfusion is complex. In vitro and in vivo studies have shown that sublethal ischemia-induced activation of NF-κB/p65 contributed to the protection of ischemic preconditioning against subsequent lethal ischemic insult [43,44]. Blondeau et al found that the protection of activated NF-κB/p65 against neuronal damage caused by following lethal stresses could be counteracted by diethyldithiocarbamate, an NF-κB/p65 specific inhibitor [44]. By contrast, other studies revealed that inhibiting the activation of NF-κB/p65 contributed to protection of tissue injury. Kin et al reported that the inhibition of myocardial apoptosis by post-

conditioning is associated with attenuation of NF-κB/p65 translocation [45]. Yin et al showed that preconditioning with mTOR inhibitor rapamycin rescued brain damage via attenuating the production of NF-κB/p65 caused by subsequent ischemia/reperfusion[46]. Although ischemic postconditioning and preconditioning might share common pathways to induce intrinsic protective mechanism such as modulation of ASIC1a, notch signaling and neuroinflammation, [47,48,31], our result showed that the effect of ischemic postconditioning on activation of NF-κB/p65 is inhibitive, which is opposite to the inducing effect produced by ischemic preconditioning.

It has been demonstrated that ischemic postconditioning protects transient ischemia-induced tissue damage in various organs, including heart, liver and intestine [13,49,50]. By now, the protective mechanism underlying ischemic postconditioning has been investigated widely and is found to be related to multiple factors including suppression of oxidative stress, maintaining mitochondrial function, inhibition of endoplasmic stress, attenuation of inflammation and mitigation of protein aggregation [51–54]. Different with previous reports showing that the inhibitory effect of ischemic postconditioning on cellular apoptosis is via down-regulating anti-apoptotic protein Bcl-2, up-regulating proapoptotic caspase-3, caspase-6 and caspase-9[55], and activation of ERK1/2 and Akt signaling pathway[56,57], our result suggests that inhibition of neuronal apoptosis by ischemic postconditioning is related to attenuation of the activation of neuronal NF-κB/p65.

Conclusion

Our study showed that ischemic postconditioning inhibited brain damage and neuronal apoptosis induced by transient ischemia. During the course of cerebral ischemia and reperfusion, the activation of NF-κB/p65 due to the phosphorylation of its inhibitor I-κBα and phosphorylation of NF-κB/p65 resulted in up-regulated expression of proapoptotic proteins Noxa, Bim and Bax. However, administration of ischemic postconditioning prior to the recovery of cerebral blood flow significantly inhibited these changes and rescued neuronal apoptosis. Therefore, our study indicates that ischemic postconditioning is an effective method that could protect neuronal apoptosis via attenuating the activation of NF-κB/p65 caused by focal cerebral ischemia and reperfusion.

Author Contributions

Conceived and designed the experiments: PG Y. Luo. Performed the experiments: JL Y. Luan BL HZ. Analyzed the data: JL Y. Luan HZ. Contributed reagents/materials/analysis tools: Y. Luo PG. Wrote the paper: JL PG.

References

1. Donnan GA, Fisher M, Macleod M, Davis SM (2008). Stroke. Lancet 371: 1612–1623.
2. Kirino T (1982). Delayed neuronal death in the gerbil hippocampus following ischemia. Brain Res 239: 57–69.
3. Albers GW, Caplan LR, Coull B, Fayad PB, Mohr JP, et al (2002). TIA Working Group. Transient ischemic attatck—proposal for a new definition. N Engl J Med 347: 1713–1716.
4. Clemens JA, Stephenson DT, Dixon EP, Smalstig EB, Mincy RE, et al (1997). Global cerebral ischemia activates nuclear factor-kappa B prior to evidence of DNA fragmentation. Brain Res Mol Brain Res 48: 187–196.
5. Zhang W, Potrovita I, Tarabin V, Herrmann O, Beer V, et al (2005). Neuronal activation of NF-kappaB contributes to cell death in cerebral ischemia. J Cereb Blood Flow Metab 25: 30–40.
6. Li WL, Yu SP, Chen D, Yu SS, Jiang YJ, et al (2013). The regulatory role of NF-κB in autophagy-like cell death after focal cerebral ischemia in mice. Neuroscience 244: 16–30.
7. Pizzi M, Sarnico I, Lanzillotta A, Battistin L, Spano P (2009). Post-ischemic brain damage: NF-kappaB dimer heterogeneity as a molecular determinant of neuron vulnerability. FEBS J 276: 27–35.
8. Schneider A, Martin-Villalba A, Weih F, Vogel J, Wirth T, et al (1999). NF-kappaB is activated and promotes cell death in focal cerebral ischemia. Nat Med 5: 554–559.
9. Hu J, Luo CX, Chu WH, Shan YA, Qian ZM, et al (2012). 20-Hydroxyecdysone protects against oxidative stress-induced neuronal injury by scavenging free radicals and modulating NF-κB and JNK pathways. PLoS One 7:e50764.
10. Qian Y, Guan T, Huang M, Cao L, Li Y, et al (2012). Neuroprotection by the soy isoflavone, genistein, via inhibition of mitochondria-dependent apoptosis pathways and reactive oxygen induced-NF-κB activation in a cerebral ischemia mouse model. Neurochem Int 60: 759–767.
11. Inta I, Paxian S, Maegele I, Zhang W, Pizzi M, et al (2006). Bim and Noxa are candidates to mediate the deleterious effect of the NF-kappa B subunit RelA in cerebral ischemia. J Neurosci 26: 12896–12903.
12. Wang Y, Ge P, Zhu Y (2013). TLR2 and TLR4 in the Brain injury caused by cerebral ischemia and reperfusion. Mediators of inflammation 2013: 124614.
13. Zhao H, Sapolsky RM, Steinberg GK (2006). Interrupting reperfusion as a stroke therapy: ischemic postconditioning reduces infarct size after focal ischemia in rats. J Cereb Blood Flow Metab 26: 1114–1121.
14. Wang JY, Shen J, Gao Q, Ye ZG, Yang SY, et al (2008). Ischemic postconditioning protects against global cerebral ischemia/reperfusion-induced injury in rats. Stroke 39: 983–990.
15. Ren C, Gao X, Niu G, Yan Z, Chen X, et al (2008). Delayed postconditioning protects against focal ischemic brain injury in rats. PLoS One 3:e3851.
16. Loukogeorgakis SP, Panagiotidou AT, Yellon DM, Deanfield JE, MacAllister RJ (2006). Postconditioning protects against endothelial ischemia-reperfusion injury in the human forearm. Circulation 113: 1015–1019.
17. Jang ER, Lee CS (2011).7-ketocholesterol induces apoptosis in differentiated PC12 cells via reactive oxygen species-dependent activation of NF-κB and Akt pathways. Neurochem Int 58: 52–59.
18. Li ZY, Liu B, Yu J, Yang FW, Luo YN, et al (2012). Ischaemic postconditioning rescues brain injury caused by focal ischaemia/reperfusion via attenuation of protein oxidization. J Int Med Res 40: 954–966.
19. Xing B, Chen H, Zhang M, Zhao D, Jiang R, et al (2008). Ischemic postconditioning inhibits apoptosis after focal cerebral ischemia/reperfusion injury in the rat. Stroke 39: 2362–2369.
20. Belayev L, Alonso OF, Busto R, Zhao W, Ginsberg MD (1996) Middle cerebral artery occlusion in the rat by intraluminal suture. Neurological and pathological evaluation of an improved model. Stroke 27: 1616–1623.
21. Ryu HJ, Kim JE, Yeo SI, Kim MJ, Jo SM, et al(2011). ReLA/P65-serine 536 nuclear factor-kappa B phosphorylation is related to vulnerability to status epilepticus in the rat hippocampus. Neuroscience 187: 93–102.
22. Baeuerle PA, Baltimore D (1996). NF-kappa B: ten years after. Cell 87: 13–20.
23. Li L, Wu W, Huang W, Hu G, Yuan W, et al (2013). NF-κB RNAi decreases the Bax/Bcl-2 ratio and inhibits TNF-α-induced apoptosis in human alveolar epithelial cells. Inflamm Res 62: 387–397.
24. You WC, Wang CX, Pan YX, Zhang X, Zhou XM, et al (2013). Activation of nuclear factor-κB in the brain after experimental subarachnoid hemorrhage and its potential role in delayed brain injury. PLoS One 8(3): e60290.
25. Chu W, Li M, Li F, Hu R, Chen Z, et al (2013). Immediate splenectomy down-regulates the MAPK-NF-κB signaling pathway in rat brain after severe traumatic brain injury. J Trauma Acute Care Surg 74: 1446–1453.
26. Nakai M, Qin ZH, Chen JF, Wang Y, Chase TN (2000). Kainic acid-induced apoptosis in rat striatum is associated with nuclear factor-kappaB activation. J Neurochem 74: 647–658.
27. Zeng M, Wei X, Wu Z, Li W, Li B, et al (2013). NF-κB-mediated induction of autophagy in cardiac ischemia/reperfusion injury. Biochem Biophys Res Commun 436: 180–185.
28. Xu M, Yang L, Hong LZ, Zhao XY, Zhang HL(2012). Direct protection of neurons and astrocytes by matrine via inhibition of the NF-κB signaling pathway contributes to neuroprotection against focal cerebral ischemia. Brain Res1454: 48–64.
29. Feng X, Yang S, Liu J, Huang J, Peng J, et al (2013). Electroacupuncture ameliorates cognitive impairment through inhibition of NF-κB-mediated neuronal cell apoptosis in cerebral ischemia-reperfusion injured rats. Mol Med Rep 7: 1516–1522.
30. Han HS, Karabiyikoglu M, Kelly S, Sobel RA, Yenari MA (2003). Mild hypothermia inhibits nuclear factor-kappaB translocation in experimental stroke. J Cereb Blood Flow Metab 23: 589–598.
31. Xiong J, Wang Q, Xue FS, Yuan YJ, Li S, et al (2011). Comparison of cardioprotective and anti-inflammatory effects of ischemia pre- and postconditioning in rats with myocardial ischemia-reperfusion injury. Inflamm Res 60: 547–554.
32. Chuang YC, Chen SD, Lin TK, Chang WN, Lu CH, et al (2010). Transcriptional upregulation of nitric oxide synthase II by nuclear factor-kappaB promotes apoptotic neuronal cell death in the hippocampus following experimental status epilepticus. J Neurosci Res 88: 1898–1907.
33. Engel T, Plesnila N, Prehn JH, Henshall DC (2011). In vivo contributions of BH3-only proteins to neuronal death following seizures, ischemia, and traumatic brain injury. J Cereb Blood Flow Metab 31: 1196–1210.
34. Ishihara Y, Shimamoto N (2012). Sulfaphenazole attenuates myocardial cell apoptosis accompanied with cardiac ischemia-reperfusion by suppressing the expression of BimEL and Noxa. J Pharmacol Sci 119: 251–259.
35. Kim JY, Ahn HJ, Ryu JH, Suk K, Park JH (2004). BH3-only protein Noxa is a mediator of hypoxic cell death induced by hypoxia-inducible factor 1alpha. J Exp Med 199: 113–124.
36. Sasaki CY, Barberi TJ, Ghosh P, Longo DL (2005). Phosphorylation of RelA/p65 on Serine 536 Defines an IκBα-independent NF-κB Pathway. J Biol Chem 280: 34538–34547.
37. Xu L, Zhan Y, Wang Y, Feuerstein GZ, Wang X(2002). Recombinant adenoviral expression of dominant negative IkappaBalpha protects brain from cerebral ischemic injury. Biochem Biophys Res Commun 299: 14–17.
38. Hu J, Haseebuddin M, Young M, Colburn NH (2005). Suppression of p65 phosphorylation coincides with inhibition of IκBα polyubiquitination and degradation. Mol Carcinog 44: 274–284.
39. Song YS, Kim MS, Kim HA, Jung BI, Yang J, et al (2010). Oxidative stress increases phosphorylation of IkappaB kinase-alpha by enhancing NF-kappaB-inducing kinase after transient focal cerebral ischemia. J Cereb Blood Flow Metab 30: 1265–1274.
40. Shen WH, Zhang CY, Zhang GY (2003). Antioxidants attenuate reperfusion injury after global brain ischemia through inhibiting nuclear factor-kappa B activity in rats. Acta Pharmacol Sin 24: 1125–1130.
41. Fischer UM, Antonyan A, Bloch W, Mehlhorn U (2006). Impact of antioxidative treatment on nuclear factor kappa-B regulation during myocardial ischemia-reperfusion. Interact Cardiovasc Thorac Surg 5: 531–535.
42. Danielisová V, Némethová M, Gottlieb M, Burda J (2006). The changes in endogenous antioxidant enzyme activity after postconditioning. Cell Mol Neurobiol 26: 1181–1191.
43. Kim EJ, Raval AP, Hirsch N, Perez-Pinzon MA (2010). Ischemic preconditioning mediates cyclooxygenase-2 expression via nuclear factor-kappa B activation in mixed cortical neuronal cultures. Transl Stroke Res 1: 40–47.
44. Blondeau N, Widmann C, Lazdunski M, Heurteaux C (2001). Activation of the nuclear factor-kappaB is a key event in brain tolerance. J Neurosci 21: 4668–4677.
45. Kin H, Wang NP, Mykytenko J, Reeves J, Deneve J, et al (2008). Inhibition of myocardial apoptosis by postconditioning is associated with attenuation of oxidative stress-mediated nuclear factor-kappa B translocation and TNF alpha release. Shock 29: 761–768.
46. Yin J, Ye S, Chen Z, Zeng Y(2012). Rapamycin preconditioning attenuates transient focal cerebral ischemia/reperfusion injury in mice. Int J Neurosci 122: 748–756.
47. Zhou XL, Wan L, Xu QR, Zhao Y, Liu JC (2013). Notch signaling activation contributes to cardioprotection provided by ischemic preconditioning and postconditioning. J Transl Med 11: 251.
48. Pignataro G, Cuomo O, Esposito E, Sirabella R, Di Renzo G, et al (2011). ASIC1a contributes to neuroprotection elicited by ischemic preconditioning and postconditioning. Int J Physiol Pathophysiol Pharmacol 3: 1–8.
49. Guo JY, Yang T, Sun XG, Zhou NY, Li FS, et al (2011). Ischaemic postconditioning attenuates liver warm ischaemia-reperfusion injury through Akt-eNOS-NO-HIF pathway. J Biomed Sci 18: 79.
50. Liu KX, Li YS, Huang WQ, Chen SQ, Wang ZX, et al (2009). Immediate postconditioning during reperfusion attenuates intestinal injury. Intensive Care Med 35: 933–942.
51. Liang JM, Xu HY, Zhang XJ, Li X, Zhang HB, et al (2013). Role of mitochondrial function in the protective effects of ischaemic postconditioning on ischaemia/reperfusion cerebral damage. J Int Med Res 41: 618–627.
52. Yuan Y, Guo Q, Ye Z, Pingping X, Wang N, et al (2011). Ischemic postconditioning protects brain from ischemia/reperfusion injury by attenuating endoplasmic reticulum stress-induced apoptosis through PI3K-Akt pathway. Brain Res 1367: 85–93.
53. Kong Y, Rogers MR, Qin X (2013). Effective neuroprotection by ischemic postconditioning is associated with a decreased expression of RGMa and inflammation mediators in ischemic rats. Neurochem Res 38: 815–825.

54. Liang J, Yao J, Wang G, Wang Y, Wang B, et al (2012). Ischemic postconditioning protects neuronal death caused by cerebral ischemia and reperfusion via attenuating protein aggregation. Int J Med Sci 9: 923–932.

55. Ding ZM, Wu B, Zhang WQ, Lu XJ, Lin YC,et al (2012). Neuroprotective Effects of Ischemic Preconditioning and Postconditioning on Global Brain Ischemia in Rats through the Same Effect on Inhibition of Apoptosis. Int J Mol Sci 13: 6089–6101.

56. Darling CE, Jiang R, Maynard M, Whittaker P, Vinten-Johansen J, et al (2005). Postconditioning via stuttering reperfusion limits myocardial infarct size in rabbit hearts: role of ERK1/2. Am J Physiol Heart Circ Physiol 289:H1618–1626.

57. Gao X, Zhang H, Takahashi T, Hsieh J, Liao J, et al (2008). The Akt signaling pathway contributes to postconditioning's protection against stroke; the protection is associated with the MAPK and PKC pathways. J Neurochem 105: 943–955.

14

Efficacy and Safety of Vitamin K-Antagonists (VKA) for Atrial Fibrillation in Non-Dialysis Dependent Chronic Kidney Disease

Judith Kooiman[1]*, Nienke van Rein[1,2], Bas Spaans[1], Koen A. J. van Beers[1], Jonna R. Bank[1], Wilke R. van de Peppel[1], Antonio Iglesias del Sol[3], Suzanne C. Cannegieter[4], Ton J. Rabelink[5], Gregory Y. H. Lip[6], Frederikus A. Klok[1], Menno V. Huisman[1]

1 Department of Thrombosis and Hemostasis, Leiden University Medical Center, Leiden, The Netherlands, 2 Einthoven Laboratory of Experimental Vascular Medicine, Leiden University Medical Center, Leiden, The Netherlands, 3 Department of Internal Medicine, Rijnland Hospital, Leiderdorp, The Netherlands, 4 Department of Clinical Epidemiology, Leiden University Medical Center, Leiden, The Netherlands, 5 Department of Nephrology, Leiden University Medical Center, Leiden, The Netherlands, 6 Haemostasis, Thrombosis, and Vascular Biology Unit, University of Birmingham Centre for Cardiovascular Sciences, City Hospital, Birmingham, United Kingdom

Abstract

Background: Essential information regarding efficacy and safety of vitamin K-antagonists (VKA) treatment for atrial fibrillation (AF) in non-dialysis dependent chronic kidney disease (CKD) is still lacking in current literature. The aim of our study was to compare the risks of stroke or transient ischemic attack (TIA) and major bleeds between patients without CKD (eGFR >60 ml/min), and those with moderate (eGFR 30–60 ml/min), or severe non-dialysis dependent CKD (eGFR <30 ml/min).

Methods: We included 300 patients without CKD, 294 with moderate, and 130 with severe non-dialysis dependent CKD, who were matched for age and sex. Uni- and multivariate Cox regression analyses were performed reporting hazard ratios (HRs) for the endpoint of stroke or TIA and the endpoint of major bleeds as crude values and adjusted for comorbidity and platelet-inhibitor use.

Results: Overall, 6.2% (45/724, 1.7/100 patient years) of patients developed stroke or TIA and 15.6% (113/724, 4.8/100 patient years) a major bleeding event. Patients with severe CKD were at high risk of stroke or TIA and major bleeds during VKA treatment compared with those without renal impairment, HR 2.75 (95%CI 1.25–6.05) and 1.66 (95%CI 0.97–2.86), or with moderate CKD, HR 3.93(1.71–9.00) and 1.86 (95%CI 1.08–3.21), respectively. These risks were similar for patients without and with moderate CKD. Importantly, both less time spent within therapeutic range and high INR-variability were associated with increased risks of stroke or TIA and major bleeds in severe CKD patients.

Conclusions: VKA treatment for AF in patients with severe CKD has a poor safety and efficacy profile, likely related to suboptimal anticoagulation control. Our study findings stress the need for better tailored individualised anticoagulant treatment approaches for patients with AF and severe CKD.

Editor: Kathrin Eller, Medical University of Graz, Austria

Funding: The authors have no support or funding to report.

Competing Interests: The authors have declared that no competing interests exist.

* E-mail: j.kooiman@lumc.nl

Introduction

About one-third of atrial fibrillation (AF) patients suffer from chronic kidney disease (CKD) [1–3], a condition that by itself increases the risk of stroke, even in the absence of AF. Inversely, AF in CKD patients is associated with progression of CKD, cardiovascular morbidity and mortality [4–6].

Antithrombotic treatment is very effective in preventing stroke or a transient ischemic attack (TIA) in patients with AF, both in patients with normal renal function and in those with CKD in terms of a relative risk reduction [7–9]. However, CKD increases a patient's risk of major bleeding complications during antithrombotic treatment [8,10]. The extent to which non-dialysis depen-

dent CKD increases the risk of stroke and major bleeds in AF patients during VKA treatment is understudied, as the main focus in research in this area has been on patients with end-stage-renal disease requiring dialysis. However, these patients comprise less than 1% of the AF population [8,11]. The few studies that have focussed on risks of stroke and/or major bleeding in AF patients with non-dialysis dependent CKD were limited by their small sample size [10,12,13], the absence of information on eGFR levels [8], exclusion of patients with severe CKD [7], or a divergent patient cohort with various indications for VKA treatment [14]. Knowledge about these risks would most certainly provide relevant insights into treatment outcomes in a patient group that frequently attends both cardiology and internal medicine practices. More-

over, with the emergence of novel oral anticoagulants, understanding the risks of stroke and major bleeding events in AF
patients with various stages of CKD is essential when evaluating
whether these new agents would provide a more favourable risk-
benefit ratio than the traditional vitamin K-antagonists (VKA) for
this specific patient population [11].

Therefore, the aim of our study was to compare risks of stroke
or TIA and major bleeds in patients with moderate or severe CKD
and AF treated with VKAs with patients without renal impairment. Second, we assessed the influence of quality of anticoagulation control on the risks of stroke or TIA and major bleeds.

Methods

Patients diagnosed with new onset valvular or non-valvular AF
starting VKA treatment between 1997 and 2005 at the Leiden
anticoagulation clinic were included in a previously described
study cohort [3]. This anticoagulation clinic serves one academic
(Leiden University Medical Center, Leiden) and two non-
academic teaching hospitals (Diaconessenhuis, Leiden, and Rijnland Hospital, Leiderdorp). Within this cohort of 5039 AF
patients, 3316 had no CKD (eGFR >60 ml/min), 1557 (eGFR
30–60 ml/min) had moderate CKD, and 166 patients severe
CKD (eGFR <30 ml/min), as measured at start of VKA therapy.
For the current analysis, we excluded fourteen patients from the
severe CKD group who had acute kidney injury at time of VKA
therapy initiation, after which renal function recovered to a less
critical CKD stage, thus leaving 152 patients with severe CKD.
Since reviewing medical records of all 1557 moderate and 3316
non-CKD patients would be an effort not offsetting the statistical
gain, we sampled 300 patients without CKD and 294 patients with
moderate CKD for inclusion, matched for age and gender to those
with severe CKD. Patients treated with VKA via the Leiden
anticoagulation clinic for <7 days were excluded from the study
cohort and replaced by others of the same age, gender, and level of
renal impairment. Patients on dialysis at start of VKA therapy
were also excluded, but were not replaced. Patients were treated
with either phenprocoumon (Marcoumar) or acenocoumarol. The
study was approved by the ethics committee of the three
participating hospitals (ethics committee Leiden University Medical Center, Leiden, the Netherlands) that waived the need for
informed consent.

Chart review

Medical records from two sources (i.e. the participating hospitals
and the Leiden anticoagulation clinic) were searched for information on patient characteristics at baseline, comorbidity, use of
platelet-inhibitors, International Normalized Ratios (INRs) and
study outcomes. Renal function was assessed using the abbreviated
modification of diet in renal disease (MDRD) formula, as it
accurately estimates renal function in elderly patients and the
mean age of our study population was high [15,16].

Study outcomes and definitions

Primary outcomes of this study were the combined endpoint of
stroke or TIA and the occurrence of major bleeding events. Major
bleeding was defined by the International Society of Thrombosis
and Hemostasis criteria (i.e. fatal bleeding, any bleeding causing a
drop in hemoglobin level ≥1.24 mmol/L and/or requiring
transfusion of ≥2 units of whole blood or red cells and/or a
symptomatic bleeding in a critical area/organ (intracranial,
intraspinal, intraocular, pericardial, or intramuscular with compartment syndrome)) [17]. Secondary endpoints were major
adverse cardiovascular events (MACE), fatal MACE and fatal

bleeding. MACE was defined as stroke or TIA, myocardial
infarction, intermittent claudication, unstable angina, carotid
endarterectomy, coronary artery bypass graft, peripheral arterial
bypass or angioplasty [18]. Other variables of interest were time
within therapeutic range (TTR) and INR-variability; both
established risk factors for MACE and major bleeding complications during VKA treatment [19–23]. INR-values were measured
using HepatoQuick (Roche Diagnostics, Mannheim, Germany)
and serum creatinine values by using Roche Diagnostics Analyzers
(Mannheim, Germany).

Follow- up

Duration of follow-up was defined as time elapsed between the
day of initiation and permanent discontinuation of VKA
treatment, occurrence of the endpoint of interest, or death, or
December 31, 2010. Only the first stroke or TIA, MACE or major
bleeding event that occurred was recorded in the database,
although some patients had more than one episode of the
endpoints. For non-acute MACE such as intermittent claudication, carotid endarterectomy, coronary artery bypass graft,
peripheral arterial bypass or angioplasty, the day of diagnosis or
intervention was recorded as the date of MACE occurrence.

Statistical analysis

Incidence rates (i.e. events/100 patient years (py)) of primary
outcomes were reported with corresponding 95% confidence
intervals (CI). As patients with moderate or without CKD were
matched for age and gender to those with severe CKD, incidence
rates of our study endpoints in the first two patient groups reflect
the incidences of these endpoints for the population with this age
and sex distribution, rather than that of the overall AF population.
Nonetheless, this design allowed us to study relative risks of stroke
or TIA and major bleeds between patients with severe or
moderate CKD and those without renal impairment, which was
our main research question. This analysis was performed using
uni- and multivariate Cox regression analyses reporting hazard
ratios (HRs) as crude values and as values corrected for age,
gender, concomitant use of platelet-inhibitors or non-steroidal
anti-inflammatory drugs, hypertension, diabetes mellitus, and
congestive heart failure. As for secondary analysis, TTR and INR-
variability were calculated using the *Rosendaal* method and the
formula by *Cannegieter*, respectively [23,24]. INR-variability and
TTR were compared between patients with moderate or severe
CKD and non-CKD patients, using first a Kruskal Wallis and
second a Mann Whitney U-test, as these values had a nonparametric distribution among the population.

Mediation analysis

A mediation analysis was performed to assess whether the
expected increased risks of stroke or TIA, major bleeds and
MACE in patients with moderate and severe CKD compared with
non-CKD patients were mediated via TTR or INR-variability.
This analysis was performed for the three endpoints and the
combined endpoint of MACE and major bleeds in a nested case-
control study [24]. We chose this design as the duration of follow-
up needed to be matched for cases and controls. Cases were
patients developing the endpoint of interest. For each case, a
maximum of four controls was selected from the total study
population of 724 patients who were treated during the same
period with VKA while not developing this specific endpoint at the
time that the case did (incidence density sampling). A control could
be selected for more than one case. INR-variability and TTR were
calculated over the entire treatment period, for the last six and the
last three months prior to the outcome of interest. For each time

frame, only patients with sufficient follow-up were selected for that specific analysis [24]. Crude odds ratios (OR) were then computed for the risks of the four outcomes comparing severe and moderate CKD with non-CKD patients. Next, these ORs were first adjusted for comorbidity, and second for either INR-variability, TTR, or both for each individual time frame.

All statistical analyses were performed in SPSS 20.0 (IBM SPSS statistics, IBM Corp, Somers, NY).

Results

Serum creatinine values were available in 5039 out of 6933 patients with new onset AF at start of VKA therapy. Of those, 733 matched subjects were selected for inclusion for this present study, comprising all patients with non-dialysis depended severe CKD, and a sample of those with moderate or without CKD. Registered duration of VKA treatment in the Leiden anticoagulation clinic was less than seven days in 52 patients who were excluded and replaced by 43 patients of similar gender, age, and level of renal impairment. The remaining nine severe CKD patients could not be replaced (Figure 1). Thus, 724 patients were included in this study, 300 without CKD (eGFR >60 ml/min), 294 with moderate (eGFR 30–60 ml/min) and 130 with severe CKD (eGFR < 30 ml/min). Patient characteristics at baseline are reported in Table 1. Compared with patients without CKD, those with moderate or severe CKD were more likely to have congestive heart failure, hypertension, diabetes mellitus, or a previous episode of major bleeds before initiation of VKA therapy. Median follow-up time was 2.1 years (2.5–97.5percentile 0.0–10.0) for the

endpoint of stroke or TIA and 2.3 years (2.5–97.5percentiles 0.0–10.0) for major bleeding events.

Stroke or TIA and MACE

During follow-up for the primary endpoint, 6.2% (45/724, 1.67/100 py) of patients developed a stroke (29 patients) or TIA (16 patients). The risk of stroke or TIA was increased in those with severe CKD compared with patients without renal dysfunction (HR 2.75, 95%CI 1.25–6.05) or those with moderate CKD (HR 3.93, 95%CI 1.71–9.00, Table 2). The risk of stroke or TIA was similar for patients with moderate and without CKD.

Overall, 14.8% (107/724) of patients developed MACE of whom 28 patients had a stroke, 15 a TIA, 28 a myocardial infarction, 17 an unstable angina pectoris, 11 patients underwent coronary artery bypass grafting, and 8 patients had developed peripheral artery disease (one patient developed a stroke and another patient a TIA after the occurrence of an earlier MACE). Patients with severe CKD were at increased risk of MACE compared with non-CKD patients (adjusted HR 3.57, 95%CI 2.10–6.06) and those with moderate CKD (adjusted HR 3.40, 95%CI 2.05–5.64). MACE risk was similar for those without and with moderate CKD. Twenty-three of 724 patients had a fatal MACE, of whom 14 (60.9%) developed a myocardial infarction and 9 (39.1%) a stroke. Although non-significant, moderate and severe CKD were associated with a 60–90% increased risk of fatal MACE compared with non-CKD patients, respectively.

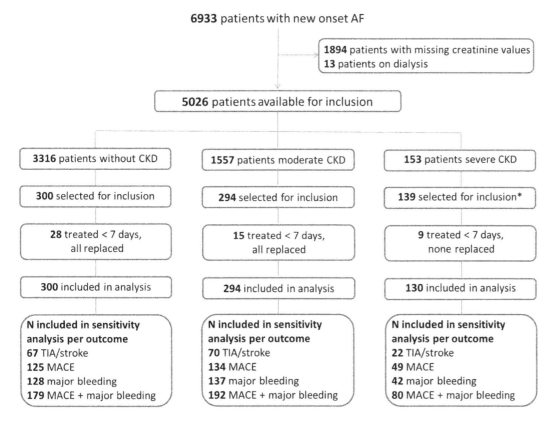

Figure 1. Flow chart. Abbreviations: CKD = Chronic kidney disease, TIA = transient ischemic attack, MACE = major adverse cardiovascular event. * Fourteen patients from the severe CKD group had acute kidney injury at time of VKA therapy initiation, after which renal function recovered to a less critical CKD stage.

Table 1. Patient characteristics at baseline of the total population.

	No CKD eGFR>60 ml/min	Moderate CKD eGFR 30–60 ml/min	Severe CKD eGFR<30 ml/min
N	**300**	**294**	**130**
Mean age (SD)	74(10)	75(10)	76(9)
Gender, m/f	171/129	165/129	73/57
Mean eGFR (SD)	92(37)	46(8)	21(7)
Diabetes Mellitus	35(11.7)	50(17.0)	38(29.2)
Hypertension	138(46.0)	181(61.6)	80(61.5)
Concomitant use of platelet inhibitors	26(8.7)	35(11.9)	7(5.4)
Previous stroke or TIA	47(15.7)	59(20.1)	21(16.2)
Previous major bleeding	14(4.7)	21(7.1)	10(7.7)
Congestive heart failure	50(17.0)	105(35.7)	54(41.5)
INR target range*			
2.0–3.0	1(0.3)	0(0.0)	1(0.8)
2.5–3.5	287(98.6)	280(97.9)	116(97.5)
3.0–4.0	3(1.0)	6(2.1)	2(1.7)
Acenocoumarol**	13(4.3)	15(5.1)	9(7.0)
Phenprocoumon	287(95.7)	278(94.6)	120(93.0)

Data is presented as n, % unless stated otherwise.
CKD = chronic kidney disease, eGFR = estimated glomerular filtration rate, SD = standard deviation, TIA = transient ischemic attack.
* Lacking in 30 patients, ** lacking in one patient.

Major bleeding complications

Major bleeding complications occurred in 15.6% of patients (113/724, 4.8/100 py). Although non-significant, severe CKD was associated with an increased risk of major bleeds compared with patients without renal impairment (adjusted HR 1.66, 95%CI0.97–2.86), and those with moderate CKD (HR 1.86, 95%CI1.08–3.21). Major bleeding risks were similar for those without and with moderate CKD. The most frequent locations of major bleeding were gastrointestinal (34.5%) and intracranial (27.4%) in the total population. Patients with severe CKD were more likely to develop gastrointestinal bleeding (63.6%), yet less frequently developed intracranial haemorrhages (13.6%).

Fatal bleeding occurred in 2.9% of patients (21/724). Severe CKD might be associated with an increased risk of fatal bleeding events compared with non-CKD patients (HR 1.52, 95%CI0.46–5.02, Table 2), and those with moderate CKD (HR 1.90, 95%CI0.57–6.41).

TTR and INR variability

Compared with patients without CKD, TTR was higher in those with moderate CKD (75.1%, p<0.01) whereas TTR was similar in patients with severe CKD (70.3%, p = 0.41, Table 3). The proportion of time spent above target range was higher for all CKD stages compared with patients without renal impairment, and higher for those with severe compared with moderate CKD. Median INR-variability during the entire treatment period significantly increased with each stage of CKD, with median values of 0.5 in patients without CKD, 0.7 (p = 0.03) in those with moderate, and 0.9 (p<0.001) in those with severe CKD. For all three groups, the degree of INR variability can be regarded as below average or unstable anticoagulant control according to previous research [25].

Mediation analysis

Mediation analyses were performed on the influence of TTR and INR-variability on the increased risks of stroke or TIA, MACE and major bleeding complications in severe CKD compared with non-CKD patients. TTR and INR-variability were analysed as continuous and categorical variables (based on 33rd and 66th percentiles) in separate models demonstrating similar results. For all four outcomes, the results demonstrated a decrease in the odds ratio towards unity in severe CKD compared with non-CKD patients, when corrected for either INR-variability or TTR (Table 4 and 5). However, the effect of INR-variability and TTR in the three months prior to combined endpoint of stroke or TIA and to the endpoint of MACE was less pronounced. This might be the result of the low number of INR measurements during this short timeframe (median 5.0, 2.5–97.5 percentile 2.0–10.5), which might not be sufficient for adequate assessment of TTR and INR-variability. Simultaneous correction for both INR-variability and TTR did not result in a further decrease towards unity for any of the endpoints comparing severe and moderate CKD to non-CKD patients, indicating no additive effect of TTR over INR-variability, and vice versa. This indicates that the increased risks in patients with severe CKD for stroke or TIA, major bleeds and MACE were mediated via suboptimal anticoagulation control.

Discussion

Our study has three important findings. First, risks of stroke or TIA, MACE and major bleeding complications during VKA therapy were high in AF patients with severe non-dialysis dependent CKD, when compared to those without renal impairment, or with moderate CKD. Second, stroke or TIA, MACE and major bleeding risks were similar for patients with moderate CKD and those with normal renal function. Third, patients with CKD spent more time above INR target range and

Table 2. Risk of stroke, TIA, MACE and major bleeding events during vitamin K-antagonist treatment stratified by renal function within the entire population.

Endpoint	No. of events	N/100 py‡ (95% CI)	Crude HR (95% CI)	Adjusted HR (95% CI)
Stroke or TIA				
No CKD	19	1.62(1.03–2.54)	ref	ref
Moderate CKD	15	1.20(0.71–1.99)	0.72(0.36–1.41)	0.70(0.35–1.41)
Severe CKD	11	4.24(2.30–7.53)	2.40(1.13–5.07)	2.75(1.25–6.05)
Overall MACE*				
No CKD	36	3.48(2.51–4.80)	ref	ref
Moderate CKD	41	3.79(2.80–5.12)	1.06(0.68–1.67)	1.05(0.66–1.67)
Severe CKD	30	15.4(10.95–21.16)	3.78(2.31–6.19)	3.57(2.10–6.06)
Fatal MACE†				
No CKD	7	0.64(0.28–1.35)	ref	ref
Moderate CKD	12	1.05(0.58–1.85)	1.68(0.66–4.27)	1.64(0.64–4.17)
Severe CKD	4	1.67(0.50–4.38)	2.09(0.60–7.23)	1.92(0.55–6.67)
Overall major bleeding*				
No CKD	46	4.45(3.34–5.89)	ref	ref
Moderate CKD	45	4.11(3.07–5.46)	0.91(0.60–1.37)	0.90(0.59–1.37)
Severe CKD	22	8.84(5.85–13.07)	1.88(1.13–3.14)	1.66(0.97–2.86)
Fatal bleeding†				
No CKD	9	0.83(0.41–1.59)	ref	ref
Moderate CKD	8	0.70(0.33–1.40)	0.85(0.33–2.21)	0.82(0.32–2.13)
Severe CKD	4	1.67(0.50–4.38)	1.62(0.49–5.33)	1.52(0.46–5.02)

Definitions: no-CKD = estimated glomerular filtration rate (eGFR) >60 ml/min, moderate CKD = eGFR 30–60 ml/min, severe CKD = eGFR <30 ml/min.
Abbreviations: CKD = chronic kidney disease, PY = patient years, CI = confidence interval, HR = hazard ratio, MACE = major adverse cardiovascular event, TIA = transient ischemic attack.
‡Reported incidences for patients with an eGFR 30–60 or eGFR >60 ml/min are influenced by sampling of patients matched for age and gender to those with an eGFR <30 ml/min.
* HR adjusted for age, gender, hypertension, the use of platelet-inhibitors, diabetes mellitus and congestive heart failure.
†HR adjusted for age and gender. Further correcting resulted in non-converging coefficients.

had a higher INR-variability. Consequently, in a nested case-control study we have shown additionally that poor anticoagulation control was associated with increased risks of stroke or TIA, MACE and major bleeds in severe CKD patients. Our study therefore provides important insights into the efficacy and safety of VKA treatment in patients with CKD and AF.

CKD is a common comorbid condition in AF patients and increases a patient's risk for both stroke and major bleeds. Suggested mechanisms for this higher stroke and bleeding risk are endothelial dysfunction, hypercoagulability, and chronic inflammation [8,11,12]. We demonstrated in a nested case-control study that impaired anticoagulation control might be an important additional determinant. Interestingly, within the total study population of 724 patients, CKD patients were spending more time above INR target range and had a higher INR variability compared with non-CKD patients, despite frequent INR monitoring. We hypothesize several explanations for this observation. CKD by itself may affect the quality of anticoagulant treatment. First, renal impairment might influence hepatic VKA metabolism, as has been shown in animal models for hepatic cytochrome P-450 metabolism [26,27]. Second, CKD influences the pharmacokinetic characteristics of VKA, as warfarin half-life was reported to be shorter in CKD compared with non-CKD patients with a greater unbound warfarin fraction [28,29]. Third, we cannot exclude that anticoagulant control is impaired in patients with CKD by poor patient compliance. Regardless of the mechanism by which CKD

influences the quality of VKA therapy, our nested case-control study indicates that the increased risks of stroke or TIA, MACE and major bleeding complications in severe CKD patients are mediated through suboptimal anticoagulation control. This suggests that although warfarin has been shown to be effective in preventing stroke in CKD patients with AF in two observational and one randomized study [7,8,12], there is a great need for better tailored anticoagulant treatment approaches for this specific population, involving either better INR control, or the use of anticoagulants other than VKAs.

The use of computer-assisted dosage programs surveying both INR-variability and TTR during VKA treatment may help to identify patients with poor anticoagulant control in order to prevent them from developing stroke, TIA or major bleeding events [30]. Further, patient education and self-monitoring of INRs might improve patient compliance [31].

The novel oral anticoagulants have demonstrated less inter- and intra-individual variability in their pharmacokinetic properties compared with VKA. Within the Phase-3 trials, subgroup analyses have been performed for the efficacy and safety of these new agents compared with standard warfarin or aspirin treatment in AF patients with moderate CKD (i.e. eGFR >25 or >30 ml/min) [32]. These analyses demonstrated either a reduced risk of stroke and systemic thromboembolism compared with warfarin (Dabigatran 150 mg twice daily) or aspirin (Apixaban 5 mg twice daily), or a similar efficacy compared with warfarin treatment for AF

Table 3. Time within therapeutic range and INR variability within the entire population of 724 patients with atrial fibrillation.

	No CKD	Moderate CKD	P-value comparison	Severe CKD	P-value comparison	P-value comparison with
	eGFR>60 ml/min	eGFR 30-60 ml/min	with no CKD patients	eGFR<30 ml/min	with no CKD patients	moderate CKD patients
Time spend within therapeutic range, %						
First six weeks of VKA therapy	39.4(13.2-73.5)	49.7(24.1-81.3)	0.01	44.1(26.4-77.9)	0.10	0.60
First eighteen weeks of VKA therapy	57.9(29.8-79.3)	65.5(42.1-83.9)	0.01	60.7(39.4-80.6)	0.37	0.19
First twenty-six weeks of VKA therapy	61.5(38.7-79.8)	67.1(46.7-82.4)	0.02	64.7(41.5-75.6)	0.92	0.07
Entire treatment period	67.0(43.1-81.1)	75.1(57.8-82.9)	<0.01	70.3(49.2-81.1)	0.41	0.10
Time under target range (entire treatment), %	8.7(2.6-35.5)	6.2(2.1-13.0)	<0.001	5.5(2.3-12.9)	0.001	0.77
Time above target range (entire treatment), %	11.7(3.9-21.2)	15.2(9.8-24.0)	<0.001	20.8(11.7-32.7)	<0.001	<0.01
INR variability (2.5-97.5 percentiles)						
First six weeks of VKA therapy	0.5(0.1-1.6)	0.6(0.2-1.6)	0.10	0.7(0.4-2.3)	0.001	0.03
First eighteen weeks of VKA therapy	0.4(0.2-1.3)	0.6(0.2-1.5)	0.08	0.8(0.4-1.8)	<0.001	0.01
First twenty-six weeks of VKA therapy	0.5(0.3-1.2)	0.7(0.4-1.2)	0.24	0.8(0.4-1.8)	<0.001	<0.01
Entire treatment period	0.5(0.3-1.2)	0.7(0.4-1.2)	0.03	0.9(0.5-1.8)	<0.001	<0.01

Data are presented as median, (Interquartile range), P-values were computed using Mann-Whitney test, after proof of significant differences between groups using a Kruskal-Wallis test. CKD = chronic kidney disease, VKA = vitamin K-antagonists, eGFR = estimated glomerular filtration rate, INR = international normalized ratio.

Table 4. Mediation analysis on effect of INR-variability on the increased risks of major adverse cardiovascular events and major bleeding complications in patients with chronic kidney disease in a nested case-control study.

Outcome	Crude OR (95% CI)	Adjusted OR 1 (95% CI)	Adjusted OR 2 (95% CI)	Adjusted OR 3 (95% CI)	Adjusted OR 4 (95% CI)
Stroke or TIA					
No CKD (N=91, of whom 67 unique)	ref	ref	ref	ref	ref
Moderate CKD (N=90, of whom 70 unique)	0.76(0.36–1.61)	0.76(0.35–1.67)	0.79(0.36–1.76)	1.06(0.41–2.75)	1.02(0.40–2.56)
Severe CKD (N=25, of whom 22 unique)	2.98(1.17–7.60)	2.56(0.92–7.10)	2.23(0.73–6.84)	1.96(0.50–7.74)	2.50(0.69–9.07)
MACE					
No CKD (N=210, of whom 125 unique)	ref	ref	ref	ref	ref
Moderate CKD (N=205, of whom 134 unique)	1.21(0.74–1.98)	1.14(0.68–1.93)	1.15(0.66–1.99)	1.05(0.58–1.91)	1.10(0.62–1.96)
Severe CKD (N=58, of whom 49 unique)	5.18(2.76–9.70)	5.07(2.57–10.02)	5.37(2.58–11.19)	3.58(1.59–8.03)	3.77(1.71–8.32)
Major bleeding					
No CKD (N=211, of whom 128 unique)	ref	ref	ref	ref	ref
Moderate CKD (N=245, of whom 137 unique)	0.81(0.51–1.28)	0.76(0.47–1.23)	0.74(0.45–1.22)	0.88(0.52–1.52)	0.83(0.49–1.40)
Severe CKD (N=60, of whom 42 unique)	2.08(1.12–3.85)	1.77(0.91–3.43)	1.82(0.93–3.56)	1.55(0.70–3.44)	1.57(0.72–3.40)
Major bleeding or MACE					
No CKD (N=361, of whom 179 unique)	ref	ref	ref	ref	ref
Moderate CKD (N=419, of whom 192 unique)	0.87(0.62–1.25)	0.85(0.59–1.24)	0.87(0.59–1.27)	0.93(0.61–1.41)	0.88(0.59–1.34)
Severe CKD (N=122, of whom 80 unique)	2.92(1.88–4.54)	2.61(1.64–4.16)	2.67(1.64–4.34)	2.49(1.40–4.41)	2.31(1.33–4.03)

Model 1 includes age, gender, hypertension, the use of platelet-inhibitors, diabetes mellitus and congestive heart failure.
Model 2 includes model 1 + INR VAR entire treatment period, Model 3 includes model 1 + INR variability over six months prior to event.
Model 4 includes model 1 + INR variability over three months prior to event.
Abbreviations: CKD = chronic kidney disease, MACE = major adverse cardiovascular event, OR = odds ratio, TIA = transient ischemic attack.

Table 5. Mediation analysis on effect of time within therapeutic range on the increased risks of major adverse cardiovascular events and major bleeding complications in patients with chronic kidney disease in a nested case-control study.

Outcome	Crude OR (95% CI)	Adjusted OR 1 (95% CI)	Adjusted OR 2 (95% CI)	Adjusted OR 3 (95% CI)	Adjusted OR 4 (95% CI)
Stroke or TIA					
No CKD (N=91, of whom 67 unique)	ref	ref	ref	ref	ref
Moderate CKD (N=90, of whom 70 unique)	0.76(0.36–1.61)	0.76(0.35–1.67)	0.94(0.41–2.13)	1.31(0.52–3.37)	1.01(0.40–2.56)
Severe CKD (N=25, of whom 22 unique)	2.98(1.17–7.60)	2.56(0.92–7.10)	1.95(0.64–5.88)	2.49(0.65–9.55)	2.46(0.68–8.88)
MACE					
No CKD (N=210, of whom 125 unique)	ref	ref	ref	ref	ref
Moderate CKD (N=205, of whom 134 unique)	1.21(0.74–1.98)	1.14(0.68–1.93)	1.16(0.67–2.01)	1.06(0.58–1.93)	1.11(0.62–1.98)
Severe CKD (N=58, of whom 49 unique)	5.18(2.76–9.70)	5.07(2.57–10.02)	4.98(2.42–10.23)	3.26(1.45–7.34)	3.42(1.55–7.55)
Major bleeding					
No CKD (N=211, of whom 128 unique)	ref	ref	ref	ref	ref
Moderate CKD (N=245, of whom 137 unique)	0.81(0.51–1.28)	0.76(0.47–1.23)	0.73(0.44–1.21)	0.87(0.51–1.50)	0.83(0.49–1.41)
Severe CKD (N=60, of whom 42 unique)	2.08(1.12–3.85)	1.77(0.91–3.43)	1.55(0.79–3.07)	1.48(0.67–3.29)	1.50(0.68–3.28)
Major bleeding or MACE					
No CKD (N=361, of whom 179 unique)	ref	ref	ref	ref	ref
Moderate CKD (N=419, of whom 192 unique)	0.87(0.62–1.25)	0.85(0.59–1.24)	0.93(0.62–1.40)	0.96(0.63–1.46)	0.93(0.62–1.40)
Severe CKD (N=122, of whom 80 unique)	2.92(1.88–4.54)	2.61(1.64–4.16)	2.22(1.27–3.88)	2.37(1.33–4.21)	2.22(1.27–3.88)

Model 1 includes age, gender, hypertension, the use of platelet-inhibitors, diabetes mellitus and congestive heart failure.
Model 2 includes model 1 + time within therapeutic range over entire treatment period, Model 3 includes model 1 + time within therapeutic range over six months prior to event, Model 4 includes model 1 + time within therapeutic range over three months prior to event.
Abbreviations: CKD = chronic kidney disease, MACE = major adverse cardiovascular event, OR = odds ratio, TIA = transient ischemic attack.

(rivaroxaban 20 mg per day, or apixaban 5 mg twice daily). In terms of safety, the Aristotle trial demonstrated a lower risk of major bleeds in the apixaban compared with the warfarin group, whereas for all other novel oral anticoagulants, bleeding risks were comparable with the risks on warfarin or aspirin treatment [32]. Though, it is unknown whether these new agents would provide a better tailored anticoagulant treatment strategy compared with warfarin in severe CKD patients as they have been excluded systematically from the Phase-3 trials [33–35]. In terms of renal clearance, apixaban (25%) and betrixaban (17%) might be most suitable for use in patients with CKD. Although betrixaban has not been studied yet in a Phase-3 trial for stroke prevention in AF, the results of the Phase-2 trial, in which only CKD patients on dialysis were excluded, were promising in terms of a lower risk of bleeding compared with standard warfarin treatment in the group receiving the lowest betrixaban dose (i.e. 40 mg daily) [36]. However, the use of novel oral anticoagulants may not be advisable when the insufficient anticoagulant control in the CKD population is caused by poor patient compliance, which might even more be difficult to manage when laboratory monitoring of anticoagulant therapy is no longer required.

Our study has limitations. First, we had no information on alterations in renal function during follow-up, which might have led to misclassification of patients and consequently a misestimation of the reported hazard ratios. Second, events were recorded from chart review given the design of the study and we cannot fully exclude that some events were missed. However, our endpoints of stroke or TIA, MACE and major bleeding were clearly defined and are both serious medical events, requiring evaluation in a hospital setting and are thus likely to be reported in medical charts. Third, our primary and secondary outcomes were not adjudicated by an independent committee. Fourth, our sample size was too small to make further subdivisions in the stages of CKD other than moderate and severe CKD, or to demonstrate statistical differences in fatal MACE and bleeding rates. Fifth, we did not investigate the influence of co-medication interacting with VKAs on study outcomes. However, the majority of medication used by severe CKD patients is not known for interactions with VKAs. Sixth, we missed serum creatinine values at time of VKA initiation in 1894 of 9633 patients (19.6%) but we selected all patients with severe CKD (for whom serum creatinine values are highly unlikely to be lacking) and sampled controls matched for age and gender with moderate or without CKD. As patients without serum creatinine values are unlikely to have severe CKD it is implausible that lacking creatinine values in 1894 patients influenced the reported HRs on study outcomes.

In conclusion, patients with severe non-dialysis dependent CKD (i.e. eGFR <30 ml/min) are at higher risk for stroke or TIA, MACE and major bleeding complications during VKA treatment for AF, compared with those with moderate CKD (i.e. eGFR 30–60), or without renal impairment. Our study suggests that suboptimal anticoagulation control is a determinant in their poor cardiovascular prognosis. These study findings stress the need for more advanced tailored anticoagulant treatment approaches for AF patients with severe CKD. Whether the use of computer-assisted VKA dosage programs monitoring both INR-variability and TTR, or the use of novel oral anticoagulants are the answer to this issue remains to be studied.

Acknowledgments

The authors thank Dr. T.J. Römer (Department of Cardiology, Diaconessenhuis, Leiden, the Netherlands) for his help with data collection.

Author Contributions

Conceived and designed the experiments: JK NVR SCC TJR GYHL MVH. Performed the experiments: JK BS KAJVB JRB WRVDP AIDS SCC. Analyzed the data: JK NVR BS KAJVB JRB WRVDP AIDS SCC TJR GYHL MVH. Contributed reagents/materials/analysis tools: JK BS KAJVB JRB WRVDP AIDS. Wrote the paper: JK NVR SCC TJR GYHL MVH FAK. Interpretation of study results: FAK.

References

1. Koren-Morag N, Goldbourt U, Tanne D (2006) Renal dysfunction and risk of ischemic stroke or TIA in patients with cardiovascular disease. Neurology 67: 224–228. 67/2/224 [pii];10.1212/01.wnl.0000229099.62706.a3 [doi].

2. Tsukamoto Y, Takahashi W, Takizawa S, Kawada S, Takagi S (2012) Chronic kidney disease in patients with ischemic stroke. J Stroke Cerebrovasc Dis 21: 547–550. S1052-3057(10)00277-6 [pii];10.1016/j.jstrokecerebrovasdis.2010.12.005 [doi].

3. Kooiman J, van de Peppel WR, van der Meer FJ, Huisman MV (2011) Incidence of chronic kidney disease in patients with atrial fibrillation and its relevance for prescribing new oral antithrombotic drugs. J Thromb Haemost 9: 1652–1653. 10.1111/j.1538-7836.2011.04347.x [doi].

4. McManus DD, Rienstra M, Benjamin EJ (2012) An update on the prognosis of patients with atrial fibrillation. Circulation 126: e143–e146. 126/10/e143 [pii];10.1161/CIRCULATIONAHA.112.129759 [doi].

5. Herzog CA, Asinger RW, Berger AK, Charytan DM, Diez J, et al. (2011) Cardiovascular disease in chronic kidney disease. A clinical update from Kidney Disease: Improving Global Outcomes (KDIGO). Kidney Int 80: 572–586. ki2011223 [pii];10.1038/ki.2011.223 [doi].

6. Winkelmayer WC (2013) More evidence on an abominable pairing: atrial fibrillation and kidney disease. Circulation 127: 560–562. 127/5/560 [pii];10.1161/CIRCULATIONAHA.112.000640 [doi].

7. Hart RG, Pearce LA, Asinger RW, Herzog CA (2011) Warfarin in atrial fibrillation patients with moderate chronic kidney disease. Clin J Am Soc Nephrol 6: 2599–2604. CJN.02400311 [pii];10.2215/CJN.02400311 [doi].

8. Olesen JB, Lip GY, Kamper AL, Hommel K, Kober L, et al. (2012) Stroke and bleeding in atrial fibrillation with chronic kidney disease. N Engl J Med 367: 625–635. 10.1056/NEJMoa1105594 [doi].

9. Camm AJ, Lip GY, De CR, Savelieva I, Atar D, et al. (2012) 2012 focused update of the ESC Guidelines for the management of atrial fibrillation: an update of the 2010 ESC Guidelines for the management of atrial fibrillation—developed with the special contribution of the European Heart Rhythm Association. Europace 14: 1385–1413. eus305 [pii];10.1093/europace/eus305 [doi].

10. Abdelhafiz AH, Myint MP, Tayek JA, Wheeldon NM (2009) Anemia, hypoalbuminemia, and renal impairment as predictors of bleeding complications in patients receiving anticoagulation therapy for nonvalvular atrial fibrillation: a secondary analysis. Clin Ther 31: 1534–1539. S0149-2918(09)00228-8 [pii];10.1016/j.clinthera.2009.07.015 [doi].

11. Ng KP, Edwards NC, Lip GY, Townend JN, Ferro CJ (2013) Atrial Fibrillation in CKD: Balancing the Risks and Benefits of Anticoagulation. Am J Kidney Dis. S0272-6386(13)00784-1 [pii];10.1053/j.ajkd.2013.02.381 [doi].

12. Lai HM, Aronow WS, Kalen P, Adapa S, Patel K, et al. (2009) Incidence of thromboembolic stroke and of major bleeding in patients with atrial fibrillation and chronic kidney disease treated with and without warfarin. Int J Nephrol Renovasc Dis 2: 33–37.

13. Roldan V, Marin F, Fernandez H, Manzano-Fernandez S, Gallego P, et al. (2013) Renal impairment in a "real-life" cohort of anticoagulated patients with atrial fibrillation (implications for thromboembolism and bleeding). Am J Cardiol 111: 1159–1164. S0002-9149(12)02648-3 [pii];10.1016/j.amjcard.2012.12.045 [doi].

14. Wieloch M, Jonsson KM, Sjalander A, Lip GY, Eriksson N, et al. (2013) Estimated glomerular filtration rate is associated with major bleeding complications but not thromboembolic events, in anticoagulated patients taking warfarin. Thromb Res 131: 481–486. S0049-3848(13)00008-X [pii];10.1016/j.thromres.2013.01.006 [doi].

15. Levey AS, Coresh J, Greene T, Stevens LA, Zhang YL, et al. (2006) Using standardized serum creatinine values in the modification of diet in renal disease study equation for estimating glomerular filtration rate. Ann Intern Med 145: 247–254. 145/4/247 [pii].

16. Pottelbergh van G, Van HL, Mathei C, Degryse J (2010) Methods to evaluate renal function in elderly patients: a systematic literature review. Age Ageing 39: 542–548. afq091 [pii];10.1093/ageing/afq091 [doi].

17. Schulman S, Kearon C (2005) Definition of major bleeding in clinical investigations of antihemostatic medicinal products in non-surgical patients. J Thromb Haemost 3: 692–694. JTH1204 [pii];10.1111/j.1538-7836.2005.01204.x [doi].

18. Klok FA, Zondag W, van Kralingen KW, van Dijk AP, Tamsma JT, et al. (2010) Patient outcomes after acute pulmonary embolism. A pooled survival analysis of different adverse events. Am J Respir Crit Care Med 181: 501–506. 200907-1141OC [pii];10.1164/rccm.200907-1141OC [doi].

19. Amouyel P, Mismetti P, Langkilde LK, Jasso-Mosqueda G, Nelander K, et al. (2009) INR variability in atrial fibrillation: a risk model for cerebrovascular events. Eur J Intern Med 20: 63–69. S0953-6205(08)00136-2 [pii];10.1016/j.ejim.2008.04.005 [doi].

20. Cannegieter SC, Rosendaal FR, Wintzen AR, van der Meer FJ, Vandenbroucke JP, et al. (1995) Optimal oral anticoagulant therapy in patients with mechanical heart valves. N Engl J Med 333: 11–17. 10.1056/NEJM199507063330103 [doi].

21. Hylek EM, Go AS, Chang Y, Jensvold NG, Henault LE, et al. (2003) Effect of intensity of oral anticoagulation on stroke severity and mortality in atrial fibrillation. N Engl J Med 349: 1019–1026. 10.1056/NEJMoa022913 [doi];349/11/1019 [pii].

22. Reynolds MW, Fahrbach K, Hauch O, Wygant G, Estok R, et al. (2004) Warfarin anticoagulation and outcomes in patients with atrial fibrillation: a systematic review and metaanalysis. Chest 126: 1938–1945. 126/6/1938 [pii];10.1378/chest.126.6.1938 [doi].

23. Rosendaal FR, Cannegieter SC, van der Meer FJ, Briet E (1993) A method to determine the optimal intensity of oral anticoagulant therapy. Thromb Haemost 69: 236–239.

24. Leeuwen van Y, Rosendaal FR, Cannegieter SC (2008) Prediction of hemorrhagic and thrombotic events in patients with mechanical heart valve prostheses treated with oral anticoagulants. J Thromb Haemost 6: 451–456. JTH2874 [pii];10.1111/j.1538-7836.2007.02874.x [doi].

25. Ibrahim S, Jespersen J, Poller L (2013) The clinical evaluation of International Normalized Ratio variability and control in conventional oral anticoagulant administration by use of the variance growth rate. J Thromb Haemost 11: 1540–1546. 10.1111/jth.12322 [doi].

26. Dreisbach AW, Lertora JJ (2003) The effect of chronic renal failure on hepatic drug metabolism and drug disposition. Semin Dial 16: 45–50. 3011 [pii].

27. Leblond F, Guevin C, Demers C, Pellerin I, Gascon-Barre M, et al. (2001) Downregulation of hepatic cytochrome P450 in chronic renal failure. J Am Soc Nephrol 12: 326–332.

28. Bachmann K, Shapiro R, Mackiewicz J (1976) Influence of renal dysfunction on warfarin plasma protein binding. J Clin Pharmacol 16: 468–472.

29. Bachmann K, Shapiro R, Mackiewicz J (1977) Warfarin elimination and responsiveness in patients with renal dysfunction. J Clin Pharmacol 17: 292–299.

30. Ibrahim S, Jespersen J, Poller L (2013) The clinical evaluation of International Normalized Ratio variability and control in conventional oral anticoagulant administration by use of the variance growth rate. J Thromb Haemost 11: 1540–1546. 10.1111/jth.12322 [doi].

31. Beyth RJ, Quinn L, Landefeld CS (2000) A multicomponent intervention to prevent major bleeding complications in older patients receiving warfarin. A randomized, controlled trial. Ann Intern Med 133: 687–695. 200011070-00010 [pii].

32. Hart RG, Eikelboom JW, Brimble KS, McMurtry MS, Ingram AJ (2013) Stroke prevention in atrial fibrillation patients with chronic kidney disease. Can J Cardiol 29: S71–S78. S0828-282X(13)00222-5 [pii];10.1016/j.cjca.2013.04.005 [doi].

33. Connolly SJ, Ezekowitz MD, Yusuf S, Eikelboom J, Oldgren J, et al. (2009) Dabigatran versus warfarin in patients with atrial fibrillation. N Engl J Med 361: 1139–1151. NEJMoa0905561 [pii];10.1056/NEJMoa0905561 [doi].

34. Patel MR, Mahaffey KW, Garg J, Pan G, Singer DE, et al. (2011) Rivaroxaban versus warfarin in nonvalvular atrial fibrillation. N Engl J Med 365: 883–891. 10.1056/NEJMoa1009638 [doi].

35. Granger CB, Alexander JH, McMurray JJ, Lopes RD, Hylek EM, et al. (2011) Apixaban versus warfarin in patients with atrial fibrillation. N Engl J Med 365: 981–992. 10.1056/NEJMoa1107039 [doi].

36. Connolly SJ, Eikelboom J, Dorian P, Hohnloser SH, Gretler DD, et al. (2013) Betrixaban compared with warfarin in patients with atrial fibrillation: results of a phase 2, randomized, dose-ranging study (Explore-Xa). Eur Heart J 34: 1498–1505. eht039 [pii];10.1093/eurheartj/eht039 [doi].

15

A Randomized Pilot Trial of Remote Ischemic Preconditioning in Heart Failure with Reduced Ejection Fraction

Michael A. McDonald[1]*, **Juarez R. Braga**[1], **Jing Li**[2], **Cedric Manlhiot**[2], **Heather J. Ross**[1], **Andrew N. Redington**[2]

1 Division of Cardiology, Peter Munk Cardiac Centre, University of Toronto, Toronto, Canada, 2 Division of Cardiology, Hospital for Sick Children, University of Toronto, Toronto, Canada

Abstract

Background: Remote ischemic preconditioning (RIPC) induced by transient limb ischemia confers multi-organ protection and improves exercise performance in the setting of tissue hypoxia. We aimed to evaluate the effect of RIPC on exercise capacity in heart failure patients.

Methods: We performed a randomized crossover trial of RIPC (4×5-minutes limb ischemia) compared to sham control in heart failure patients undergoing exercise testing. Patients were randomly allocated to either RIPC or sham prior to exercise, then crossed over and completed the alternate intervention with repeat testing. The primary outcome was peak VO2, RIPC versus sham. A mechanistic substudy was performed using dialysate from study patient blood samples obtained after sham and RIPC. This dialysate was used to test for a protective effect of RIPC in a mouse heart Langendorff model of infarction. Mouse heart infarct size with RIPC or sham dialysate exposure was also compared with historical control data.

Results: Twenty patients completed the study. RIPC was not associated with improvements in peak VO2 (15.6+/−4.2 vs 15.3+/−4.6 mL/kg/min; p = 0.53, sham and RIPC, respectively). In our Langendorff sub-study, infarct size was similar between RIPC and sham dialysate groups from our study patients, but was smaller than expected compared to healthy controls (29.0%, 27.9% [sham, RIPC] vs 51.2% [controls]. We observed less preconditioning among the subgroup of patients with increased exercise performance following RIPC (p<0.04).

Conclusion: In this pilot study of RIPC in heart failure patients, RIPC was not associated with improvements in exercise capacity overall. However, the degree of effect of RIPC may be inversely related to the degree of baseline preconditioning. These data provide the basis for a larger randomized trial to test the potential benefits of RIPC in patients with heart failure.

Trial Registration: ClinicalTrials.gov NCT01128790

Editor: Yoshihiro Fukumoto, Kurume University School of Medicine, Japan

Funding: The authors have no funding or support to report.

Competing Interests: Andrew Redington is co-holder of a patent and shareholder in a company developing an automated remote preconditioning device. There was no commercial funding or other involvement for this project and an automated device was not used in this study.

* Email: Michael.mcdonald@uhn.on.ca

Introduction

Exercise impairment in patients with chronic heart failure (HF) is associated with significant morbidity and mortality [1–4]. Objective measures of exercise capacity continue to be important predictors of clinical outcomes, and are widely used to risk stratify HF patients for advanced therapies, including cardiac transplantation [3–5]. The effects of chronic left ventricular dysfunction and HF on exercise capacity are multifactorial, and relate to diminished cardiac output and to alterations in peripheral and respiratory skeletal muscle structure and function [6–9]. Notably, improvements in skeletal muscle function and exercise capacity are associated with improvements in left ventricular function [10], reduced hospitalization [11], and better transplant-free survival [12]. It follows that interventions to improve exercise capacity may translate into significant clinical benefits in the HF population.

Remote ischemic preconditioning (RIPC) is a well-described protective mechanism in which a transient, sub-lethal reduction in blood flow to tissues in one area of the body renders other remote tissues more resistant to subsequent episodes of prolonged ischemia [13]. Although the precise mechanisms are not fully defined, the remote ischemic preconditioning stimulus appears to trigger release of circulating factors [14–16] that result in downstream effects on mitochondrial function within the target organ(s) [13]. Early clinical application of RIPC in cardiac patients has been encouraging; transient limb ischemia, typically involving 2–4 cycles of 5–10 minutes each, has been shown to limit myocardial injury in the setting of elective cardiac or vascular surgery, as well as percutaneous coronary intervention for angina or acute myocardial infarction [17–21].

To date, the impact of RIPC in HF patients has not been explored. However, 'local' ischemic preconditioning of the legs improved maximal power output and maximal oxygen consumption during subsequent bicycle ergometry in healthy volunteers [22]. Recent work from members of our group has demonstrated that RIPC can improve maximal performance in highly trained swimmers, suggesting a salutary effect on peripheral skeletal, respiratory and cardiac muscle function under conditions of exercise induced hypoxic ischemia [23]. We therefore sought to determine whether RIPC would be associated with improvements in exercise capacity in patients with HF due to left ventricular systolic dysfunction.

Methods

The protocol for this trial and supporting CONSORT checklist are available as supporting information; see Checklist S1 and Protocol S1.

Ethics Statement

All patients provided written informed consent, and the study protocol was approved by the Research Ethics Board of the University Health Network, and registered prior to initiation (Identifier: NCT01128790, registered December 2009 at ClinicalTrials.gov). The CONSORT 2010 Statement for clinical trials was followed for the reporting of our study results herein. There are currently no ongoing clinical trials of RIPC intervention from our group at this time.

Patient Population

We performed a randomized, controlled, crossover pilot trial of patients recruited from the Heart Function Clinic at the Toronto General Hospital, a University of Toronto affiliated teaching hospital. The Heart Function Clinic is a large volume multi-disciplinary clinic that manages of a broad spectrum of HF patients, including those with advanced HF referred for consideration of transplantation or mechanical circulatory support.

Ambulatory clinic patients scheduled for routine cardiopulmonary stress testing were approached for study inclusion if they met all of the following criteria: ≥18 years of age, left ventricular ejection fraction (LVEF) <40%, history of New York Heart Association (NYHA) class II–IV symptoms, HF for at least 12 weeks, and clinical stability. Patients were initially excluded for any of the following reasons: ischemic cardiomyopathy, cardiovascular related hospitalization within the preceding four weeks, diabetes, peripheral neuropathy, inability to exercise or other contraindications to stress testing, inability or unwillingness to participate in serial exercise testing. Patients were enrolled and followed from September 2009 to February 2011. Following study initiation, there were comparatively few patients from our clinic population with non-ischemic cardiomyopathy who met all other inclusion criteria, and we therefore modified our protocol to include patients with stable underlying coronary disease that were otherwise eligible. All other exclusion criteria were maintained throughout the study.

Study Protocol

Patients were approached for participation and consent was obtained prior to their scheduled cardiopulmonary exercise test. Immediately prior to testing, patients were randomized by one of the investigators (MM or JB) in a 1:1 ratio by computer generated allocation sequence, to the order in which they received either RIPC intervention or sham intervention. Patients then crossed over to receive the alternate intervention at a dedicated follow-up visit for repeat exercise testing. Where possible, patients were scheduled for a second exercise study within four weeks to minimize the potential impact of disease progression or any interim therapeutic intervention on exercise capacity. Throughout the duration of the trial, patients were unaware of the expected effects of the sham or RIPC treatment and investigators (other than those performing the intervention) remained blinded to treatment assignment.

The RIPC stimulus consisted of four cycles of 5 minutes of upper limb ischemia followed by 5 minutes of reperfusion. A blood pressure cuff was placed over the upper arm, and limb ischemia was achieved by inflating the cuff 20 mmHg above the systolic pressure. The sham intervention consisted of four cycles of 5 minutes of blood pressure cuff inflation to only 10 mmHg, interspersed with 5 minutes of cuff deflation to simulate reperfusion. After completing four cycles of either intervention, 30 mL of blood was drawn, placed on ice and transferred to the investigators' laboratory as part of the pre-specified mechanistic sub-study. Immediately thereafter, patients completed a cardiopulmonary exercise test with respiratory gas analysis according to a routine stationary bicycle ramp protocol (10 Watt per minute incremental workload). Testing was symptom limited after achieving a diagnostic workload, defined as a respiratory exchange ratio >1.05. A dedicated exercise physiologist who was unaware of the treatment assignment supervised all tests, and a blinded investigator (HR) reported the results.

The primary outcome measure was peak oxygen consumption (VO2) measured in milliliters of oxygen consumed per kilogram of body mass per minute (mL/kg/min) during peak exercise following sham intervention compared to peak VO2 following RIPC intervention. Secondary outcomes included a comparison of exercise duration, workload achieved, ventilatory anaerobic threshold, absolute peak VO2, and the slope of the minute ventilation (VE) to carbon dioxide production (VCO2) ratio. As this pilot study was exploratory in nature and undertaken for feasibility, no sample size calculations were performed. We estimated that 20 patients with paired exercise data would represent an adequate sample to inform future trial design and generate appropriate study hypotheses.

Sub-study Protocol

We conducted a pre-specified sub-study to assess whether HF patients elaborate circulating protective factor(s) in response to a RIPC stimulus. The animal protocols used for this study were approved by the Animal care and Use Committee of the Hospital for Sick Children in Toronto and conformed with the Guide for the Care and Use of Laboratory Animals published by the National Institutes of Health (publication # 85-23, revised 1996). The 30 mL of blood drawn immediately following the RIPC or sham intervention was collected in heparinized tubes and placed on ice. It was subsequently centrifuged at 3000 rpm for 20 minutes at room temperature and the plasma fraction was dialyzed against a 20 fold volume of Krebs-Henseleit solution across a 12–14 kDa dialysis membrane. The dialysate was then prepared for use in a mouse heart Langendorff model as previously described [23]. Briefly, the dialysate was made isotonic and adjusted to pH 7.4 with sodium bicarbonate and glucose. Prior to perfusion of the mouse hearts, D-glucose, NaHCO3 and EDTA were added to a final concentration of 15 mM, 25 mM and 0.5 mM in the dialysate, respectively. Mice were anesthetized with pentobarbital in standard fashion and the hearts were excised, cannulated at the aorta, and perfused with modified Krebs-Ringer buffer at 37°C. A water-filled latex balloon was inserted into the left ventricle, connected to a pressure transducer and maintained at 7–10 mmHg to allow beat to beat measurement of left ventricular pressures (PowerLab data acquisition system AD Instruments; Colorado Springs, CO, USA). Dialysate derived from each patient for both sham and RIPC conditions was used to perfuse 2–4 mouse hearts, and data from each preparation was averaged.

Following a 20 minute stabilization period, the hearts were perfused with the study patient dialysate solution and then subjected to 30 minutes of no-flow ischemia followed by 60 minutes of reperfusion. After completing the protocol, the hearts were frozen at −80°C. Each heart was then sectioned into 1 mm thick slices and stained with 1.25% 2,3,5-triphynyltetrazolium chloride to distinguish areas of infarcted tissue (white colour) from non-infarcted tissue (red colour). The slices were formalin fixed and scanned into Photoshop. Using this method, it was possible to trace the area of infarcted tissue and express this as a proportion of the total area of LV myocardium at risk. The primary endpoint of this Langendorff sub-study was infarct area in hearts perfused with sham dialysate versus infarct area in hearts perfused with RIPC dialysate. Secondary endpoints included LV developed pressure, LV end-diastolic pressure, maximum rate of systolic pressure rise (dP/dt max) and fall (dP/dt min). Infarct size observed after sham or RIPC dialysate exposure in heart failure patients described above was also compared with infarct size observed using an identical sham and RIPC procedure to prepare dialysate from 4 healthy subjects serving as historical controls (4 males, age range 25–50 years).

Statistical Analysis

Continuous data are reported as means with standard deviation, and categorical data are reported as frequencies. Normality of the distribution of continuous variables was tested using the Shapiro-Wilks test. Differences in exercise outcomes between sham control and RIPC intervention were assessed using paired t-tests. Logistic regression model was used to identify factors associated with response to RIPC, with relative difference between RIPC and Sham used as a dependent variable and each categorical variable or each tertile of continuous variables as independent predictors. A p-value of <0.05 was considered significant for all comparisons. All analyses were performed using SPSS for Windows v 11.0 (SPSS Inc., Chicago, IL).

Results

Main Study

Figure 1 outlines the patient flow through the study. In total, 22 patients consented to participate from September 2009 to January 2011, and all 22 were randomized and subsequently completed the assigned first intervention prior to undergoing the initial cardiopulmonary exercise stress test. Two patients, both allocated to the initial sham control group, withdrew from the study and declined to undergo follow-up exercise testing. Therefore, the final study population included in the analysis consisted of 20 patients who completed the protocol with both sham and RIPC interventions.

The baseline characteristics of the study patients are shown in Table 1. As outlined, the majority were males with non-ischemic

cardiomyopathy. All patients were treated with beta blockers and ACE inhibitors, 70% required loop diuretics, and a large proportion of patients had received a defibrillator and/or cardiac resynchronization therapy. Although all patients had previously been characterized as NYHA class II, III, or IV, most were minimally symptomatic at the time of enrollment.

The majority of patients in this study (16/20) completed sequential cardiopulmonary exercise tests within 30 days as planned. Two patients were unable to return for scheduled follow-up testing for logistical reasons and completed the protocol within 90 days, and an additional two patients completed follow-up by 180 days. There were no adverse effects observed for any of our study patients. The results for the primary outcome, peak VO2 for RIPC compared to sham intervention, are shown in Figure 2 and Table 2. Overall, RIPC prior to cardiopulmonary exercise testing was not associated with improvements in peak VO2 in this population (15.6+/−4.2 mL/kg/min vs 15.3+/−4.6 mL/kg/min; p = 0.53, for sham and RIPC, respectively). With respect to the secondary outcomes, there was no observed benefit of RIPC on exercise duration, workload achieved, anaerobic threshold, or VE/CO2 slope (Table 2). Excluding patients that did not complete the protocol within 30 days had no impact on our results. Moreover, post-hoc exploratory analysis did not identify any baseline clinical characteristics, (including age, gender, duration of heart failure, functional class, BNP level) associated with an improved peak VO2 following RIPC intervention. Finally, the sequence of testing did not appear to have an effect on our results, as there were no significant differences in peak VO2 from the initial exercise study compared to the follow-up study, irrespective of the treatment allocation.

Langendorff Sub Study

In the Langendorff study, there was no significant difference in infarct area between mouse hearts perfused with sham dialysate and those perfused with RIPC dialysate (29.0+/−7.9% versus 27.9+/−6.8%; p = 0.62). Additionally, the secondary endpoint hemodynamic measurements were not significantly different at any stage following perfusion with either sham or RIPC derived dialysate.

Using this Langendorff model, we undertook a further exploratory comparison of infarct size following perfusion with dialysate derived from our heart failure study population versus infarct size following perfusion with dialysate derived from plasma from healthy controls undergoing sham/RIPC intervention. The infarct size observed in hearts perfused with dialysate from our heart failure patients was nearly 45% less than the infarct size observed in hearts perfused with healthy control dialysate following sham intervention. Moreover, the infarct area seen in our study approximates the infarct area seen with exposure to dialysate from healthy control subjects following RIPC intervention (Figure 3).

In order to determine whether the apparent lack of effect of RIPC in our study population could be explained by a high degree of baseline preconditioning, we assessed infarct size in the Langendorff model according to clinical response to RIPC treatment. In this post hoc analysis, mouse infarct size was significantly smaller among the subgroup of patients who had no improvement in exercise capacity following RIPC intervention, suggesting that the overall absence of a clinical response to RIPC in our study population may relate to a higher degree of preconditioning at baseline for the majority of patients (Figure 4).

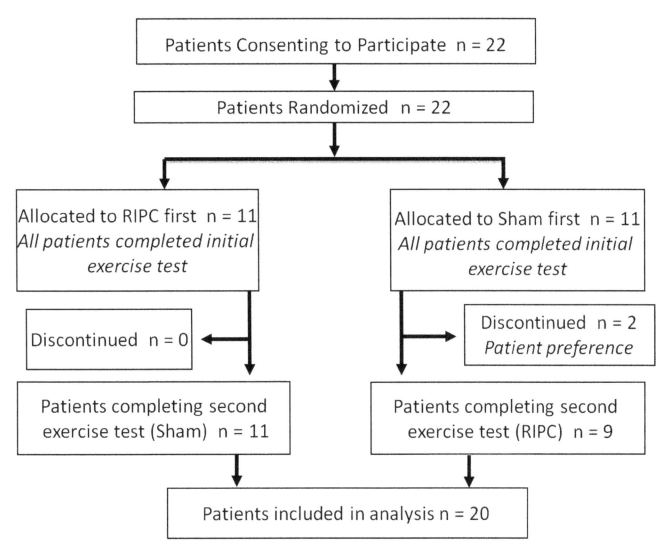

Figure 1. Patient flow through the study. 22 patients consented to participate in the study. Two patients declined repeat testing and were excluded from the analysis; 20 patients complete the study protocol with paired testing.

Discussion

In this randomized crossover pilot study, RIPC was not associated with improvements in objective measures of exercise capacity in ambulatory HF patients with left ventricular dysfunction. Specifically, there was no overall benefit with respect to any of the prognostically important exercise variables, including peak VO2, exercise duration, workload achieved or VE/VCO2 slope during cardiopulmonary stress testing. A principle finding from our Langendorff sub-study was that RIPC in this study population does not appear to confer additional protection against ischemia reperfusion injury through release of circulating preconditioning factor(s). This observation is in contrast with the effects of RIPC in a healthy control population [23]; moreover our results suggest that patients with chronic HF may already be relatively preconditioned.

To our knowledge, this is the first clinical trial to evaluate the effect of RIPC in a heart failure population. There is a growing body of evidence that suggests RIPC induced by transient limb ischemia, similar to the protocol used in our study, is associated with a significant reduction in end organ injury due to a variety of

ischemic stressors. One of the earliest clinical studies of RIPC was a randomized controlled trial of 37 pediatric patients undergoing cardiopulmonary bypass for corrective cardiac surgery [17]. In this study, four 5-minute cycles of limb ischemia and reperfusion resulted in less troponin elevation, lower inotrope requirements, and better lung function in the early post-operative setting. RIPC with lower limb ischemia was also shown to attenuate myocardial and renal injury in a randomized controlled trial of 82 patients undergoing elective abdominal aortic aneurysm repair [19]. These early trials have supported the observation that RIPC confers multisystem protection in an ischemic environment.

Maximal exercise performance is limited by 'relative' ischemia of skeletal muscle and is associated with tissue hypoxia and lactic acid accumulation, and thus can be considered a form of ischemic stress. Recently, the potential benefits of ischemic preconditioning have extended into the domain of exercise performance in healthy individuals. de Groot and colleagues showed that ischemic preconditioning of each leg prior to bicycle exercise testing improved both maximal workload and maximal oxygen consumption [22] in healthy volunteers. Members of our group have shown that RIPC induced by transient upper limb ischemia immediately

Table 1. Baseline characteristics of the study population.

Age (years)	56.3+/−11.8
Male	18 (90)
Duration of heart failure (months)	71.3+/−63.4
Etiology:	
Ischemic	4 (20)
Non-ischemic	16 (80)
LVEF (%)	29.3+/−6.8
NYHA functional class:	
I	5 (25)
II	10 (50)
III	5 (25)
IV	-
HTN*	3 (15)
Smoking history:	
Never	11 (55)
Prior	8 (40)
Current	1 (5)
Atrial fibrillation	6 (30)
Medications:	
ACE inhibitor/ARB[†]	20 (100)
Beta blocker	20 (100)
Spironolactone	10 (50)
Digoxin	7 (35)
Loop diuretic	14 (70)
Nitrate	2 (10)
AICD[‡]	12 (60)
CRT[ι]	5 (25)
Systolic blood pressure (mmHg)	105.7+/−12.8
Diastolic blood pressure (mmHg)	69+/−9.9
Heart rate (beats/min)	64.8+/−7.8
Height (cm)	178.6+/−8.6
Weight (kg)	94.7+/−22.5
Hemoglobin (g/L)	145.4+/−14.8
Serum creatinine (μmol/L)	94+/−22.5
Serum sodium (mmol/L)	138.5+/−2.7
BNP[#] (pg/mL)	Range 10.0–1616.0

(N = 20).
Values are expressed as means +/− standard deviation, or numbers and percentages.
*HTN: hypertension.
[†]ARB: angiotensin receptor blocker.
[‡]AICD: automated implantable cardioverter-defibrillator.
[ι]CRT: cardiac resynchronization therapy.
[#]BNP: B-type natriuretic peptide.

prior to exercise was associated with significant improvements in competitive swim times in elite athletes [23]. Furthermore, dialyzed serum taken from the swimmers following RIPC (but not serum taken before) was shown to carry a circulating "protective factor" that significantly reduced infarct size in a mouse Langendorff model of ischemia-reperfusion [23], confirming the importance of humoral-mediated pathways discussed earlier [14–16]. Prior to performing our study, we hypothesized that RIPC may have a favorable impact on exercise capacity of HF patients who are subject to musculoskeletal and cardiac

ischemia as they reach an anaerobic state at peak exercise. These patients have poor exercise tolerance secondary to reduced cardiac output, abnormalities in myocyte fibre composition, and reduced mitochondrial density [7–9]. Any intervention to improve exercise performance in a HF population with various physiologic limitations could potentially translate into important clinical benefits.

Why then was there no overall impact of RIPC on exercise capacity in this study, despite using a conventional preconditioning protocol? The answer to this question may be multifactorial, but

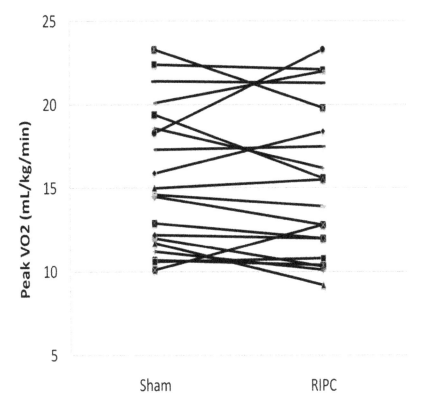

Figure 2. Individual exercise test results for sham versus RIPC intervention. Peak VO2 is shown for all study subjects undergoing exercise stress testing immediately following sham and RIPC interventions.

our Langendorff study provides important new evidence to suggest that these patients may already be in a 'preconditioned state'. Indeed, our results show that plasma obtained after sham intervention already contained dialyzable circulating cardioprotective factors characteristic of those liberated by remote preconditioning stimuli [14–16]. Consequently, overall the level of cardioprotection observed in control dialysate from the heart failure patients was similar to that seen after RIPC in normal volunteers, and was unaffected by additional RIPC. The reason for this is less clear however. There is emerging evidence that vigorous exercise in healthy subjects itself is a stimulus for release of cardioprotective factors [24]. We speculate that daily activities

in HF patients may act as a similar stimulus to the release of cardioprotective factors as a result of skeletal muscle ischemia. It is also possible that the heart may act as a paracrine organ for the release of cardioprotective factors. For example, Dickson and colleagues have shown that coronary effluent from hearts subjected to brief periods of ischemia is cardioprotective in an untreated acceptor heart [25].

Irrespective of where the circulating factors originate, our data do suggest that there may be a subgroup of heart failure patients that might respond to RIPC. Although the numbers were small, when we compared those that had significantly improved exercise performance with RIPC, versus those that did not, there was also a

Table 2. Exercise performance of Sham control versus RIPC intervention.

	Sham	RIPC	P value
Peak VO2 (ml/kg/min)	15.6+/−4.2	15.3+/−4.6	0.53
Secondary Endpoints:			
Exercise duration (minutes)	10.3+/−3.0	11.0+/−3.0	0.13
Workload (watts)	108.5+/−29.8	103.0+/−32.6	0.07
AT* (ml/kg/min)	9.6+/−2.6	9.6+/−3.0	0.98
Peak VO2[†] (L/min)	1.45+/−0.36	1.42+/−0.42	0.39
VE/VECO2[‡] slope	28.7+/−4.3	29.9+/−5.4	0.06

(N = 20).
Values expressed as means +/− standard deviation.
*AT: anaerobic threshold.
[†]VO2: oxygen uptake.
[‡]VE/VCO2: minute ventilation - carbon dioxide production ratio.

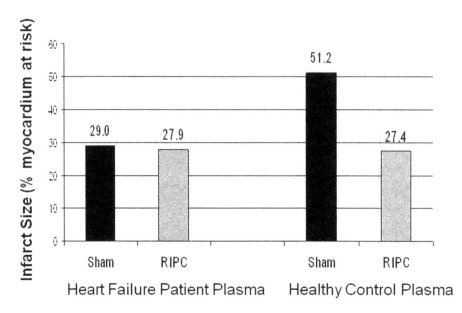

Figure 3. Langendorff mouse heart infarct size after perfusion with dialysate from heart failure patients versus healthy controls. Heart failure patient dialysate, irrespective of RIPC or sham treatment, reduced infarct to the same extent as the dialysate from RIPC-treated healthy controls, as compared to sham treated healthy controls.

significant difference in the level of cardioprotection afforded by their plasma dialysate in the mouse Langendorff studies. Plasma from patients that showed improvement in exercise capacity had lower baseline protection against ischemia, suggesting that their degree of baseline preconditioning was lower, and hence their capacity to respond to RIPC was higher.

It is also important to note, that while we were able to demonstrate the presence of circulating cardioprotective factors in vitro, we cannot confirm that they are the same as those induced by RIPC, nor can we confirm that they have any effect in-vivo in our HF patients. In pre-clinical studies, older age and underlying cardiac dysfunction have been shown to result in abnormal mitochondrial permeability transition pore and kATP channel

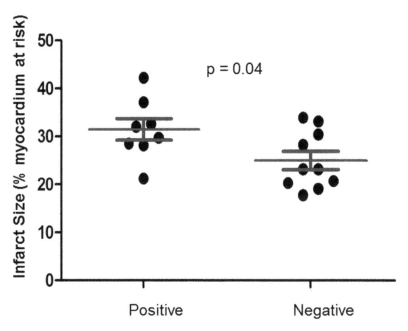

Difference in peak VO2 between RIPC and Sham Intervention

Figure 4. Infarct size stratified by the effect of RIPC on exercise performance. In the Langendorff model, mean infarct size was significantly smaller after perfusion with dialysate from the subgroup of patients who had no improvement in exercise performance following RIPC treatment. Data are presented as mean +/− SD % of infarcted myocardium.

function that may blunt the effects of RIPC [26,27]. There are also well documented ultrastructural changes in peripheral skeletal muscle associated with impairments in oxidative capacity [7–9,28], and the implications for ischemic preconditioning remain unclear. Failing myocardium also undergoes ultrastructural adaptation characterized by fetal gene reprogramming, with a decreased rate of aerobic metabolism and relative resistance to ischemia [29,30]. Coupled with the observation that mitochondrial kATP channels are endogenously activated in heart failure [27], all of this data suggest that in the clinical domain, RIPC may not yield significant additional protection from ischemic stress in a relatively 'preconditioned' HF state. While our pilot data show that there appears to be a subgroup of patients that benefit most from RIPC (those with low baseline preconditioning), in the absence of a clinical test of 'pre-existing preconditioning' the widespread adoption of RIPC as a clinical tool will require demonstration of effect in large, unselected, cohort studies. In this regard, it is likely that our study was underpowered to detect a small, but still meaningful difference in peak VO2 between RIPC intervention and sham control exercise tests. Based on the results from our pilot data, future trials would need an approximately 4–5 fold our sample size to have at least 80% power to detect a clinically important difference of 1–2 mL/kg/min in peak VO2. Smaller degrees of improvement would not likely translate into better transplant free survival [12].

Our study has a number of important limitations that may warrant caution in the interpretation of our results. Our post-hoc subgroup analysis of 'responders' versus 'non-responders' to RIPC, is not only somewhat artificial in terms of examining responses in a binary fashion, but also does not allow meaningful analysis of factors associated with those response, beyond the reported differences in cardioprotective activity of their plasma. A number of comorbidities and medications have been associated with either blunted or enhanced responses to ischemia-reperfusion injury and preconditioning [31,32]. As we did not exclude patients with comorbidities such as hypertension, dyslipidemia or left ventricular hypertrophy, and we did not perform a medication washout prior to testing, it is possible that our results may have been confounded. The impact of residual medications such as ACE inhibitors and statins in the Langendorff perfusate is indeterminate, and it is conceivable that these therapies may have modified the preconditioning response in the mouse heart. Although our model has previously been used to demonstrate the presence of a humoral mediator of RIPC [23], it is also possible that some of the larger sized key mediators of preconditioning were filtered from plasma

while preparing the dialysate. For example, Giricz and colleagues recently demonstrated that extracellular vesicles (exosomes and microvesicles) may be necessary to confer protection in a rat heart Langendorff model of ischemic preconditioning [33]. Furthermore, we did not measure lactic acid levels to confirm a state of relative hypoxia with anaerobic metabolism at peak exercise. However, our cardiopulmonary exercise protocol with respiratory gas analysis did allow for an estimation of anaerobic threshold as a surrogate for lactic acidosis. Finally, patients in our trial had considerable variability in their inter-test intervals. Although we attempted to repeat paired exercise tests within 4 weeks from enrollment, we were unable to achieve this for all patients, providing the opportunity for bias due to changes in treatment or clinical status between tests.

In summary, we conducted the first randomized controlled trial of RIPC in ambulatory patients with HF and left ventricular systolic dysfunction. In this study, RIPC was not associated with improvements in objective measures of exercise capacity. The apparent absence of an effect of RIPC may relate to a high degree of baseline preconditioning in our patient population, and those with lesser degrees may be benefit with RIPC. However large, adequately powered clinical trials and further mechanistic translational studies are needed before the effects of RIPC in HF can be established definitively.

Acknowledgments

We wish to thank Michael Walker for his expertise in exercise physiology and cardiopulmonary stress testing

Author Contributions

Conceived and designed the experiments: MM HR AR. Performed the experiments: MM JB JL. Analyzed the data: MM JB JL CM. Contributed reagents/materials/analysis tools: JL HR AR. Wrote the paper: MM CM AR.

References

1. McElroy PA, Janicki JS, Weber KT (1988) Cardiopulmonary exercise testing in congestive heart failure. Am J Cardiol 62: 35A–40A.
2. Mancini DM, Eisen H, Kussmaul W, Mull R, Edmunds LH Jr, et al (1991) Value of peak exercise oxygen consumption for optimal timing of cardiac transplantation in ambulatory patients with heart failure. Circulation 83: 778–86.
3. Pardaens K, Van Cleemput J, Vanhaecke J, Fagard RH (2000) Peak oxygen uptake better predicts outcome than submaximal respiratory data in heart transplant candidates. Circulation 101: 1152–57.
4. O'Neill JO, Young JB, Pothier CE, Lauer MS (2005) Peak oxygen consumption as a predictor of death in patients with heart failure receiving beta-blockers. Circulation 111: 2313–18.
5. Aaronson KD, Schwartz JS, Chen TM, Wong KL, Goin JE, et al (1997) Development and prospective validation of a clinical index to predict survival in ambulatory patients referred for cardiac transplant evaluation. Circulation 95: 2660–67.
6. Wilson JR, Martin JL, Ferraro N (1984) Impaired skeletal muscle nutritive flow during exercise in patients with congestive heart failure: role of cardiac pump dysfunction as determined by the effect of dobutamine. Am J Cardiol 53: 1308–15.
7. Mancini DM, Coyle E, Coggan A, Beltz J, Ferraro N, et al (1989) Contribution of intrinsic skeletal muscle changes to 31P NMR skeletal muscle metabolic abnormalities in patients with chronic heart failure. Circulation 80: 1338–46.
8. Duscha BD, Kraus WE, Keteyian SJ, Sullivan MJ, Green HJ, et al (1999) Capillary density of skeletal muscle: a contributing mechanism for exercise intolerance in class II–III chronic heart failure independent of other peripheral alterations. J Am Coll Cardiol 33: 1956–63.
9. Hambrecht R, Fiehn E, Yu J, Niebauer J, Weigl C, et al (1997) Effects of endurance training on mitochondrial ultrastructure and fibre type distribution in skeletal muscle of patients with stable chronic heart failure. J Am Coll Cardio 29: 1067–73.
10. Haykowsky MJ, Liang Y, Pechter D, Jones LW, McAlister FA, et al (2007) A meta-analysis of the effect of exercise training on left ventricular remodeling in heart failure patients. The benefit depends on the type of training performed. J Am Coll Cardiol 49: 2329–36.
11. O'Connor CM, Whellan DJ, Lee KL, Keteyian SJ, Cooper LS, et al (2009) Efficacy and safety of exercise training in patients with chronic heart failure: HF-ACTION randomized controlled trial. JAMA 301: 1439–50.
12. Stevenson LW, Steimle AE, Fonarow G, Kermani M, Kermani D, et al (1995) Improvement in exercise capacity of candidates awaiting heart transplantation. J Am Coll Cardiol 25: 163–70.
13. Kharbanda RK, Nielsen TT, Redington AN (2009) Translation of remote ischaemic preconditioning into clinical practice. Lancet 374: 1557–65.
14. Shimizu M, Tropak M, Diaz RJ, Suto F, Surendra H, et al (2009) Transient limb ischaemia remotely preconditions through a humoral mechanism acting

directly on the myocardium ; evidence suggesting cross-species protection. Clin Sci (Lond) 117: 191–200.

15. Steensrud T, Li J, Dai X, Manlhiot C, Kharbanda RK, et al (2010) Pretreatment with the nitric oxide donor SNAP or nerve transection blocks humoral preconditioning by remote limb ischemia or intra-arterial adenosine. Am J Physiol 299: H1598–603.

16. Redington KL, Disenhouse T, Strantzas SC Gladstone R, Wei C, et al (2012) Remote cardioprotection by direct peripheral nerve stimulation and topical capsaicin is mediated by circulating humoral factors. Basic Res Cardiol 107: 1–10.

17. Cheung MM, Kharbanda RK, Konstantinov IE, Shimitzu IE, Shimizu M, et al (2006) Randomized controlled trial of the effects of remote ischemic preconditioning on children undergoing cardiac surgery: first clinical application in humans. J Am Coll Cardiol 47: 2277–82.

18. Venugopal V, Hausenloy DJ, Ludman A, Di Salvo C, Kolvekar S, et al (2009) Remote ischaemic preconditioning reduces myocardial injury in patients undergoing cardiac surgery with cold-blood cardioplegia: a randomised controlled trial. Heart 95: 1567–71.

19. Ali ZA, Callaghan CJ, Lim E, Ali AA, Nouraei SA, et al (2007) Remote ischemic preconditioning reduces myocardial and renal injury after elective abdominal aortic aneurysm repair: a randomized controlled trial. Circulation 116(11 Suppl): I98–105.

20. Hoole SP, Heck PM, Sharples L, Khan SN, Duehmke R, et al (2009) Cardiac remote ischemic preconditioning in coronary stenting (CRISP Stent) study: a prospective randomized control trial. Circulation 119: 820–7.

21. Botker HE, Kharbanda R Schmidt MR, Bottcher M, Kaltoft AK, et al (2010) Remote ischaemic conditioning before hospital admission, as a complement to angioplasty, and effect on myocardial salvage in pateints with acute myocardial infarction: a randomized trial. Lancet 375: 727–34.

22. de Groot PC, Thijssen DH, Sanchez M, Ellenkamp R, Hopman MT (2010) Ischemic preconditioning improves maximal performance in humans. Eur J Appl Physio 108: 141–6.

23. Jean-St-Michel E, Manlhiot C, Li J, Tropak M, Michelsen MM, et al (2011) Remote preconditioning improves maximal performance in highly-trained athletes. Med Sci Sports Exerc 43: 1280–6.

24. Michelsen MM, Stottrup NB, Schmidt MR, Lofgren B, Jensen RV, et al (2012) Exercise induced cardioprotection is medicated by a bloodborne, transferable factor. Basic Res Cardiol 107: 1–9.

25. Dickson EW, Lorbar M, Porcaro WA, Lee WJ, Blehar DJ, et al (1999) Rabbit heart can be "preconditioned" via transfer of coronary effluent. Am J Physiol 277:H2451–7.

26. Zhu J, Rebecchi MJ, Tan M, Glass PS, Brink PR, et al (2010) Age-associated differences in activation of Akt/GSK-3beta signaling pathways and inhibition of mitochondrial permeability transition pore opening in the rat heart. J Gerontol A Biol Sci Med Sci 65: 611–9.

27. Maack C, Dabew ER, Hohl M, Schafers HJ, Hohm M (2009) Endogenous activation of mitochondrial katp channels protects human failing myocardium from hydroxyl radical-induced stunning. Circ Res 105: 811–7.

28. Hambrecht R, Niebauer J, Fiehn E, Kalberer B, Offner B, et al (1995) Physical training in patients with stable chronic heart failure: effects on cardiorespiratory fitness and ultrastructural abnormalities of leg muscles. J Am Coll Cardiol 25: 1239–49.

29. Rajabi M, Kassiotis C, Razeghi P, Taegtmeyer H (2007) Return to the fetal gene program protects the stressed heart: a strong hypothesis. Heart Fail Rev 12: 331–43.

30. Ostadal B, Ostadalova I, Kolar F, Charvatova Z, Netuka I (2009) Ontogenetic development of cardiac tolerance to oxygen deprivation – possible mechanisms. Physiol Res 58 Suppl 2: S1–12.

31. Hausenloy DJ, Botker HE, Condorelli G, Ferdinandy P, Garcia-Dorado D, et al (2013) Translating cardioprotection for patient benefit: position paper from the Working Group of Cellular Biology of the Heart of the European Society of Cardiology. Cardiovasc Res 98: 7–27.

32. Ferdinandy P, Schultz R, Baxter GF (2007) Interaction of cardiovascular risk factors with myocardial ischemia/reperfusion injury, preconditioning, and postconditioning. Pharmcol Rev 59: 418–58.

33. Giricz A, Varga ZV, Baranyai T, Sipos P, Paloczi K, et al (2014) Cardioprotection by remote ischemic preconditioning of the rat heart is mediated by extracellular vesicles. J Mol Cell Cardiol 68: 75–78.

16

Delphi-Consensus Weights for Ischemic and Bleeding Events to Be Included in a Composite Outcome for RCTs in Thrombosis Prevention

Agnes Dechartres[1,2,3,4], Pierre Albaladejo[5,6], Jean Mantz[7,8], Charles Marc Samama[3,9], Jean-Philippe Collet[10,11], Philippe Gabriel Steg[8,12,13], Philippe Ravaud[1,2,3,4], Florence Tubach[1,2,8,14,15]*

1 UMR-S 738, INSERM, Paris, France, 2 UMR-S 738, Université Paris Diderot, Paris, France, 3 Université Paris Descartes, Paris, France, 4 Centre d'Epidémiologie Clinique, Hôpital Hôtel-Dieu, APHP, Paris, France, 5 Pôle d'Anesthésie et de Réanimation, Centre Hospitalier Universitaire, Grenoble, France, 6 Université Joseph Fourier, Grenoble, France, 7 Service d'anesthésie réanimation et SMUR, Hôpital Beaujon, APHP, Clichy, France, 8 Université Paris Diderot, Paris, France, 9 Service d'anesthésie réanimation, Hôpital Hôtel-Dieu, APHP, Paris, France, 10 Service de cardiologie, Hôpital Pitié-Salpétrière, APHP, Paris, France, 11 Université Pierre et Marie Curie, France, 12 INSERM U-698, Paris, France, 13 Service de cardiologie, Hôpital Bichat-Claude Bernard, APHP, Paris, France, 14 CIE 801, INSERM, Paris, France, 15 Département d'Epidémiologie, Biostatistique et Recherche Clinique, Hôpital Bichat-Claude Bernard, APHP, Paris, France

Abstract

Background and Objectives: To weight ischemic and bleeding events according to their severity to be used in a composite outcome in RCTs in the field of thrombosis prevention.

Method: Using a Delphi consensus method, a panel of anaesthesiology and cardiology experts rated the severity of thrombotic and bleeding clinical events. The ratings were expressed on a 10-point scale. The median and quartiles of the ratings of each item were returned to the experts. Then, the panel members evaluated the events a second time with knowledge of the group responses from the first round. Cronbach's a was used as a measure of homogeneity for the ratings. The final rating for each event corresponded to the median rating obtained at the last Delphi round.

Results: Of 70 experts invited, 32 (46%) accepted to participate. Consensus was reached at the second round as indicated by Cronbach's a value (0.99 (95% CI 0.98-1.00)) so the Delphi was stopped. Severity ranged from under-popliteal venous thrombosis (median = 3, Q1 = 2; Q3 = 3) to ischemic stroke or intracerebral hemorrhage with severe disability at 7 days and massive pulmonary embolism (median = 9, Q1 = 9; Q3 = 9). Ratings did not differ according to the medical specialty of experts.

Conclusions: These ratings could be used to weight ischemic and bleeding events of various severity comprising a composite outcome in the field of thrombosis prevention.

Editor: Rochelle E. Tractenberg, Georgetown University Medical Center, United States of America

Funding: The authors have no support or funding to report.

Competing Interests: P. Albaladejo: Research grants (to the institution) from Bristol Myers Squibb, Pfizer, Daiichi Sankyo, Eli-Lilly, Boehringer Ingelheim, LFB, consulting or lecture fees from Bayer, Bristol-Myers Squibb, Pfizer, Daiichi-Sankyo, Eli-Lilly, Boehringer Ingelheim, Sanofi-Aventis, LFB, and Vifor. J. Mantz: Consulting fees from Baxter, Pall Medical and Orionpharma. C.M. Samama: Research grants (to the institution) from LFB, NovoNordisk, CSL Behring, SanofiAventis, Bayer, consulting or lecture fees from AstraZeneca, Bayer, Bristol-Myers Squibb, Daichi-Sankyo, Eli-Lilly, Sanofi-Aventis Group, Pfizer, Boehringer-Ingelheim, and GSK. J.P. Collet: Research grants (to the institution) from Abbott Vascular, Bristol-Myers Squibb, Boston Scientific, Cordis, Eli-Lilly, Fédération Française de Cardiologie, Fondation de France, Guerbet Medical, INSERM, Medtronic, Sanofi-Aventis Group, Société Française de Cardiologie, consulting or lecture fees from Zsra-Zeneca, Bayer, Bristol-Myers Squibb, Daichi-Sankyo, Eli-Lilly, Sanofi-Aventis Group, and Servier. P.G. Steg: Hamilton Health Services Astellas, AstraZeneca, Boerhinger-Ingelheim, Bristol-Myers Squibb, GSK, Daiichi-Sankyio/Eli-Lilly Alliance, Medtronic, Merck Sharpe Dohme, Roche, Sanofi-Aventis, Servier, The Medicines Company, and Aterovax. P. Ravaud: None. F. Tubach: Research grants (to the institution) from Abbott, AstraZeneca, Pfizer, and Schering Plough.

* E-mail: florence.tubach@bch.aphp.fr

Introduction

A composite outcome consists of two or more component outcomes. Patients who have experienced any one of the events specified by the components are considered to have experienced the composite outcome[1,2]. The use of composite outcomes in RCTs is common, particularly in cardiology[3] having the advantage of reducing sample size requirement, costs and time because of higher event rates. Composite outcomes estimate the net clinical benefit of treatment and enable to avoid an arbitrary choice between a number of important outcomes[2,4–7] so they may be used to summarize the risk/benefit profile of an intervention[8,9]. In the field of thrombosis prevention where treatments aim to decrease the rate of ischemic events but may cause hemorrhagic side effects of various severity, using composite outcomes including both ischemic and hemorrhagic events may be particularly appropriate to capture the net clinical benefit. Many authors have argued that all components of a composite outcome should be of similar importance to adequately interpret treatment effect[1–4,6–8,10–12] which is not frequently the case. Cordoba showed that the components were not of similar importance in 70% of RCTs reporting a binary composite outcome[1]. Choosing individual components of the same importance might also be irrelevant if the aim is to capture the overall impact of treatment. This is why some authors have proposed to assign each component a weight reflecting severity[8,12–14]. Since weighting may be somewhat arbitrary, it should be subjected to consensus panel[12,13,15].

STRATAGEM is a multicenter, randomized, double-blind, placebo-controlled trial whose objective was to compare low-dose aspirin therapy versus placebo (stopping anti platelet therapy) in the perioperative period in patients treated with antiplatelet therapy as secondary prevention (with documented symptomatic stable atherothrombotic disease) who undergo non-coronary surgery (registration number: NCT00190307, IRB authorization from the "Comité Consultatif de Protection des Personnes se prêtant à la Recherche Biomédicale (CCPPRB) de Paris Bichat" (Ref 2004/18, authorization obtained the 10th of Novembre 2004). The composite outcome took into account the balance of risk and benefit associated with maintaining antiplatelet therapy in the peri-operative period including both ischemic events (e.g., ischemic stroke, non-fatal myocardial infarction, acute limb ischemia, clinical deep venous thrombosis) and bleeding events (e.g., life-threatening bleeding or conducive to revision, or redo surgery, cerebral hemorrhage, intra- or retroperitoneal bleeding, bleeding requiring the transfusion of more than 3 units of packed red blood cells) in addition to overall mortality within one month following surgery. Since the individual components of this composite outcome clearly do not have the same value and severity, the aim of the present project was to attribute consensus-driven weights to ischemic and bleeding events according to their severity to be used in a composite outcome in RCTs in the field of thrombosis prevention.

Methods

Study design

The Delphi method was used to synthesize expert opinion [16,17]. It is a well-recognized method to reach consensus, relying on the following principles: anonymity, iteration, controlled feedback, and statistical aggregation of group responses [18–20].

Staff

A steering committee was initiated to perform this study and included all authors. The committee was responsible for the selection of events to be evaluated and experts, the analysis of the responses and the presentation of results.

Selection of experts

Experts were recruited from clinical disciplines involved in the management of patients with atherothrombotic disease in the perioperative period. In France, both cardiologists and anesthesiologists are involved in this field. Experienced academic experts were identified from different centers all over the country within national organizations such as the French Society of Anesthesia and Intensive Care or the French Society of Cardiology. The selected experts had also to be involved in design, execution and evaluation of clinical trials. Thirty cardiologists and 40 anaesthesiologists were invited to participate in the study. The experts were sent a standardized information package containing a synopsis of the study and a description of the Delphi process. The experts were informed that the consensus-driven ratings would be used as weights in a composite outcome.

Selection of events to be evaluated

Events to be evaluated were identified from the Common Terminology Criteria for Adverse Events (CTCAE) v3.0[21] which is a descriptive terminology that can be used for Adverse Event (AE) reporting. A grading (severity) scale is provided for each AE term. One author (F.T.) identified 28 ischemic and bleeding events that were then submitted to the steering committee for validation to enter the first Delphi round. They covered all the fields addressed by the STRATAGEM composite endpoint, in a more detailed way (for instance myocardial infarction was addressed by 3 different events corresponding to 3 different levels of severity in accordance with the CTCAE). We did not include death among the events to be assessed since the steering committee decided to attribute it automatically the worse rating (i.e., 10). The items involved in the Delphi process are reported in table 1.

Delphi consensus

The steering committee planned to perform at least two Delphi rounds. If consensus was not reached after 2 rounds, it was planned to perform additional rounds until a consensus was reached. The consensus process was conducted via email. Two reminders were sent at each round in case of non response.

In the first Delphi round, each member of the panel evaluated the severity of each of the 28 events on a 10-point scale. For each event, the experts were asked to answer the following question: "According to you, how severe is this event?". A 10-point scale with the anchors "not severe at all" at 0 and "extremely severe" at 9 was used to record the responses. The experts had the possibility to suggest events that were missing. They were added at the following round provided that they were not redundant with the other events. The median rating (1st quartile-3rd quartile (Q1–Q3)) for the whole group was established for each individual event.

In the second round, the experts considered the same event, and were also informed of each event rating at the first round by reporting of the median ((Q1–Q3)) rating on the scale for each event. The experts were asked to rate each event again in light of the responses at the first round.

Analysis

For each event, the experts' ratings were summarized as median (Q1–Q3). We applied a Last Observation Carried Forward (LOCF) strategy for missing data after the first round that is to say that, if an expert did not answer the second round, we considered his answers at the first round.

The concept of consensus within a group was defined as homogeneity or consistency opinion among the experts. Assuming that each event was characterized by a constant but unknown severity, the ratings of the experts could be considered as multiple measures of this characteristic. We used Cronbach's a to measure internal consistency among the experts for the set of events reflects the extent of consensus within the group for the severity of the set of events. When Cronbach's a is close to 1.0, it can be argued that there is consistency in the responses of the index panel, suggesting consensus. According to the recommendation of Bland and Altman [22], we considered that a consensus would be reached for a Cronbach's a value of 0.95. We also calculated intra-class correlation coefficient as a measure of the overall agreement between experts [23]. Ninety five percent confidence intervals for both Cronbach's a and intra-class correlation coefficient were calculated with bootstraps (1000 simulations). We planned to stop the Delphi consensus after the second round if the Cronbach's a value was superior to 0.95. The final weight for each event was the median rating obtained at the last Delphi round.

All analyses were performed on R version 2.10.0[24].

Table 1. Delphi panel events.

Clinical events	Definition
Ischemic events	
Transient ischemic attack	Transient ischemic event q 24 hrs duration
Ischemic stroke with no symptom at 7 days	Defined by a modified Rankin scale of 0–1
Ischemic stroke with slight disability at 7 days	Defined by a modified Rankin scale of 2
Ischemic stroke with moderate disability at 7 days	Defined by a modified Rankin scale of 3
Ischemic stroke with severe disability at 7 days	Defined by a modified Rankin scale of 4–5
Limb ischemia not requiring heparin or intervention	Brief (q 24 hrs) episode of ischemia managed non surgically and without permanent deficit
Limb ischemia requiring heparin or intervention	Recurring or prolonged (> 24 hrs) requiring medical or surgical intervention
Limb ischemia requiring amputation*	Life-threatening, disabling limb ischemia requiring end organ damage (i.e., limb loss)
Increased level of troponin	Without new Q wave or heart failure
Non-fatal myocardial infarction without heart failure	Killip 1
Non-fatal myocardial infarction with heart failure	Killip ≥2
Under-popliteal deep venous thrombosis	Under-popliteal deep venous thrombosis
Deep venous thrombosis with iliac extension	Deep venous thrombosis with iliac extension
Venous thrombosis of the pectoral limb	Venous thrombosis of the pectoral limb
Venous thrombosis other	Venous thrombosis other
Pulmonary embolism	Pulmonary embolism
Massive pulmonary embolism	Clinical or echographical acute pulmonary heart and/or impact on hepatic biology and/or more than half obstruction at angiography
Hemorrhagic events	
Intracerebral hemorrhage with no symptom at 7 days	Defined by a modified Rankin scale of 0–1
Intracerebral hemorrhage with slight disability at 7 days	Defined by a modified Rankin scale of 2
Intracerebral hemorrhage with moderate disability at 7 days	Defined by a modified Rankin scale of 3
Intracerebral hemorrhage with severe disability at 7 days	Defined by a modified Rankin scale of 4–5
Bleeding with increased length of stay	Mild bleeding not requiring intervention other than iron supplements
Bleeding requiring redo surgery or endoscopic sclerosis	
Bleeding requiring both redo surgery and interventions to maintain cardiac output	Bleeding with life-threatening consequences requiring urgent and major interventions
Bleeding requiring transfusion of 3 U or more packed red blood cells	Bleeding requiring transfusion of 3 U or more packed red blood cells
Bleeding requiring both transfusion of 3 U or more packed red blood cells and interventions to increase cardiac output	Bleeding with life-threatening consequences requiring urgent and major interventions
Intra or retroperitoneal bleeding	Intra or retroperitoneal bleeding
Intra or retroperitoneal bleeding requiring interventions to maintain cardiac output	Bleeding with life-threatening consequences requiring urgent and major interventions

Mesenteric ischaemia is considered as peripheral ischemia and then classified as "Life-threatening, disabling limb ischemia requiring end organ damage (i.e., limb loss)" and thus with limb ischemia requiring amputation.

Results

Delphi process

Of the 70 experts invited (30 cardiologists and 40 anaesthesiologists), 32 (46%) accepted to participate in the survey and completed the first round (9 cardiologists (30%) and 23 anesthesiologists (57%)). Twenty five experts (78%) completed the second round (6 cardiologists and 19 anesthesiologists). One event suggested by an expert was added at the second round.

At the second round, Cronbach's a was 0.99 (95% CI 0.98–1.00) showing a high internal consistency indicating consensus between the experts and therefore the end of the Delphi process. Overall agreement between experts was good with an intra-class correlation coefficient at 0.72 (95% CI: 0.59–0.80).

Consensus

A summary of experts' rating for each event and for each Delphi round is presented in Table 2. The ranking of the events slightly changed between the 1st and 2nd round. Events with the lowest rating of severity were: increased Troponin level (median = 3, Q1 = 3; Q3 = 4) and infra-popliteal venous thrombosis (median = 3, Q1 = 2; Q3 = 3). Events with the highest rating of importance were: ischemic stroke with severe disability at 7 days (median = 9, Q1 = 9; Q3 = 9), non-fatal myocardial infarction with heart failure (median = 9, Q1 = 8; Q3 = 9), massive pulmonary embolism (median = 9, Q1 = 9; Q3 = 9) and intra-cerebral hemorrhage with severe disability at 7 days (median = 9, Q1 = 9; Q3 = 9). Delphi-consensus weights are presented in Table 3. Ratings did not differ according to the specialty of experts (Appendix S1). Ratings at the first Delphi round did not differ

Table 2. Summary of experts' rating at each Delphi round for the assessment of severity on a 10-point scale of events deriving from individual components of a composite outcome.

Events	Median (Q1–Q3) 1st Delphi round	Median (Q1–Q3) 2nd Delphi round
Thombotic events:		
Transcient ischemic attack	5 (3–6)	5 (4–5)
Ischemic stroke with no symptom at 7 days	6 (5–6)	6 (5–6)
Ischemic stroke with slight disability at 7 days	7 (6–7)	7 (6–7)
Ischemic stroke with moderate disability at 7 days	8 (7–8)	8 (8–8)
Ischemic stroke with severe disability at 7 days	9 (9–9)	9 (9–9)
Limb ischemia not requiring heparin or intervention	5 (4–6)	5 (4–5)
Limb ischemia requiring heparin or intervention	7 (6–7)	6 (6–7)
Limb ischemia requiring amputation	9 (8–9)	9 (8–9)
Increased level of troponin	4 (3–5)	4 (3–4)
Non-fatal myocardial infarction without heart failure	7 (6–8)	7 (6–7)
Non-fatal myocardial infarction with heart failure	8 (8–9)	9 (8–9)
Under-popliteal deep venous thrombosis	3 (2–4)	3 (2–3)
Deep venous thrombosis with iliac extension	6 (5–6)	6 (6–6)
Venous thrombosis of the pectoral limb	5 (4–6)	5 (4–5)
Venous thrombosis other	7 (6–8)	7 (6–7)
Pulmonary embolism	7 (6–8)	8 (7–8)
Massive pulmonary embolism	9 (8–9)	9 (9–9)
Hemorrhagic events:		
Intracerebral hemorrhage with no symptom at 7 days	6 (5–6)	6 (5–6)
Intracerebral hemorrhage with slight disability at 7 days	7 (7–7)	7 (7–7)
Intracerebral hemorrhage with moderate disability at 7 days	8 (8–8)	8 (8–8)
Intracerebral hemorrhage with severe disability at 7 days	9 (9–9)	9 (9–9)
Bleeding with increased length of stay		3 (2–4)
Bleeding requiring redo surgery or endoscopic sclerosis	5 (4–6)	5 (5–6)
Bleeding requiring both redosurgery and interventions to maintain cardiac output	7 (6–8)	7 (7–8)
Bleeding requiring transfusion of 3 U or more packed red blood cells	5 (4–7)	5 (4–6)
Bleeding requiring both transfusion of 3 U or more packed red blood cells and nterventions to increase cardiac output	7 (6–8)	7 (7–8)
Intra or retroperitoneal bleeding	6 (4–7)	6 (5–7)
Intra or retroperitoneal bleeding requiring interventions to maintain cardiac output	7 (6–8)	8 (7–8)

Table 3. Delphi-consensus weights for ischemic and bleeding events comprising a composite outcome in the field of thrombosis prevention.

Event	Rating
Death	10
Ischemic stroke with severe disability at 7 days	9
Limb ischemia requiring amputation	9
Non-fatal myocardial infarction with heart failure	9
Massive pulmonary embolism	9
Intracerebral hemorrhage with severe disability at 7 days	9
Ischemic stroke with moderate disability at 7 days	8
Pulmonary embolism	8
Intracerebral hemorrhage with moderate disability at 7 days	8
Intra or retroperitoneal bleeding requiring interventions to maintain cardiac output	8
Ischemic stroke with slight disability at 7 days	7
Non-fatal myocardial infarction without heart failure	7
Venous thrombosis other	7
Intracerebral hemorrhage with slight disability at 7 days	7
Bleeding requiring both redosurgery and interventions to maintain cardiac output	7
Bleeding requiring both transfusion of 3 U or more packed red blood cells and interventions to increase cardiac output	7
Ischemic stroke with no symptom at 7 days	6
Limb ischemia requiring heparin or intervention	6
Deep venous thrombosis with iliac extension	6
Intracerebral hemorrhage with no symptom at 7 days	6
Intra or retroperitoneal bleeding	6
Transcient ischemic attack	5
Limb ischemia not requiring heparin or intervention	5
Venous thrombosis of the pectoral limb	5
Bleeding requiring redo surgery or endoscopic sclerosis	5
Bleeding requiring transfusion of 3 U or more packed red blood cells	5
Increased level of troponin	4
Under-popliteal deep venous thrombosis	3
Bleeding with increased length of stay	3
No event	0

between experts who responded at the second Delphi round and those who did not respond (Appendix S2).

Discussion

Before introducing a new treatment or strategy to common practice, or in comparative effectiveness research, capturing the overall impact of a therapeutic strategy in term of benefit and risk is important[25]. This is a well-recognized advantage of composite outcomes, but their use relies on the underlying assumption that patients will attach similar importance to each component [5]. However, this is rarely true. As outlined by Ferreira-Gonzalez[4] and cordoba[1], most composite end points showed either a large or moderate gradient in importance to patients. Weighting composite outcomes according to severity or importance to patients has been suggested to deal with this issue[8,12–14]. This approach is possible only if a consensus can be reached on the importance of each individual component[15]. We report in this study how consensus-driven severity ratings were obtained for a wide range of ischemic and bleeding events comprising a composite outcome. The Delphi method was used to assign each individual component of the composite outcome a rating reflecting its severity. This well-recognized method to reach consensus in health care research[18–20] presents major advantages : it can be conducted via mail or email which improves feasibility and lowers costs and it can be completely anonymous which limits the influence of a single expert. Experts presented a high level of agreement so the Delphi was stopped at the second round.

All individual components of the composite outcome were ranked from the most (i.e., death) to the least severe (i.e., absence of event) considering the final median rating attributed by the experts for each event. There are several possibilities to deal with the fact that a single patient may present several events of interest during the follow-up period. As proposed by Braunwald[13], the score for each patient may represent the score of the most serious event encountered by this patient regardless of the number of events having occurred what we planned to do in this study. Another possibility could be to use the sum of the ratings for all outcomes encountered[14]. We believe that presenting both a transient ischemic attack (weight = 5) and increased level of troponin (weight = 4) during the follow-up period is not equivalent to ischemic stroke with severe disability at 7 days (weight = 9). Furthermore, we believe that death from myocardial infarction should not account for a higher rating than death from unknown cause occurring at home, which might also be due to myocardial infarction. Rating multiple events was not possible in our study given the number of possible combinations so the consensus was limited to severity ratings for each event and did not relate to their combination.

Felker proposed an alternative method[26]: all patients who met the worst event (i.e., death) during the follow-up would be assigned the worst ranks, in order to their time to event (e.g., the patient who died first would have the worst rank, the second patient who died the second worst rank). Patient not dying during study follow-up would be evaluated for the second worst endpoint and ranked above those who died, using the same methodology. Those patients not experiencing any of the event components during follow-up would be ranked according to quality of life scores from baseline to last follow-up. After all study subjects are ranked, the comparative efficacy of the 2 treatments is evaluated by comparing the ranks between the 2 groups.

Events rated by the experts to be included in the final composite outcome can be considered as patient important outcomes (which was previously defined as death, morbidity or, patient reported outcomes[27]). Nevertheless, a potential limitation of this study is the absence of involvement of patients to assess the severity of clinical events which may be differently perceived than by physicians. We believed that explaining clearly all events with their possible consequences to make the judgment of patients possible would have been difficult.

Whatever the way to use the ratings to build the composite outcome, there is no evidence that such a composite outcome represents a clinically meaningful endpoint. A validation study should be undertaken with comparison of the different strategies for integrating the ratings. Important questions may be also raised about which between-arm difference will be relevant, with implications for interpretation of results and sample size calculation. Calculating sample size is generally difficult for composite outcomes since information for the control group may be available for one or several components separately but rarely for the overall outcome. The most important problem pertains to the interpretation of results, which is not intuitive using this approach. Which between-arm difference for the final composite outcome corresponds to a clinically relevant difference is an issue.

It has to be noted that the severity ratings were ordinal and not true interval so the composite outcome should not theorically be treated as a continuous variable. We also made the assumption that the experts not responding at the second round would have had identical answers in the second round and applied a LOCF strategy. We compared the ratings at the first round between the experts having responded at the second round and those who did not and checked that there was no difference in the ratings (appendix S2). Third, we made the assumption that cardiologists and anesthesiologists would be consistent in their ratings, which we verified by comparing their ratings (appendix S1).

In conclusion, the consensus-driven ratings that were obtained could be used to weight ischemic and bleeding events of various severity comprising a composite outcome in the field of thrombosis prevention. This approach could be reproduced for other types of treatment and medical areas.

Supporting Information

Appendix S1 Summary of experts' rating for the assessment of importance on a 10-point scale of events deriving from individual components of a composite outcome at the second Delphi round according to the specialty of experts.

Appendix S2 Comparison of summary of experts' rating at the first Delphi round between experts who responded at the second round and those who did not.

Acknowledgments

We would like to thank all experts who participated in this study: Michel Bertrand, Emmanuel Teiger, Emile Ferrari,Yves Juillière, Marie-Claude Morice, Pierre Aubry, Gérald Roul, Jeanne Barré, Vincent Piriou, Bernard Cholley, Souhayl Dahmani, Jean-Paul Depoix, Hawa Keita, Gilles Lebuffe, Hervé Dupont, Benoit Plaud, Jean-François Payen, Paul Zufferey, Benjamin Tremey, Philippe Vanderlinden, Sylvain Belisle, Jean François Hardy, Samir Jaber, Jean Luc Fellahi, Gérard Janvier, Vincent Minville, Karim Asehnoune, Sylvie Schlumberger.

Author Contributions

Conceived and designed the experiments: AD PA JM J-PC CMS PGS PR FT. Performed the experiments: AD JM CS J-PC PGS FT. Analyzed the data: AD FT. Contributed reagents/materials/analysis tools: FT JM PA CS J-PC PGS PR. Wrote the paper: AD FT. Drafting the manuscript: AD FT. Critical revision of the manuscript for important intellectual content: PA JM CS J-PC PGS PR.

References

1. Cordoba G, Schwartz L, Woloshin S, Bae H, Gotzsche PC (2010) Definition, reporting, and interpretation of composite outcomes in clinical trials: systematic review. BMJ 341: c3920.
2. Ferreira-Gonzalez I, Permanyer-Miralda G, Busse JW, Bryant DM, Montori VM, et al. (2007) Methodologic discussions for using and interpreting composite endpoints are limited, but still identify major concerns. J Clin Epidemiol 60: 651-657; discussion 658-662.
3. Lim E, Brown A, Helmy A, Mussa S, Altman DG (2008) Composite outcomes in cardiovascular research: a survey of randomized trials. Ann Intern Med 149: 612-617.
4. Ferreira-Gonzalez I, Busse JW, Heels-Ansdell D, Montori VM, Akl EA, et al. (2007) Problems with use of composite end points in cardiovascular trials: systematic review of randomised controlled trials. BMJ 334: 786.
5. Freemantle N, Calvert M, Wood J, Eastaugh J, Griffin C (2003) Composite outcomes in randomized trials: greater precision but with greater uncertainty? JAMA 289: 2554-2559.
6. Freemantle N, Calvert MJ (2010) Interpreting composite outcomes in trials. BMJ 341: c3529.
7. Ross S (2007) Composite outcomes in randomized clinical trials: arguments for and against. Am J Obstet Gynecol 196: 119 e111-116.

8. Pogue J, Thabane L, Devereaux PJ, Yusuf S (2010) Testing for heterogeneity among the components of a binary composite outcome in a clinical trial. BMC Med Res Methodol 10: 49.

9. Tugwell P, Judd MG, Fries JF, Singh G, Wells GA (2005) Powering our way to the elusive side effect: a composite outcome 'basket' of predefined designated endpoints in each organ system should be included in all controlled trials. J Clin Epidemiol 58: 785–790.

10. Ferreira-Gonzalez I, Permanyer-Miralda G, Busse JW, Devereaux PJ, Guyatt GH, et al. (2009) Composite outcomes can distort the nature and magnitude of treatment benefits in clinical trials. Ann Intern Med 150: 566–567.

11. Montori VM, Permanyer-Miralda G, Ferreira-Gonzalez I, Busse JW, Pacheco-Huergo V, et al. (2005) Validity of composite end points in clinical trials. BMJ 330: 594–596.

12. Neaton JD, Gray G, Zuckerman BD, Konstam MA (2005) Key issues in end point selection for heart failure trials: composite end points. J Card Fail 11: 567–575.

13. Braunwald E, Cannon CP, McCabe CH (1992) An approach to evaluating thrombolytic therapy in acute myocardial infarction. The 'unsatisfactory outcome' end point. Circulation 86: 683–687.

14. Sampson UK, Metcalfe C, Pfeffer MA, Solomon SD, Zou KH (2010) Composite outcomes: weighting component events according to severity assisted interpretation but reduced statistical power. J Clin Epidemiol 63: 1156–1158.

15. Califf RM, Harrelson-Woodlief L, Topol EJ (1990) Left ventricular ejection fraction may not be useful as an end point of thrombolytic therapy comparative trials. Circulation 82: 1847–1853.

16. Dalkey NC, Helmer O (1963) An experimental application of the Delphi method to the use of experts. Manage Sci.

17. Delbecq AL, van de Ven AH, Gustafson DH (1975) Group techniques for program planning; a guide to nominal group and Delphi processes. Glenview: Scott, Foresman.

18. Dalkey NC (1969) The delphi method: an experimental study of group opinion. Santa MonicaCA: RAND Corporation.

19. Fink A, Kosecoff J, Chassin M, Brook RH (1984) Consensus methods: characteristics and guidelines for use. Am J Public Health 74: 979–983.

20. Pill J (1971) The Delphi method: substance, context, a critique and an annotated bibliography. Socio-Econ Plan Sci 5: 57–71.

21. Program CTE (2006) Common Terminology Criteria for Adverse Events, Version 3.0, DCTD, NCI, NIH, DHHS. March 31, 2003 (http://ctep.cancer.gov)..

22. Bland JM, Altman DG (1997) Cronbach's alpha. BMJ 314: 572.

23. Bravo G, Potvin L (1991) Estimating the reliability of continuous measures with Cronbach's alpha or the intraclass correlation coefficient: toward the integration of two traditions. J Clin Epidemiol 44: 381–390.

24. R Development Core Team (2009) R: A language and environment for statistical computing. R Foundation for Statistical Computing, Vienna, Austria ISBN 3-900051-07-0, URL http://wwwR-project.org.

25. Kraemer HC, Frank E (2010) Evaluation of comparative treatment trials: assessing clinical benefits and risks for patients, rather than statistical effects on measures. JAMA 304: 683–684.

26. Felker GM, Anstrom KJ, Rogers JG (2008) A global ranking approach to end points in trials of mechanical circulatory support devices. J Card Fail 14: 368–372.

27. Rahimi K, Malhotra A, Banning AP, Jenkinson C (2010) Outcome selection and role of patient reported outcomes in contemporary cardiovascular trials: systematic review. BMJ 341: c5707.

17

Overexpression of Mitochondrial Uncoupling Protein 2 Inhibits Inflammatory Cytokines and Activates Cell Survival Factors after Cerebral Ischemia

Bryan Haines[1], P. Andy Li[2]*

1 The Buck Institute for Research on Aging, Novato, California, United States of America, 2 Department of Pharmaceutical Sciences, Biomanufacturing Research Institute and Technological Enterprise (BRITE), North Carolina Central University, Durham, North Carolina, United States of America

Abstract

Mitochondria play a critical role in cell survival and death after cerebral ischemia. Uncoupling proteins (UCPs) are inner mitochondrial membrane proteins that disperse the mitochondrial proton gradient by translocating H^+ across the inner membrane in order to stabilize the inner mitochondrial membrane potential ($\Delta\Psi_m$) and reduce the formation of reactive oxygen species. Previous studies have demonstrated that mice transgenically overexpressing UCP2 (UCP2 Tg) in the brain are protected from cerebral ischemia, traumatic brain injury and epileptic challenges. This study seeks to clarify the mechanisms responsible for neuroprotection after transient focal ischemia. Our hypothesis is that UCP2 is neuroprotective by suppressing innate inflammation and regulating cell cycle mediators. PCR gene arrays and protein arrays were used to determine mechanisms of damage and protection after transient focal ischemia. Our results showed that ischemia increased the expression of inflammatory genes and suppressed the expression of anti-apoptotic and cell cycle genes. Overexpression of UCP2 blunted the ischemia-induced increase in IL-6 and decrease in Bcl2. Further, UCP2 increased the expression of cell cycle genes and protein levels of phospho-AKT, PKC and MEK after ischemia. It is concluded that the neuroprotective effects of UCP2 against ischemic brain injury are associated with inhibition of pro-inflammatory cytokines and activation of cell survival factors.

Editor: Christoph Kleinschnitz, Julius-Maximilians-Universität Würzburg, Germany

Funding: Work was funded by the National Institutes of Health R01DK075476-06. The BRITE program is partially funded by the Golden Leaf Foundation. The funders had no role in study design, data collection and analysis, decision to publish, or preparation of the manuscript.

Competing Interests: The authors have declared that no competing interests exist.

* E-mail: pli@nccu.edu

Introduction

Hyperpolarization of the mitochondrial membrane potential precedes reactive oxygen species production and cell death in cultured neurons and astrocytes exposed to oxygen and/or glucose deprivation [1,2]. Inhibiting hyperpolarization protected neuronal cells from oxidative stress-induced cell death [3]. It is likely that mitochondrial hyperpolarization places pressure on the electron transport chain increasing the chance for incomplete oxygen reduction when there is a persistent flow of electrons from NADH and FADH2. This condition occurs after recirculation or re-oxygenation following stroke in vivo or hypoxia in vitro.

Uncoupling proteins (UCPs) are located in the inner mitochondrial membrane and function to transport protons into the mitochondrial matrix. UCPs were first described for the ability to generate heat without shivering in brown adipose tissue (BAT) [4]. Subsequent studies revealed that reduction of the proton motor force across the mitochondrial inner membrane by UCP2 decreased the formation of reactive oxygen species [5]. A small reduction in the mitochondrial membrane potential induced by mild uncoupling has a significant effect in attenuating reactive oxygen species (ROS) production [6]. UCP2 is ubiquitously expressed in all tissues with more levels in the brain and skeletal muscle at levels up to 1000 times less than UCP1 in BAT [7,8].

Proposed functions of UCP2 include preventing the formation of ROS and atherosclerosis, participation in inflammation, body weight regulation, adaptive thermogenesis and aging [9].

The majority of studies have demonstrated increasing UCP2 is neuroprotective; however, it is still a matter of debate. Up-regulation of UCP2 has been reported to reduce neuronal damage in cerebral stroke, traumatic brain injury, epilepsy and Parkinson's models [10–13]. Neuroprotective ischemic pre-conditioning and ischemic post-conditioning up-regulate UCP2 expression [14]. Neuroprotection by ischemic post-conditioning is partially dependent on AKT phosphorylation and involves the mitogen-activated protein kinase (MAPK) and protein kinase-C (PKC) pathways [15]. Neuroprotection by ischemic pre-conditioning and hypothermia is dependent on phosphorylated AKT [16,17]. The role of ERK1/2 in the MAPK pathway during cerebral ischemia is in debate; however, ERK1/2 is transiently increased in response to neuroprotective estrogen, hypothermia, ischemic pre-conditioning and post-conditioning [18,19]. Ischemic pre-conditioning and post-conditioning prevent the decrease in phosphorylated εPKC after stroke [15].

Oxidative stress and delayed inflammation are critical factors in facilitating neuronal death after cerebral ischemia-reperfusion injury [20]. It has been established that ROS production is increased after cerebral ischemia and reperfusion and such increases initiate expression of inflammatory cytokines [21]. These, in turn, stimulate innate inflammation to generate more ROS, creating a positive feedback mechanism. Tumor necrosis factor-α (TNF-α) and interleukin-6 (IL-6) are up-regulated after ischemic injury [22]. TNF-α has a divergent role in brain injury. Blocking TNF-α by antibodies, TNF binding protein or genetic knockout protects against cerebral ischemia [22,23]. In contrast to those findings, administering TNF-α before cerebral ischemia is neuroprotective, and ischemic pre-conditioning increases levels of TNF-α to activate the neuroprotective functions behind Nf-κB [22,23].

The goals of this study were to explore the mechanisms behind UCP2-mediated neuroprotection after transient focal ischemia. We evaluated changes in gene and protein expression related to inflammation and p53 associated proteins. One hour of middle cerebral arterial occlusion with 24 hours of reperfusion was utilized to determine infarct volumes, changes in gene expression and changes in protein expression. Our results confirmed previous studies that demonstrated up-regulating UCP2 reduces infarction after transient focal ischemia [12]. Overexpressing UCP2 reduces the levels of IL-6 mRNA, but not Tnf-α after ischemia. UCP2 Tg mice had increased protein levels of phospho-Ser AKT 473, Heat Shock Protein 90, Protein Kinase C, MAP Kinase Kinase, and MAP Kinase Kinase 4 compared with wild-type controls after ischemia.

Materials and Methods

Animals

Fifty-seven mice (30 wild-type and 27 UCP2 Tg) were randomly assigned into control and ischemic group for cerebral vasculature examination, infarct volume measurement, PCR array and protein array studies. Number of animals used in each experiment is given in figure legend. All procedures were performed in strict compliance with the National Institutes of Health guidelines for animal research and were approved by the Institutional Animal Care and Use Committee. UCP2/3 transgenic overexpressing mice were generated by overexpressing human UCP2 and UCP3 within the native promoter [24]. Uncoupling proteins 2, 4 and 5 are the predominant endogenous isoforms found in brain the brain [8]. Because the current experiments were performed in brain tissue and UCP3 is not expressed in brain,, this mouse genotype will be referred to as UCP2 Tg. Mice were backcrossed onto a C57/Bl6 background. Mice were fasted overnight with free access to water. Anesthesia was induced with 3% and maintained at 1–1.5% isoflurane in 30% oxygen and 70% nitrous oxide. Body and head temperatures were maintained between 36.5–37.5°C by a combination of a heating blanket and a lamp. Animals with a fasting blood glucose level between 4–6 mM were used for the experiment. Pre-ischemic blood pressure was 100–120 mmHg with no statistical difference between UCP2 Tg and wild-type animals.

Anatomy of the Middle Cerebral Artery and Circle of Willis

Naïve wild-type and UCP2 Tg mice (n = 3 in each group) were deeply anesthetized and transcardially perfused with 2% India ink in 20% gelatin in saline. Mice were decapitated after 30 seconds and brains were removed and fixed with 4% paraformaldehyde. Brain images were captured using a Leica dissecting scope (Leica Microsystems, Wetzlar, Germany).

Ischemic model

Transient middle cerebral artery occlusion (MCAO) was induced in 9 wild-type and 7 UCP2 Tg mice as described before

[25]. Briefly, a nylon monofilament (Doccol, Redlands, CA, USA) coated with silicon, size 6-0, was inserted into the common carotid artery to the internal carotid artery in order to block the middle cerebral artery. Mice were revived and behavior was observed for neurological defect to confirm the successfulness of MCAO. The degree of functional deficit at 30 min post occlusion was scored using a 5-point Bederson's scale [26]. Briefly, scale 0, no deficit; 1, mild forelimb weakness; 2, severe forelimb weakness and consistently turns to side of deficit when lifted by tail;3, compulsory circling; 4, unconscious; and 5, dead. Three wild-type and 2 UCP2 Tg mice with a Bederson's score less than 2 were excluded from the study. After 1 hour of ischemia, mice were re-anesthetized and the filament was removed to restore blood flow.

Measuring Brain Infarction

Infarct volume was determined by using 2% 2, 3, 5-Triphenyltetrazolium chloride (TTC) staining. After 1 hour of MCAO and 24 hours of reperfusion, mice were deeply anesthetized with 5% isoflurane and transcardially perfused with ice cold saline. The brains were removed and sectioned coronally at 1 mm thick using a brain matrix (Harvard Apparatus, Holliston, MA, USA), and incubated in 2% TTC for 15 minutes at room temperature. Brain slices were then fixed in 4% paraformaldehyde, scanned (Hewlett Packard, Palo Alto, CA, USA) into a computer, and quantified using NIH imaging software (rsb.info. nih.gov/nih-image).

PCR Array

At 24 hours reperfusion, both control and ischemic animals from wild-type and UCP2 Tg (n = 4 in each group) were decapitated after being deeply anesthetized with 5% isoflurane. The brains were extracted within 30 seconds, frozen in liquid nitrogen and stored at −80°C for later dissection. A peripheral area of the ipsilateral cortex (equivalent to the ischemic penumbra area in this model) was dissected in a −20°C glove box. RNA was isolated by Mini RNeasy Columns (Qiagen, Rockville, MD, USA), treated with DNase 1for 30 minutes at 37°C and, then, deactivated with 25 mM EDTA and incubation at 65°C and stored at −80°C. cDNA was synthesized using 1 μg of RNA Superscript III and oligo dT (Invitrogen, Carlsbad, CA, USA). RNA and primers were annealed at 65°C for 5 min. The Superscript enzyme was added and incubated for 50 min at 50°C. The reaction was terminated by incubating at 85°C for 5 min and stored at −20°C. Ninety-six-well PCR plates pre-spotted with oligonucleotides for p53 associated genes (Super-Array, Frederick, MD, USA) were used with SYBR Green RT-PCR master mix (Invitrogen) and run on the ABI 9600 (Applied Biosystems, Foster City, CA, USA). One cDNA prep was used for each array plate. The sample was denatured and polymerase enzyme was heat activated for 10 min at 95°C, 40 cycles of 15 sec 95°C and 1 min at 60°C amplified the transcript and data was collected at each cycle. Crossing threshold (Ct) values were manually set at 2.0 and were normalized to the housekeeping genes β-actin and HPRT1. The PCR array included control wells with no template and wells with no primers.

p53 Protein Array

A separate set of animals was used for the antibody protein array study. At 24 hours reperfusion, mice were decapitated under deep anesthesia with 5% isoflurane. The brains were excised (n = 4 in each group), frozen in liquid nitrogen and stored at −80°C for later dissection. A peripheral area of the ipsilateral cortex was dissected in a −20°C glove box. The brains were homogenized using a tissue homogenizer (Cole-Palmer, Vernon Hills, IL, USA) at 14,000 rpm in the Sigma Protein Isolation Buffer (Sigma, St. Louis, MO, USA) containing 1 m M EDTA (Sigma), 5 mM DTT (Sigma) and protease inhibitors (Thermo Scientific, Rockford, IL, USA). The homogenates were centrifuged at 750 g for 15 min to separate the nuclear fraction from the cytosolic and mitochondrial fractions. The supernatant containing the cytosolic and mitochondrial proteins was used for cytokine quantification. Protein was quantified using the A280 protein quantification program on the NanoDrop 2000 (Thermo Scientific). 1 mg of total protein (at 1 mg/mL) was directly labeled with Cy5 dye reagent (Sigma) in 100 mM carbonate-bicarbonate buffer pH 9.6, excess dye was removed by a SigmaSpin column, incubated on the protein array slide (Sigma), and signal was detected using a fluorescent array reader (Agilent, Santa Clara, CA, USA). Protein levels were normalized to cytoketerin on the array.

Data analysis

Experiments were carried out by BH and data were analyzed by PAL without knowing the experimental conditions. T-test was used to analyze infarct volume between the two species of animals. PCR data were analyzed using analysis RT^2 Profiler^{TM} PCR Array Data Analysis Excel Template provided by SuperArray and protein array data were analyzed using Data Analysis Workbook for the Panorama p53 Array provided by Sigma. P value<0.05 was considered statistically significant.

Results

Cerebral Vasculature

To evaluate if transgenically overexpressing UCP2 in the brain caused a phenotypic change in the cerebral vasculature, we transcardially injected carbon black ink and imaged the cerebral blood vessels (**Fig. 1**). Both wild-type and UCP2 Tg mice demonstrated intact and correct alignment of the Circle of Willis,

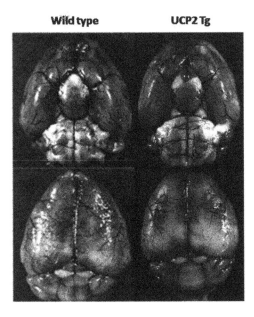

Figure 1. Major cerebral vasculature detected by perfusion of carbon black in wild-type and UCP2 Tg mice. The Circle of Willis, anterior cerebral arteries, middle cerebral arteries and posterior arteries all appear normal in both wild-type and UCP2 Tg animals (n = 3 for each group).

anterior cerebral arteries, middle cerebral arteries and posterior arteries with no remarkable difference.

Infarct volume

One hour middle cerebral arterial occlusion with 24 hours reperfusion induced a mild brain damage located predominantly in the caudate-putamen in wild-type mice. Infarct volume was measured as a percentage per hemisphere. Mice overexpressing UCP2 in the brain had significantly less damage after transient focal ischemia (**Fig. 2**). Thus the infarct volume was reduced from 18% in wild-type to 12% in UCP2 Tg mice (33% reduction, p<0.01).

Alteration of Gene Expression

To determine the mRNA expression profile in the ischemic penumbra area of wild-type and UCP2 Tg mice after transient focal ischemia, the p53 PCR array (Qiagen, Frederick, MD) was used to measure transcript levels of 84 genes using quantitative PCR (ABI 7300). Housekeeping genes Hprt1 and β-actin were used to normalize results. The original comparisons were made by comparing wild-type MCAO over wild-type sham, UCP2 Tg MCAO over UCP2 Tg sham, and UCP2 Tg sham over wild-type sham. Because of no significant change in gene expression between UCP2Tg sham and wild-type sham and variation in the UCP2Tg sham, we decided to use wild-type sham as controls. Data are summarized in Table 1. After transient focal ischemia in wild-type mice compared with wild-type sham controls,, cytokines IL-6 (23.36 fold, p=0.05) and Tnf-α (20.19 fold, p<0.001) are increased significantly. Cell cycle genes: Chek1 (1.78, p=0.024), Esr1 (3.35 fold, p=0.022), Myc (3.93 fold, p=0.039), and RelA (1.77 fold, p=0.046), were also increased less profoundly. The anti-apoptotic gene Bcl-2 (−1.98 fold p=0.021) was decreased in the wild-type ischemic penumbra compared with sham controls. Cell cycle genes Cdk4 (−5.00 fold, p=0.18), Cnng2 (−1.76 fold, p=0.014) and Ccnh (−1.42, p=0.074) were also decreased in the wild-type ischemic penumbra. In UCP2 Tg mice, the cytokines IL-6 (7.34 fold, p=0.037) and Tnf-α (24.04 fold, p=0.001) were increased after MCAO compared to wildtype sham controls, but the increase in IL-6 was much less profound than in wild-type animals (7.3-fold versus 23.4-fold). Chek1 (2.24 fold, p=0.008), Esr1 (1.39 fold, p=0.64), Myc (4.28 fold, p=0.0001), and RelA (1.48 fold, p=0.019) were increased in UCP2 Tg mice after MCAO. There was no significant decrease in the anti-apoptotic gene Bcl2 (p=0.226) after MCAO in UCP2 Tg mice. The cell cycle genes Ccng2 (−1.44 fold, p=0.092) and Ccnh (−1.40 fold, p=0.028) were all decreased after MCAO in UCP2 Tg mice. In summary, ischemia in wild-type mice increased the expression of inflammatory genes and suppressed the expression of anti-apoptotic and a few cell cycle genes. Overexpression of UCP2 ameliorated the increase in IL-6, the decrease in Bcl2, and increased the expression of cell cycle genes as well.

2.4 Change in Cell Signaling Proteins

A protein array focused on p53 associated proteins was used to measure the change in protein levels in the ischemic penumbra between UCP2 Tg and wild-type mice after 1 hour MCAO and 24 hours of reperfusion. Protein levels were normalized to pan-cytokeratin before a comparison was made between the two groups (Table 2). In comparing UCP2 Tg to wild-type after MCAO, cell survival related proteins HSP-90, MEK, phospho-serine 473 AKT, protein p300/CBP, p300/CBP associated protein and protein kinase C were significantly increased. Cdc25A, which is a phosphotase mediating c-myc induced apoptosis, was decreased in UCP2 Tg mice. In addition,

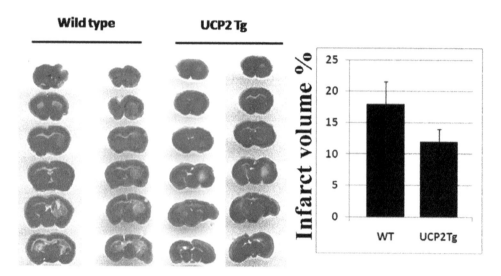

Figure 2. Infarct volume at 24 hours of recovery after 1 hour MCAO. A, Representative TTC stained brain sections depict the infarct area (white color). **B,** percentage of infarct volume per hemisphere. Data were collected from 6 wild-type and 5 UCP2 Tg mice. * P<0.05, Student t test.

overexpression of UCP2 increased non-cleaved caspase 3 but decreased non-cleaved caspase 9 levels.

Discussion

In this study, we first confirmed that overexpression of UCP2 is neuroprotective against transient focal ischemia induced brain damage, which is consistent to previous publication [12]. This protection was independent from any abnormalities in the cerebral vasculature. We then investigated the potential mechanisms of UCP2 mediated neuroprotection.

Decreases in inflammatory cytokines appear to contribute to the neuroprotection provided by UCP2. Transient focal ischemia caused 23 and 20 fold increases in IL-6 and Tnf-α mRNA respectively, suggesting that ischemia induces neuroinflammatory responses in the brain. Overexpression of UCP2 significantly reduced the IL-6 expression to less than one third of the levels

observed in wild-type animals after being challenged with ischemia, suggesting that UCP2 suppresses neuroinflammation in the brain after stroke. Reports have shown that expression of IL-6 in human patients after ischemic stroke is associated with the size of infarction [27]. IL-6 is increased in brain injury and is directly up-regulated by IL-1β and TNF-α [28].Mice transgenically overexpressing the antioxidant enzyme glutathione peroxidase had reduced expression of IL-6 after transient focal ischemia [29]. It is possible that suppression of IL-6 lessens inflammatory response. This is supported by studies showing that UCP2/3 overexpressing mice have reduced inflammatory responses after endotoxin challenges and decreased IL-6 and IL-4 levels after lipopolysaccharide challenge [24] and that UCP2 homozygous knockout (UCP2$^{-/-}$) mice have increased expression of IL-6 after listeria infection compared with wild-type controls [30].

Ischemia in wild-type mice suppressed Bcl2 and overexpression of UCP2 alleviated the suppression. Bcl2 is a well-known anti-

Table 1. Results of PCR Array.

Symbol	Full name	Fold Difference WT MCAO/WT sham	P value	Fold Difference TG MCAO/Sham	p value
Bcl2	B-cell leukemia/lymphoma 2	−1.98	0.021	−1.43	0.226
Ccng2	Cyclin G2	−1.17	0.031	−1.44	0.092
Ccnh	Cyclin H	−1.42	0.074	−1.40	0.028
Chek1	Checkpoint kinase 1 homolog	1.78	0.024	2.24	0.008
Esr1	Estrogen receptor 1 alpha	3.35	0.022	1.39	0.639
Il6	Interleukin 6	23.36	0.050	7.34	0.037
Mcl1	Myeloid cell leukemia sequence 1	−2.24	0.362	4.52	0.152
Myc	Myelocytomatosis oncogene	3.93	0.039	4.28	<0.001
RelA	V-rel reticuloendothe-liosis viral oncogene homolog A	1.77	0.046	1.48	0.019
Tnf	Tumor necrosis factor	20.19	<0.001	24.04	0.001

After being normalized against house-keeping gene, the average delta Ct values of targets genes were compared between the test samples and control samples (n = 4 in each group) and presented as fold change. Negative value indicates decrease and positive value indicates increase compared to control. Data were analyzed using RT^2 Profiler^{TM} PCR Array Data Analysis Excel Template provided by SuperArray.

Table 2. P53 Protein Array.

Protein	UCP2 Tg	WT MCAO	p value
Caspase-3	8.56±1.95	5.82±0.64	0.001
Caspase-9**	5.82±0.39	6.75±0.46	0.038
Cdc25a	3.99±0.18	5.04±0.61	0.016
Heat Shock Protein 90	4.96±0.48	4.14±0.46	0.049
JNK	4.97±0.16	5.94±0.01	0.001
MAP Kinase Kinase (MEK)	8.24±1.13	5.73±0.47	0.006
AKT Phospho Ser 473	6.57±0.24	4.82±0.53	0.024
p300/CBP associated factor (PCAF)	7.13±0.34	5.97±0.41	0.035
p300/CBP	4.67±0.63	3.76±0.38	0.048
Protein Kinase C	8.92±1.36	6.36±0.77	0.016

Mean and s.d values are derived from 4 samples in each group after being normalized against the housekeeping protein. Data were analyzed using Data Analysis Workbook for the Panorama p53 Array provided by Sigma.

apoptotic gene that inhibits the mitochondria-initiated cell death pathway. Bcl-2 provides protection from oxidative stress [31] and cerebral ischemia [32]. Transgenically overexpressing Bcl-2 reduced infarction from permanent focal ischemia [33]. Upregulation of Bcl-2 is associated with several neuroprotective strategies including ischemic pre-conditioning [34]. Our studies confirmed previous findings that cerebral ischemia reduces the transcript levels of Bcl-2 [35] and showed that upregulation of UCP2 in transgenic mice ameliorated ischemia-induced Bcl2 suppression. Similarly, Mcl-1, a Bcl-2 family protein [36,37]. is suppressed by ischemia and its suppression is elevated by UCP2 overexpression. These data suggest that the neuroprotective effects of UCP2 may be associated with prevention of Bcl2 family suppression induced by cerebral ischemia. This is supported by the study showing that upregulation of UCP2 by ghrelin protects hypoxia-induced damage by increasing Bcl-2/Bax ratios [38].

Ischemia resulted in cell arrest as reflected by the suppression of cell cycle genes cyclin G2 and cyclin H,, which stimulate cell proliferation and survival [39,40]. UCP2 overexpression alleviated ischemia-induced suppression on cyclin G2 and cyclin H, suggesting that the neuroprotective effects of UCP2 may be associated with cell cycle regulation.

Estrogen receptor alpha (Esr1) and checkpoint kinase 1 (Check1) are involved in neuroprotection, DNA repair and regulation of cell proliferation [40,41]. In the present study, Esr1 increased after ischemia and reperfusion injury, suggesting ischemia activates cell protective machinery. However, since UCP2 did not increase Esr1, its neuroprotetive effects may not be associated with Esr1. Two oncogenes, Myc and RelA, are pregluated by ischemia. This is consistent with previous publication showing increased Myc in brain after cerebral ischemia [42]. While the role of these two genes in ischemic brain damage has not been established, persistent expression of Myc induces apoptosis [43]. RelA is a major component of NF-κB transcription factor [44]. Since Myc and RelA are both upregluated after focal ischemia in both wild-type and UCP2 Tg mice, UCP2 mediated neuroprotection may not be associated with these two genes.

UCP2 activates cell survival signaling pathways. The protein levels of HSP90, phospho-AKT, PKC, p300/CBP, p300/CBP associated factor (PCAF), and MEK were significantly increased in the ischemic penumbra of UCP2 Tg mice after transient focal ischemia compared to wild-type ischemic mice. Ischemic preconditioning is known to increase HSP90 [45]. Inhibiting HSP90 with geldanamycin increased oxidative stress and cell death in PC12 cells [46]. Neuroprotective hypothermia, ischemic pre-conditioning and ischemic post-conditioning cause phosphorylation of AKT 473 [17,18] and PKC [47]. Inhibiting phosphorylation of AKT blocks the beneficial effects of hypothermia, ischemic pre- and post-conditioning [17,18]. Upregulating UCP2 by ghrelin provides neuroprotection by activating ERK and PKC pathways [38]. MEK phosphorylates MAP kinase (ERK) and promotes cell proliferation. MEK protects from glutamate-induced damage in neuronal cultures [19]. Inhibiting MEK blocked neuroprotection by ischemic pre-conditioning [18]. p300/CBP plays a critical role in transcriptional regulation of hypoxia responsive genes, including hypoxia-inducing factor and its downstream vascular endothelial growth factor (VEGF) and erythropoietin [48]. Both VEGF and erythropoietin protect brain against ischemic injury [49,50]. Our results suggest that UCP2 protects against ischemia-induced brain damage by activating cell survival signals.

UCP2 decreases protein levels of Cdc25A in the ischemic penumbra region. Cdc25A is a phosphatase with significant roles in cell cycle progression by activating cyclin dependent kinases [51]. It is regulated post-translational by the ubiquitin-proteasome pathway [52]. Cdc25A is necessary for c-myc induced apoptosis. Cdc25a activity is increased in degenerating neurons of patients who died with Alzheimer's disease [51]. Blocking Cdc25a inhibits c-myc mediated apoptosis [53]. UCP2 decreases the levels of Cdc25a, therefore it may reduce apoptotic cell death induced by ischemia.

The protein levels of caspase-3 increased and caspase-9 decreased in the ischemic penumbra of UCP2 Tg mice. Since the measured caspase-3 and caspase-9 are the uncleaved form, it is not clear whether the increase in caspase3 or decrease in capspase-9 has any pathogenic meaning.

Our results confirmed overexpressing UCP2 is neuroprotective from transient focal ischemia. Overexpressing UCP2 suppresses mRNA levels of inflammatory cytokine and elevated the ischemia-induced suppression of cell cycle genes. Furthermore, overexpression of UCP2 increases the protein levels of cell survival factors.

Author Contributions

Conceived and designed the experiments: BH PAL. Performed the experiments: BH PAL. Analyzed the data: BH PAL. Contributed reagents/materials/analysis tools: BH PAL. Wrote the paper: BH PAL.

References

1. Iijima T, Mishima T, Akagawa K, Iwao Y (2003) Mitochondrial hyperpolarization after transient oxygen-glucose deprivation and subsequent apoptosis in cultured rat hippocampal neurons. Brain Res 993: 140–145.

2. Ouyang YB, Xu LJ, Sun YJ, Giffard RG (2006) Overexpression of inducible heat shock protein 70 and its mutants in astrocytes is associated with maintenance of mitochondrial physiology during glucose deprivation stress. Cell Stress Chaperones 11: 180–186.

3. Choi K, Kim J, Kim GW, Choi C (2009) Oxidative stress-induced necrotic cell death via mitochondira-dependent burst of reactive oxygen species. Curr Neurovasc Res 6: 213–222.

4. Nicholls DG, Bernson VS (1977) Inter-relationships between proton electrochemical gradient, adenine-nucleotide phosphorylation potential and respiration, during substrate-level and oxidative phosphorylation by mitochondria from brown adipose tissue of cold-adapted guinea-pigs. Eur J Biochem 75: 601–612.

5. Mehta SL, Li PA (2009) Neuroprotective role of mitochondrial uncoupling protein 2 in cerebral stroke. J Cereb Blood Flow Metab 29: 1069–1078.

6. Teshima Y, Akao M, Jones SP, Marban E (2003) Uncoupling protein-2 overexpression inhibits mitochondrial death pathway in cardiomyocytes. Circ Res 93: 192–200.

7. Yoshitomi H, Yamazaki K, Tanaka I (1999) Mechanism of ubiquitous expression of mouse uncoupling protein 2 mRNA: control by cis-acting DNA element in 5′-flanking region. Biochem J 340: 397–404.

8. Lengacher S, Magistretti PJ, Pellerin L (2004) Quantitative rt-PCR analysis of uncoupling protein isoforms in mouse brain cortex: methodological optimization and comparison of expression with brown adipose tissue and skeletal muscle. J Cereb Blood Flow Metab 24: 780–788.

9. Jezek P (2002) Possible physiological roles of mitochondrial uncoupling proteins– UCPn. Int J Biochem Cell Biol 34: 1190–1206.

10. Bechmann I, Diano S, Warden CH, Bartfai T, Nitsch R, et al. (2002) Brain mitochondrial uncoupling protein 2 (UCP2): a protective stress signal in neuronal injury. Biochem Pharmacol 64: 363–367.

11. Kim HS, Park KG, Koo TB, Huh S, Lee IK (2007) The modulating effects of the overexpression of uncoupling protein 2 on the formation of reactive oxygen species in vascular cells. Diabetes Res Clin Pract 77 Suppl 1: S46–48.

12. Mattiasson G, Shamloo M, Gido G, Mathi K, Tomasevic G, et al. (2003) Uncoupling protein-2 prevents neuronal death and diminishes brain dysfunction after stroke and brain trauma. Nat Med 9: 1062–1068.

13. Nakase T, Yoshida Y, Nagata K (2007) Amplified expression of uncoupling proteins in human brain ischemic lesions. Neuropathology 27: 442–447.

14. Liu Y, Chen L, Xu X, Vicaut E, Sercombe R (2009) Both ischemic preconditioning and ghrelin administration protect hippocampus from ischemia/reperfusion and upregulate uncoupling protein-2. BMC Physiol 9: 17.

15. Zhao H (2009) Ischemic postconditioning as a novel avenue to protect against brain injury after stroke. J Cereb Blood Flow Metab 29: 873–885.

16. Yano S, Morioka M, Fukunaga K, Kawano T, Hara T, et al. (2001) Activation of Akt/protein kinase B contributes to induction of ischemic tolerance in the CA1 subfield of gerbil hippocampus. J Cereb Blood Flow Metab 21: 351–360.

17. Zhao H, Shimohata T, Wang JQ, Sun G, Schaal DW, et al. (2005) Akt contributes to neuroprotection by hypothermia against cerebral ischemia in rats. J Neurosci 25: 9794–9806.

18. Pignataro G, Meller R, Inoue K, Ordonez AN, Ashley MD, et al. (2008) In vivo and in vitro characterization of a novel neuroprotective strategy for stroke: ischemic postconditioning. J Cereb Blood Flow Metab 28: 232–241.

19. Sawe N, Steinberg G, Zhao H (2008) Dual roles of the MAPK/ERK1/2 cell signaling pathway after stroke. J Neurosci Res 86: 1659–1669.

20. Chan PH (1996) Role of oxidants in ischemic brain damage. Stroke 27: 1124–1129.

21. Minami M, Katayama T, Satoh M (2006) Brain cytokines and chemokines: roles in ischemic injury and pain. J Pharmacol Sci 100: 461–470.

22. Sriram K, O'Callaghan JP (2007) Divergent roles for tumor necrosis factor-alpha in the brain. J Neuroimmune Pharmacol 2: 140–153.

23. Shohami E, Ginis I, Hallenbeck JM (1999) Dual role of tumor necrosis factor alpha in brain injury. Cytokine Growth Factor Rev 10: 119–130.

24. Horvath TL, Diano S, Miyamoto S, Barry S, Gatti S, et al. (2003) Uncoupling proteins-2 and 3 influence obesity and inflammation in transgenic mice. Int J Obes Relat Metab Disord 27: 433–442.

25. Li PA, Gisselsson L, Keuker J, Vogel J, Smith ML, et al. (1998) Hyperglycemia-exaggerated ischemic brain damage following 30 min of middle cerebral artery occlusion is not due to capillary obstruction. Brain Res 804: 36–44.

26. Bederson JB, Pitts LH, Tsuji M, Nishimura MC, Davis RL, et al. (1986) Rat middle cerebral artery occlusion: evaluation of the model and development of a neurologic examination. Stroke 17: 472–476.

27. Acalovschi D, Wiest T, Hartmann M, Farahmi M, Mansmann U, et al. (2003) Multiple levels of regulation of the interleukin-6 system in stroke. Stroke 34: 1864–1869.

28. Tuttolomondo A, Di Raimondo D, di Sciacca R, Pinto A, Licata G (2008) Inflammatory cytokines in acute ischemic stroke. Curr Pharm Des 14: 3574–3589.

29. Ishibashi N, Prokopenko O, Reuhl KR, Mirochnitchenko O (2002) Inflammatory response and glutathione peroxidase in a model of stroke. J Immunol 168: 1926–1933.

30. Rousset S, Emre Y, Join-Lambert O, Hurtaud C, Ricquier D, et al. (2006) The uncoupling protein 2 modulates the cytokine balance in innate immunity. Cytokine 35: 135–142.

31. Fiskum G, Rosenthal RE, Vereczki V, Martin E, Hoffman GE, et al. (2004) Protection against ischemic brain injury by inhibition of mitochondrial oxidative stress. J Bioenerg Biomembr 36: 347–352.

32. Ouyang YB, Giffard RG (2004) Cellular neuroprotective mechanisms in cerebral ischemia: Bcl-2 family proteins and protection of mitochondrial function. Cell Calcium 36: 303–311.

33. Martinou JC, Dubois-Dauphin M, Staple JK, Rodriguez I, Frankowski H, et al. (1994) Overexpression of BCL-2 in transgenic mice protects neurons from naturally occurring cell death and experimental ischemia. Neuron 13: 1017–1030.

34. Liu XQ, Sheng R, Qin ZH (2009) The neuroprotective mechanism of brain ischemic preconditioning. Acta Pharmacol Sin 30: 1071–1080.

35. Lu D, Jiang D (1997) [The expression of hsp70 and BCL-2 genes in hippocampus of the rats exposed to cerebral ischemia and reperfusion]. Zhongguo Ying Yong Sheng Li Xue Za Zhi 13: 224–227.

36. Craig RW (2002) MCL1 provides a window on the role of the BCL2 family in cell proliferation, differentiation and tumorigenesis. Leukemia 16: 444–454.

37. Mori M, Burgess DL, Gefrides LA, Foreman PJ, Opferman JT, et al. (2004) Expression of apoptosis inhibitor protein Mcl1 linked to neuroprotection in CNS neurons. Cell Death Differ 11: 1223–1233.

38. Chung H, Kim E, Lee DH, Seo S, Ju S, et al. (2007) Ghrelin inhibits apoptosis in hypothalamic neuronal cells during oxygen-glucose deprivation. Endocrinology 148: 148–159.

39. Li Y, Chopp M, Powers C, Jiang N (1997) Immunoreactivity of cyclin D1/cdk4 in neurons and oligodendrocytes after focal cerebral ischemia in rat. J Cereb Blood Flow Metab 17: 846–856.

40. Gao Q, Zhou J, Huang X, Chen G, Ye F, et al. (2006) Selective targeting of checkpoint kinase 1 in tumor cells with a novel potent oncolytic adenovirus. Mol Ther 13: 928–937.

41. Elzer JG, Muhammad S, Wintermantel TM, Regnier-Vigouroux A, Ludwig J, et al. Neuronal estrogen receptor-[alpha] mediates neuroprotection by 17[beta]-estradiol. J Cereb Blood Flow Metab 30: 935–942.

42. Nakagomi T, Asai A, Kanemitsu H, Narita K, Kuchino Y, et al. (1996) Up-regulation of c-myc gene expression following focal ischemia in the rat brain. Neurol Res 18: 559–563.

43. Macdonald K, Bennett MR (1999) cdc25A is necessary but not sufficient for optimal c-myc-induced apoptosis and cell proliferation of vascular smooth muscle cells. Circ Res 84: 820–830.

44. Palgrave CJ, Gilmoour L, Lowden CS, Lillico SG, Mellencamp MA, et al. (2011) Species-specific variation in RELA underlies differences in NF-κB activity: a potential role in African swine fever pathogenesis. J Virol 85: 6008–6014.

45. Dhodda VK, Sailor KA, Bowen KK, Vemuganti R (2004) Putative endogenous mediators of preconditioning-induced ischemic tolerance in rat brain identified by genomic and proteomic analysis. J Neurochem 89: 73–89.

46. Clark CB, Rane MJ, El Mehdi D, Miller CJ, Sachleben LR, Jr., et al. (2009) Role of oxidative stress in geldanamycin-induced cytotoxicity and disruption of Hsp90 signaling complex. Free Radic Biol Med 47: 1440–1449.

47. Ginsberg MD, Sternau LL, Globus MY, Dietrich WD, Busto R (1992) Therapeutic modulation of brain temperature: relevance to ischemic brain injury. Cerebrovasc Brain Metab Rev 4: 189–225.

48. Arany Z, Huang LE, Eckner R, Bhattacharya S, Jiang C, et al. (1996) An essential role for p300/CBP in the cellular response to hypoxia. Proc Natl Acad Sci U S A 93: 12969–12973.

49. Kaya D, Gursoy-Ozdemir Y, Yemisci M, Tuncer N, Aktan S, et al. (2005) VEGF protects brain against focal ischemia without increasing blood-brain permeability when administered intracerebroventricularly. J Cereb Blood Flow Metab 25: 1111–1118.

50. Dang S, Liu X, Fu P, Gong W, Fan F, et al. (2011) Neuroprotection by local intra-arterial infusion of erythropoietin after focal cerebral ischemia in rats. Neurol Res 33: 520–528.

51. Ding XL, Husseman J, Tomashevski A, Nochlin D, Jin LW, et al. (2000) The cell cycle Cdc25A tyrosine phosphatase is activated in degenerating postmitotic neurons in Alzheimer's disease. Am J Pathol 157: 1983–1990.

52. Bernardi R, Liebermann DA, Hoffman B (2000) Cdc25A stability is controlled by the ubiquitin-proteasome pathway during cell cycle progression and terminal differentiation. Oncogene 19: 2447–2454.

53. Macdonald K, Bennett MR (1999) cdc25A is necessary but not sufficient for optimal c-myc-induced apoptosis and cell proliferation of vascular smooth muscle cells. Circ Res 84: 820–830.

18

Growth Hormone Secretagogues Protect Mouse Cardiomyocytes from *in vitro* Ischemia/Reperfusion Injury through Regulation of Intracellular Calcium

Yi Ma[1], Lin Zhang[2], Joshua N. Edwards[1], Bradley S. Launikonis[1], Chen Chen[1]*

1 School of Biomedical Sciences, University of Queensland, Brisbane, Queensland, Australia, **2** School of Biological Sciences, University of Auckland, Auckland, New Zealand

Abstract

Background: Ischemic heart disease is a leading cause of mortality. To study this disease, ischemia/reperfusion (I/R) models are widely used to mimic the process of transient blockage and subsequent recovery of cardiac coronary blood supply. We aimed to determine whether the presence of the growth hormone secretagogues, ghrelin and hexarelin, would protect/improve the function of heart from I/R injury and to examine the underlying mechanisms.

Methodology/Principal Findings: Isolated hearts from adult male mice underwent 20 min global ischemia and 30 min reperfusion using a Langendorff apparatus. Ghrelin (10 nM) or hexarelin (1 nM) was introduced into the perfusion system either 10 min before or after ischemia, termed pre- and post-treatments. In freshly isolated cardiomyocytes from these hearts, single cell shortening, intracellular calcium ($[Ca^{2+}]_i$) transients and caffeine-releasable sarcoplasmic reticulum (SR) Ca^{2+} were measured. In addition, RT-PCR and Western blots were used to examine the expression level of GHS receptor type 1a (GHS-R1a), and phosphorylated phospholamban (p-PLB), respectively. Ghrelin and hexarelin pre- or post-treatments prevented the significant reduction in the cell shortening, $[Ca^{2+}]_i$ transient amplitude and caffeine-releasable SR Ca^{2+} content after I/R through recovery of p-PLB. GHS-R1a antagonists, [D-Lys3]-GHRP-6 (200 nM) and BIM28163 (100 nM), completely blocked the effects of GHS on both cell shortening and $[Ca^{2+}]_i$ transients.

Conclusion/Significance: Through activation of GHS-R1a, ghrelin and hexarelin produced a positive inotropic effect on ischemic cardiomyocytes and protected them from I/R injury probably by protecting or recovering p-PLB (and therefore SR Ca^{2+} content) to allow the maintenance or recovery of normal cardiac contractility. These observations provide supporting evidence for the potential therapeutic application of ghrelin and hexarelin in patients with cardiac I/R injury.

Editor: Alfred Lewin, University of Florida, United States of America

Funding: This work was supported by funding from the Australian National Health and Medical Research Council and the University of Queensland. The funders had no role in study design, data collection and analysis, decision to publish, or preparation of the manuscript.

Competing Interests: The authors have declared that no competing interests exist.

* E-mail: chen.chen@uq.edu.au

Introduction

Cardiac ischemia is one of the leading causes of mortality in the world. It is caused by a temporary interruption of blood flow in the arteries of the heart [1]. The primary clinical therapeutic strategy for treatment of cardiac ischemia is reperfusion. However, reperfusion can cause additional injury to the heart [1,2]. Recovery of cardiac function following ischemia is critically dependent on the time spent under ischemic conditions and reperfusion [3].

In vitro global and *in vivo* regional ischemia/reperfusion (I/R) models have been developed to examine experimentally cardiac ischemia and subsequent reperfusion of the ischemic heart. The *in vivo* regional I/R model mimics atherosclerosis by ligating the left anterior descending coronary artery. The global I/R model for *in vitro* study blocks all perfusion of the heart for a given period. The latter can be easily implemented and affects a larger area with a less variability among different regions [4]. It is used to mimic the process of cardiac arrest and cardiac surgery [5]. This model is

also more appropriate for obtaining isolated cells which have been through similar ischemia conditions without the regional differences often observed in regional I/R models.

In the past 50 years, great progress has been made to clarify the metabolic changes that occur following I/R [1,2,6,7]. During ischemia, depletion of oxygen and ATP inhibits SR Ca^{2+} ATPase (SERCA2a) and Na^+-K^+ ATPase activities. This results in an accumulation of intracellular Ca^{2+} ($[Ca^{2+}]_i$) and Na^+ ($[Na^+]_i$) [1,2,6,7]. The subsequent reintroduction of oxygen during reperfusion leads to the generation of large amounts of reactive oxygen species (ROS), causing increased oxidative stress and subsequent damage to the plasma and SR membranes resulting in further increases in $[Ca^{2+}]_i$. The combined effects of ROS and $[Ca^{2+}]_i$ overload also favor the opening of the mitochondrial permeability transition pore (mPTP), which induces cardiomyocyte apoptosis and necrosis [1,2,6,7].

Ghrelin is a 28 amino acid peptide produced in the stomach and is an endogenous ligand of the growth hormone secretagogue

(GHS) receptor type 1a (GHS-R1a) [8]. A synthetic analogue of ghrelin, hexarelin, also binds and activates the GHS-R1a [9,10,11]. Ghrelin mainly exists in the pituitary and gastrointestinal system [8,12], while the distribution of its receptor GHS-R1a is ubiquitous and has been confirmed in the myocardium [12,13]. Although ghrelin may bind to receptors other than GHS-R1a [14,15,16], its main target is GHS-R1a.

Previous studies have confirmed the protective effects of GHS on whole heart function after I/R. Administration of ghrelin *in vitro* to I/R rat hearts was shown to reduce the infarct size [17], and enhance cardiac function [18] through the activation of PKC [17]. These effects are likely initiated by the binding of ghrelin to its receptor, GHS-R1a [18]. Further studies in rats pre-treated with GHS for 7 days *in vivo* prior to *in vitro* I/R injury showed an improvement in cardiac function [10] and attenuation of myocardial injury and apoptosis through the inhibition of endoplasmic reticulum (ER) stress [19]. Similarly, hexarelin has also been shown to play a cardioprotective role in I/R hearts from rodents [10,17,20].

As discussed above, whole heart functional studies employing the *in vivo* and *in vitro* I/R models have revealed some potential mechanisms of the cardioprotective effects of GHS. Detailed cellular and molecular pathways employed by GHS through activation of GHS-R1a after cardiac I/R remain elusive. Since $[Ca^{2+}]_i$ plays a critical role in cardiomyocyte contraction and I/R injury, in this study we investigated the alterations in and regulation of $[Ca^{2+}]_i$ homeostasis in isolated mouse cardiomyocytes with or without I/R and GHS treatment.

Methods

Animals and Chemicals

All experiments conformed to the Guide for the Care and Use of Laboratory Animals published by the US National Institutes of Health (NIH Publication No.85-23, revised 1996), and the protocol was approved by the Animal Ethics Committee of the University of Queensland (AEC # SBMS/814/07/NHMRC). All surgeries were performed under sodium pentobarbital anesthesia, and all efforts were made to minimize suffering.

Human ghrelin was obtained from Auspep (Parkville, Australia). Hexarelin was obtained from GL Biochem (Shanghai, China). Pentobarbital sodium was purchased from Virbac Pty Ltd (Australia). Heparin sodium salt was purchased from Sigma Aldrich (St. Louis, MO, USA). Fura 2-AM was purchased from Invitrogen (Eugene, Oregon, USA). [D-Lys3]GHRP-6 was purchased from Anaspec Inc. (San Jose, CA). BIM28163 was kindly provided by Michael D. Culler (Ipsen Pty Ltd, Australia). Other chemicals for recording solutions were purchased from Sigma (St. Louis, MO, USA).

In vitro Ischemia/Reperfusion Model and Preparation of Ventricular Myocytes

Adult male C57/Bl mice (7 to 9 weeks old) weighing between 34 g and 36 g were anesthetized with sodium pentobarbitone (40 mg/kg, ip) containing heparin (500 Units, ip). The heart was rapidly excised, cannulated and perfused retrogradely via the aorta with Tyrode solution at 3 ml/min on a Langendorff perfusion apparatus (composition in mM: 10 HEPES, 143 NaCl, 5.4 KCl, 0.5 MgCl$_2$, 10 Glucose, 20 Taurine, 1.5 CaCl$_2$; pH 7.4; bubbled with 100% O$_2$ at 37°C).

The times for stabilization, ischemia and reperfusion were similar to previous studies [3], and are generally considered the most appropriate for functional studies using an *in vitro* I/R model. After 20 min of stabilization, the heart was subjected to 20 min of no-flow global ischemia followed by 30 min of reperfusion. Control hearts were continuously perfused for 70 min. Ghrelin (10 nM) or hexarelin (1 nM) was administered in the perfusion solution before or after ischemia for 10 min [13], termed GHS pre-treatment and post-treatment respectively. In some experiments, the GHS-R1a antagonist [D-Lys3]-GHRP-6 (200 nM) or BIM28163 (100 nM) was introduced into the perfusion system 5 min before the onset of ischemia and remained present throughout (15 min in total).

Following perfusion, cardiomyocytes were isolated from the left ventricle of each heart with Tyrode solution containing 100 μM CaCl$_2$, 0.6 mg/ml collagenase Type II (Worthington, NJ, USA) and 0.1 mg/ml proteinase type XXIV (Sigma, MO, USA). The Ca^{2+} level was gradually increased to 1.5 mM over 30 min. The yield of this isolation was usually around 60 – 70%. Only cardiomyocytes that were quiescent with a rod shape, sharp edges and clear striations were used in this investigation. At least 3 hearts were used in each group.

Measurement of Sarcomere Shortening

Sarcomere shortening was measured as previously described [21]. In brief, cardiomyocytes were electrically stimulated at 0.5 Hz until contractions became uniform. Following this, 10 – 20 consecutive contractions were recorded. The percentage of sarcomere shortening, time-to-peak shortening and time-to-90% relaxation were determined by IonWizard software (IonOptix Corporation, MA).

Measurement of Intracellular Ca^{2+} Transients and SR Ca^{2+} Content

The isolated and Ca^{2+}-tolerant cardiomyocytes were loaded with 5 μM Fura-2 AM (Invitrogen, CA, USA) for 10 min at room temperature. Cardiomyocytes were observed through a Nikon fluor ×40 oil immersion objective and positioned for recording of Fura-2 fluorescence signals. During field stimulation at 0.5 Hz, cytoplasmic Fura-2 was excited by an IonOptix Hyperswitch dual-excitation light source (IonOptix Corporation, MA) at 340 and 380 nm and emitted light collected in a photomultiplier tube. $[Ca^{2+}]_i$ concentration was inferred from the ratio (R) of the intensity of the emitted fluorescence signals. Amplitude, time-to-peak, time-to-90% decay, and rate of rise (dR/dt) of the derived $[Ca^{2+}]_i$ transients were determined by IonWizard software.

For estimation of SR Ca^{2+} content, cardiomyocytes with cytoplasmic Fura-2 were paced at least 15 times at 0.5 Hz and then stopped. About 30s later, 10 mM caffeine was added to induce SR Ca^{2+} release. The area under the caffeine-induced $[Ca^{2+}]_i$ transient (area under curve, AUC) and its amplitude were used as a reflection of the SR Ca^{2+} content [22]. Time-to-90% decay of caffeine-induced increase in $[Ca^{2+}]_i$ was also measured to estimate the Ca^{2+} clearance ability of Na$^+$-Ca^{2+} exchanger (NCX).

RT–PCR

Total cellular RNA was extracted from left ventricle, septum and right ventricle of mouse hearts using a TRIzol Plus RNA Purification kit (Invitrogen, CA, USA). Single-stranded cDNA was synthesized from 2 μg total RNA with an iScript cDNA Synthesis kit (Bio-Rad Laboratories, CA, USA) following the manufacturer's instructions.

PCR was performed using JumpStart *Taq* DNA polymerase (Sigma, MO, USA), the cDNA generated above and the corresponding primers for GHS-R1a [23] (Forward: TCATC-GATCACAGCCATGT; Reverse: AAGCCAAACTGAC-CATGT; Tm = 64°C, 40 cycles). Mouse 18s rRNA was amplified as a control. Following our previous report [13], liver and pituitary were chosen as negative and positive controls respectively for GHS-R1a. PCR products were separated by agarose gel electrophoresis (2%), stained with ethidium bromide and visualized under UV light.

Western Blotting

Protein expression of the GHS receptor GHS-R1a and the phosphorylated phospholamban (p-PLB)/phospholamban (PLB) that are essential for SERCA2a activity were examined by Western blot analysis according to previous reports [24,25]. In brief, proteins were extracted from isolated cardiomyocytes (GHS-R1a) or minced mouse left ventricles (p-PLB and PLB) in lysis buffer. Extracted proteins (100 μg) were denatured at 37°C for 30 min (p-PLB and PLB) or 70°C for 10 min (GHS-R1a) in 2× sample buffer, separated on 10–15% SDS-polyacrylamide gels and transferred to nitrocellulose membranes. After blocking, the membrane was incubated with polyclonal rabbit anti- mouse phospholamban (phospho S16,1:1000; abcam, Cambridge, MA, USA), polyclonal rabbit anti- mouse phospholamban (1:1000; abcam) or polyclonal goat anti-human GHS-R1a (1:1000; Santa Cruz Biotechnology, Inc., Santa Cruz, CA, USA) primary antibodies overnight at 4°C before incubation with the corresponding secondary antibodies (1:5000) and detection with enhanced chemiluminescence (Pierce) according to the manufacturer's instructions. Mouse GAPDH (1:2000; Milipore, Billerica, MA, USA) was used as the internal control to allow semi-quantitative densitometry analysis on scanned films using ImageJ software [24].

Statistical Analysis

All data were expressed as mean ± S.E.M. One-way ANOVA with Tukey post hoc test was carried out for multiple comparisons as appropriate. In all comparisons, the differences were considered to be statistically significant at a value of $P < 0.05$.

Results

GHS-R1a Expression in Mouse Heart

The mRNA and protein expression of GHS-R1a, a GHS receptor in the mouse heart, was examined by RT-PCR and Western blots. As shown in FIG.1, GHS-R1a mRNA and protein is distributed in different regions of mouse heart, including left ventricle, septum and right ventricle. However, the protein expression level was relatively low compared to the breast cancer cell line used as positive control [24].

Effect of Ghrelin and Hexarelin on Sarcomere Shortening and Intracellular Ca^{2+} Transients after I/R

To determine the effects of ghrelin and hexarelin on cardiomyocyte function after I/R, cell shortening (FIG. 2A and E) and [Ca^{2+}]$_i$ transients (FIG. 3A and 3F) were recorded during stimulation at 0.5 Hz.

Sarcomere shortening was expressed as percentage of the resting sarcomere length (FIG. 2). It was found that relative sarcomere shortening was significantly reduced after I/R. However, the presence of 10 nM ghrelin or 1 nM hexarelin during pre- and post-treatments protected cardiomyocytes against this negative effect of I/R (FIG. 2B and F). The amplitude of the corresponding [Ca^{2+}]$_i$ transients decreased in the I/R group, as determined by the cytoplasmic fura-2 ratio changes shown in FIG. 3. Again, GHS treatment showed protective effects in cardiomyocytes against I/R-induced reductions in [Ca^{2+}]$_i$ transients (FIG. 3).

Basal [Ca^{2+}]$_i$ levels were significantly increased after 20 min ischemia (control vs ischemia: 1.63 ± 0.03, n = 72 cells vs 1.80 ± 0.05, n = 80 cells; $P < 0.01$), which is consistent with previous reports describing increased cytoplasmic Ca^{2+} and possible Ca^{2+} overload after ischemia [1,2]. The increased basal [Ca^{2+}]$_i$ after I/R was not reversed by either ghrelin pre- (1.99 ± 0.04, n = 90 cells, $P < 0.05$) and post-treatment (2.23 ± 0.05, n = 103 cells, $P < 0.001$), or hexarelin pre- (2.24 ± 0.05, n = 63 cells, $P < 0.001$) and post-treatment (2.20 ± 0.06, n = 66 cells, $P < 0.001$).

GHS treatment also influenced the time course of sarcomere shortening (FIG. 2) and [Ca^{2+}]$_i$ transients after I/R (FIG. 3). First, ghrelin post-treatment (FIG. 2C) and hexarelin pre-treatment (FIG. 2G) further prolonged the increased time-to-peak shortening following I/R. In addition, the corresponding time-to-peak of [Ca^{2+}]$_i$ transients in the ischemic group was also delayed by hexarelin pre-treatment (FIG. 3H). Furthermore, the time-to-90% decay of the [Ca^{2+}]$_i$ transients after GHS treatments (FIG. 3D and I) was similar to that in the ischemic group without GHS treatment, but nearly all GHS treatments except ghrelin pre-treatment (FIG. 2D and H) shortened the time-to-90% relaxation of the force compared to the I/R group. This indicates a lusitropic effect of GHS. As shown in FIG. 3E and J, the decrease in the rising rates of [Ca^{2+}]$_i$ transients after I/R was also diminished by all GHS treatments, which may indicate the effect of GHS on Ca^{2+} influx through L type Ca^{2+} current (I_{CaL}), Ca^{2+} release from SR through ryanodine receptors (RyR2s) or both.

Effect of Ghrelin and Hexarelin on SR Ca^{2+} Content after I/R

A possible explanation for the decrease in the [Ca^{2+}]$_i$ transient amplitude (FIG. 3B and G) and the rate of increase in dR/dt of Ca^{2+} transients (FIG. 3E and J) after I/R may be a consequence of reductions in SR Ca^{2+} content [22,26]. In order to estimate the SR Ca^{2+} content, we used caffeine (10 mM) to activate RyR2s and thoroughly deplete the SR, resulting in a significant rise in [Ca^{2+}]$_i$ (see the details in Methods and FIG. 4A [27]). The amplitude of caffeine-induced [Ca^{2+}]$_i$ transients and area under the transient curve can be used as estimates of the amount of Ca^{2+} stored in the SR [22]. Prior to caffeine application, cells were stimulated at 0.5Hz for 30s to normalize and replenish the SR Ca^{2+} content [22]. As shown in FIG.4B and C, there was a reduction in SR Ca^{2+} content after I/R that was restored by all GHS treatments.

To confirm whether GHS has an effect on the SR Ca^{2+} content of normal cardiomyocytes without ischemia, we performed ghrelin post-treatment on control hearts. We selected ghrelin post-treatment because it was the most effective at increasing SR Ca^{2+} content in I/R cardiomyocytes. The results (FIG. 4B and C) show no significant differences in area under the curve and amplitude of caffeine-induced Ca^{2+} transients between the control and ghrelin post-treated non-ischemic cardiomyocytes.

The time-to-90% decay of caffeine-induced Ca^{2+} transients mainly reflects the Ca^{2+} clearance ability of the NCX with a lesser contribution of sarcolemmal Ca^{2+} ATPase and mitochondrial uniporter [28], as the function of SERCA2a was counteracted by the opening of RyR2 in the presence of caffeine. As shown in FIG. 4D, the shortened time-to-90% decay of caffeine-induced Ca^{2+} transients after I/R indicates an accelerated Ca^{2+} clearance by the NCX. Therefore, this may suggest exaggerated NCX activity after I/R. GHS treatment prevented the reduction in the time-to-90% decay of caffeine-induced Ca^{2+} transients after I/R, which may suggest a normalization of NCX activity.

In order to further confirm whether these changes in the SR Ca^{2+} store were partially due to alterations in the uptake of Ca^{2+} into SR, the protein expression level of p-PLB and total PLB were

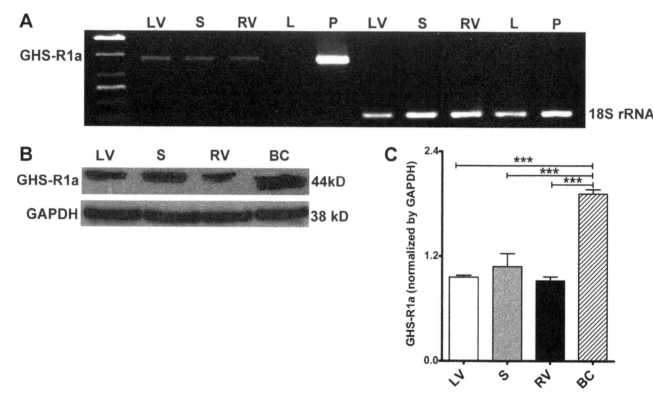

Figure 1. mRNA (A) and protein (B and C) expression of GHS-R1a in mouse heart. (A) Liver (L) and pituitary gland (P) were used as the negative and positive controls respectively. Mouse 18s rRNA was chosen as an internal control. (B) A breast cancer (BC) cell line was used as the positive control. (C) n = 3 for Western blots, data are shown as means ± S.E.M. and analyzed by One-way ANOVA with *Tukey's post hoc* test. ***$P <$ 0.001 vs BC group. GHS-R1a mRNA and protein are expressed in the left ventricle (LV), septum (S) and right ventricle (RV) of the mouse heart.

examined by Western blotting (FIG. 4E). PLB and its phosphorylated form p-PLB have opposing effects on SERCA2a, as PLB inhibits SERCA2a activity and p-PLB releases this inhibition [28]. As shown in FIG. 4F, a significant decrease in p-PLB/PLB ratio after I/R was reversed by GHS treatment. This change corresponds with the recovery of SERCA2a activity after I/R by all GHS treatments. Taken together, these results further support our assertion that the protective effect of ghrelin on Ca^{2+} transients was achieved at least in part by the recovery of SERCA2a activity and SR Ca^{2+} content.

GHS-R1a Mediates the Cardioprotective Effect of GHS

To investigate whether the GHS-induced effect on cardiomyocytes exposed to I/R injury was mediated by GHS receptors, we tested the GHS-R1a antagonists [D-Lys3]-GHRP-6 and BIM28163 [29,30] in ghrelin and hexarelin post-treatment groups. [D- Lys3]-GHRP-6 (200 nM) or BIM28163 (100 nM) was introduced into the perfusion system 5 min before GHS posttreatment for a total of 15 min. Alone, neither of these antagonists showed any effect on the sarcomere shortening or [Ca^{2+}]$_i$ transients. However, both antagonists completely blocked the protective effects of ghrelin and hexarelin on sarcomere shortening (FIG. 5A) and [Ca^{2+}]$_i$ transients (FIG. 5B). These observations suggest that the protective effect of GHS is mediated by the GHS-R1a.

Discussion

In the present study, we have confirmed that reduced cell shortening in mouse cardiomyocytes exposed to *in vitro* I/R injury

is attributable to a reduction in both the amplitude and rising rate of [Ca^{2+}]$_i$ transients, which may be due to a reduced SR Ca^{2+} content caused by decreased SERCA2a activity. We have also demonstrated for the first time that GHS such as ghrelin and hexarelin, produce a protective effect on cardiomyocytes exposed to *in vitro* I/R injury. Normal cardiac myocyte contractility was maintained by a normal amplitude and rising rate of [Ca^{2+}]$_i$ transients after GHS treatment, which may be attributed to normalized SERCA2a activity and SR Ca^{2+}content.

The mechanisms underlying cardiac ischemia are multifaceted, including ATP depletion, ROS generation, [Ca^{2+}]$_i$ overload amongst others. The disruption of Ca^{2+} homeostasis can cause inappropriate activation of Ca^{2+} dependent proteases and phospholipases essential for various cardiac functions, which may lead to further damage of the cardiomyocytes [2]. A tighter regulation of Ca^{2+} might therefore be an effective way to protect cardiomyocytes from I/R injury [6,7].

As shown in our study, reduced heart function after I/R exists at the single cell level, as reflected by reduced cardiomyocyte contractility (FIG. 2) accompanied by a decrease in the [Ca^{2+}]$_i$ transient amplitude (FIG. 3) and an increase in the basal [Ca^{2+}]$_i$ (details in Results). In addition, the prolonged time for maximal sarcomere shortening after I/R (FIG. 2C and G) with unchanged time-to-peak Ca^{2+} transients (FIG. 3C and H) may reflect impairment of the contractile machinery essential for cell contraction, such as the degradation of the regulatory protein troponin [31]. Moreover, the reduction observed in the amplitude (FIG. 3B and G) and rising rate of [Ca^{2+}]$_i$ transients after I/R (FIG. 3E and J) could be due to decreases in voltage-gated L type Ca^{2+} current (I_{CaL}) [32], SR Ca^{2+} content (FIG. 4B and C) or

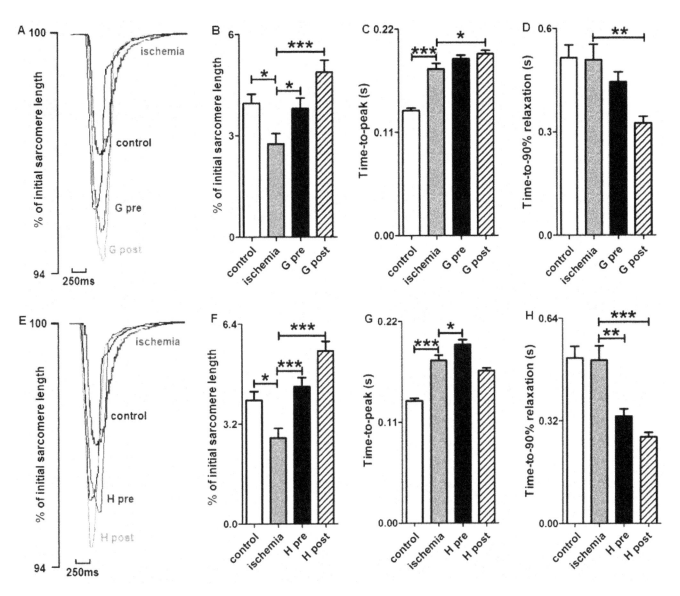

Figure 2. Effects of GHS on the contractile properties of mouse cardiomyocytes exposed to ischemia/reperfusion. (A) and (E) are representative superimposed traces of sarcomere shortening after ghrelin (G) or hexarelin (H) pre-treatment (pre) and post-treatment (post). Both hexarelin and ghrelin improved the reduction in sarcomere shortening (B and F), but not the prolonged time-to-peak shortening (C and G). The time-to-peak shortening was further prolonged in G post- and H pre-treatment groups. The time for relaxation (D and H) was shortened in G post-, H pre- and post-treatment groups. n = 99, 84, 84, 95, 106 and 100 cells/3 mice in control, ischemia, G pre, G post, H pre and H post groups, respectively. Data are shown as means ± S.E.M. and analyzed by One-way ANOVA with *Tukey's post hoc* test. *$P < 0.05$, ** $P < 0.01$, *** $P < 0.001$ vs ischemic group.

both. Any combination of these would reduce the magnitude of the SR Ca^{2+} release and subsequently alter the shortening phase of contraction. Our results certainly support the concept of a reduction in SR Ca^{2+} loading ability. This is shown by the reduced caffeine-induced Ca^{2+} transients, the reduction in the ratio of p-PLB to total PLB at the protein level and therefore the reduced activity of SERCA2a (FIG. 4). The reduced activity of SERCA2a is indicated by our data where we compared the time-to-90% decay of $[Ca^{2+}]_i$ transients under normal twitch with the time-to-90% decay of caffeine-induced Ca^{2+} transients. Under normal twitch, there was no significant difference in the time-to-90% decay of Ca^{2+} transients among experimental groups (FIG. 3D and I), however, the time-to-90% decay of caffeine-induced Ca^{2+} transients was shortened in ischemic group

(FIG. 4D). Taken together, this suggests increased NCX activity but decreased SERCA2a activity after IR, with the decreased SERCA2a activity contributing to the decreased SR Ca^{2+} content. Nevertheless, the reduction in SR Ca^{2+} content may also be caused by an increase in the RyR2s-dependent and -independent Ca^{2+} leak from SR, as reported in cardiomyocytes from the failing rabbit heart [33].

A previous study from our laboratory has found that ghrelin and hexarelin exert a positive inotropic effect on normally perfused rat hearts [34] and isolated adult rat ventricular cardiomyocytes [21] through GHS-R1a [34], the reported functional receptor for GHS. This study also demonstrated that ghrelin and hexarelin pre- or post-treatments exert a protective effect on adult mouse ventricular cardiomyocytes during *in vitro* I/R injury via a positive

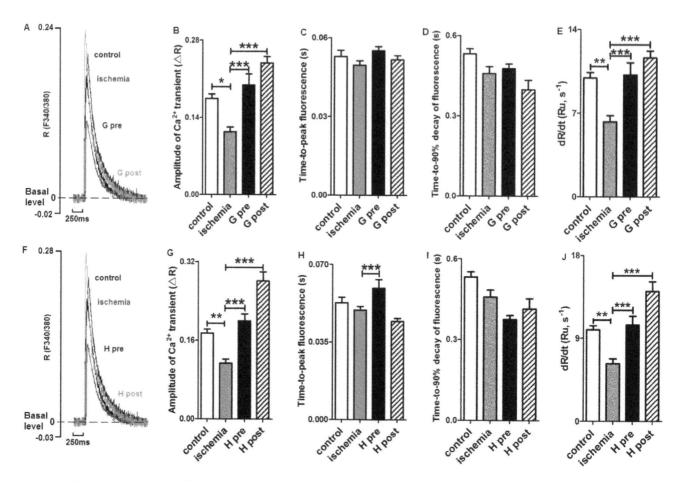

Figure 3. Effects of GHS on $[Ca^{2+}]_i$ transients in cardiomyocytes exposed to ischemia?reperfusion. (A) and (F) are representative superimposed traces of $[Ca^{2+}]_i$ transient after ghrelin (G) or hexarelin (H) pre-treatment (pre) and post-treatments (post). R represents the emission fluorescence ratio of fura-2 from excitation at 340 and 380nm, and Ru represents the ratio unit. Both hexarelin and ghrelin improved the reduced amplitude of $[Ca^{2+}]_i$ transients (B and G). The time-to-peak fluorescence was prolonged in ghrelin and hexarelin pre-treatment (C and H) groups, but the decreased rate of rise of $[Ca^{2+}]_i$ transients after ischemia was reversed to control level by all H and G pre- and post-treatments (E and J). Ghrelin and hexarelin had no effect on the time-to-90% decay of $[Ca^{2+}]_i$ transient (D and I). n = 72, 80, 90, 103, 63 and 66 cells/3 mice in control, ischemia, G pre, G post, H pre and H post groups, respectively. Data are shown as means ± S.E.M. and analyzed by One-way ANOVA with Tukey's post hoc test. *$P < 0.05$, **$P < 0.01$, *** $P < 0.001$ vs ischemic group.

inotropic effect and lusitropic effect (FIG. 2 and 3). Our results are consistent with those from previous studies using whole heart after I/R. Administrations of 20 nM ghrelin/1 µM hexarelin by Frascarelli et al. [17] or 0.1 nM-10 nM ghrelin by Chang et al. [18] protected the *in vitro* I/R rat heart from a reduction in cardiac function. Treatment with 320 µg/kg ghrelin or 80 µg/kg hexarelin (daily for 7 days) [10], or 10 nM/kg ghrelin (2 doses 12 h apart, the hearts were removed 1h after the last dose) [19] prevented I/R injury in the isolated rat heart by ameliorating the damaged heart function and attenuating the myocardial apoptosis. It has been suggested that ghrelin and hexarelin may exert their protective effects on rat heart I/R models through the activation of protein kinase C (PKC) [17] and/or inhibition of ER stress [19].

For the first time, we have demonstrated that the positive inotropic effect of GHS is at least partially due to the recovery or maintenance of normal SERCA2a activity (FIG. 4E and F) and therefore normal SR Ca^{2+} content (FIG. 4B and C). This is supported by the increased p-PLB/PLB protein ratio (FIG. 4F) after GHS treatment. Furthermore, when comparing the time-to-90% decay of $[Ca^{2+}]_i$ transients under normal twitch (FIG. 3D and I) and the time-to-90% decay of caffeine-induced Ca^{2+} transients (FIG. 4D), it suggests that SERCA2a activity was

recovered after GHS treatment since the time-to-90% decay of caffeine-induced Ca^{2+} transients was restored back to control levels (normalization of NCX) by GHS treatment, whereas the time-to-90% decay of $[Ca^{2+}]_i$ transients under normal twitch had no significant change.

Ca^{2+} overload, which has been reported as the main damaging factor causing cardiac dysfunction after ischemia [2], was also observed in this study (see results for details). The basal level of $[Ca^{2+}]_i$ was increased in ischemic cells with or without GHS treatment. The basal level of $[Ca^{2+}]_i$ would reflect the activity of both SERCA2a and RyR2s [35]. Following the recovery of SERCA2a activity by GHS treatment (FIG. 4F), SR Ca^{2+} content was also restored. If the sensitivity of RyR2s to Ca^{2+} is changed in ischemia (Ca^{2+} leak from SR), increased Ca^{2+} leak from SR may occur. Such a presumption seems consistent with an even greater increase in the basal level of $[Ca^{2+}]_i$ after GHS treatment. Moreover, the increased basal $[Ca^{2+}]_i$ in GHS treated groups may also be due to the increased Ca^{2+} influx into the cell through I_{CaL}, which has been reported previously by our group [21]. To what extent this effect contributes to the improvements in Ca^{2+} homeostasis and cardiomyocyte function seen in the current study requires further investigation.

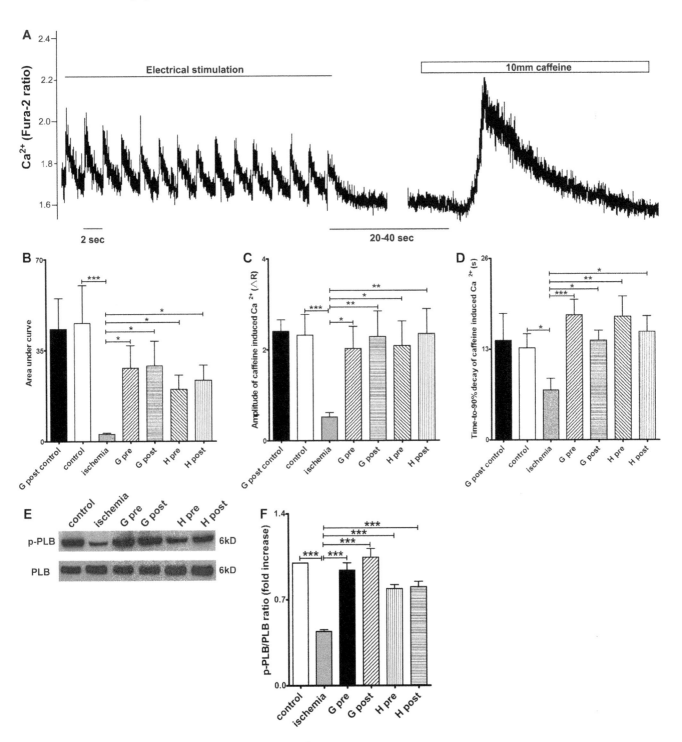

Figure 4. Effects of GHS on sarcoplasmic reticulum (SR) Ca²⁺ content and phospho-phospholamban (p-PLB)/phospholamban (PLB) expression. (A) Illustration of the SR Ca^{2+} content measurement protocol (data from cardiomyocytes exposed to ischemia/reperfusion). R represents the emission fluorescence ratio of fura-2 from excitation at 340 and 380nm. Cardiomyocytes were perfused with Tyrode solution containing 1.5 mM $CaCl_2$ and paced at 0.5 Hz for at least 30 s. 10 mM caffeine was then added to induce SR Ca^{2+} release. SR Ca^{2+} content, as determined by both (B) Area under curve and (C) amplitude of the caffeine-induced Ca^{2+} release, significantly decreased after 20 min ischemia compared with the control group. Ghrelin (G) or hexarelin (H) pre-treatment (pre) and post-treatment (post) significantly increased the SR Ca^{2+} content after 20 min ischemia (B and C), but introduction of ghrelin into the perfusion system at 40 min and lasting for 10 min (G post control) had no effect on the SR Ca^{2+} content of the cells isolated from the normal perfused heart. (D) The time-to-90% decay of caffeine-induced increases in $[Ca^{2+}]_i$ mainly reflect the Ca^{2+} clearance ability of the Na^+/Ca^{2+} exchanger (NCX). n = 18, 44, 44, 33, 38, 41 and 38 cells/3 mice in G post control, control, ischemia, G pre, G post, H pre and H post, respectively. (E) Representative western blots of the total phospholamban (PLB) and the phosphorylated PLB (p-PLB) in 6 groups and (F) the densitometric quantification of ratio of p-PLB/PLB (expressed as fold increase relative to control). n = 5 mice in each group. Data are shown as means ± S.E.M. and analyzed by one-way ANOVA with *Tukey's post hoc* test. *$P < 0.05$, **$P < 0.01$, *** $P < 0.001$ vs ischemic group.

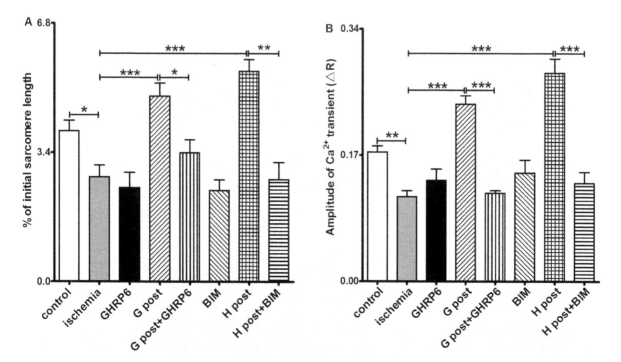

Figure 5. Role of GHS-R1a in the cardiac effects of hexarelin (H) and ghrelin (G). R represents the emission fluorescence ratio of fura-2 from excitation at 340 and 380nm. The GHS-R1a antagonists, [D-Lys3]-GHRP-6 (GHRP6, 200 nM) and BIM28163 (BIM,100 nM), completely blocked the effects of 1 nM hexarelin (H) and 10 nM ghrelin (G) post-treatment (post) on sarcomere shortening (A) and [Ca^{2+}]$_i$ transients (B). These peptides alone did not produce any noticeable change in sarcomere shortening (A) and [Ca^{2+}]$_i$ transients (B). For sarcomere shortening experiments, n = 99, 84, 52, 95, 46,100, 50 and 61 in control, ischemic, GHRP6, G post, G post +GHRP6, BIM, H post and H post+BIM groups, respectively. For [Ca^{2+}]$_i$ transient experiments, n = 72, 80, 55, 103, 69, 60, 66 and 68 in control, ischemic, GHRP6, G post, G post +GHRP6, BIM, H post and H post+BIM groups, respectively. Data were analyzed by one-way ANOVA with *Tukey's post hoc* test, and expressed as means ± S.E.M. *$P < 0.05$, ** $P < 0.01$, *** $P < 0.001$.

We show here the expression of GHS-R1a in the mouse heart at both the mRNA and protein level (FIG.1). In order to determine whether the protective effect of GHS on cardiomyocytes after I/R injury was mediated by GHS-R1a, we administrated the GHS-R1a antagonists [D-Lys3]-GHRP-6 or BIM28163 along with GHS in I/R hearts. There is no report of non-specific effects of BIM28163 and [D-Lys3]-GHRP-6, and both reagents are widely applied as selective GHS-R1a antagonists in different cell types (eg neurons) [36], organs (stomach, small intestine) [37,38,39], and species (rodents [36,38], dogs [37]). The GHS-R1a antagonists alone showed no effect on cardiomyocytes, but completely blocked the effects of ghrelin or hexarelin on sarcomere shortening and [Ca^{2+}]$_i$ transients of cardiomyocytes after I/R injury (FIG. 5). This suggests that the effects of GHS, especially their actions on the contractile properties of cardiomyocytes and the corresponding increases in [Ca^{2+}]$_i$ transients, are mediated by GHS-R1a.

In summary, ghrelin and hexarelin pre- and post-treatments protected mouse cardiomyocytes from *in vitro* I/R injury and

preserved the cell shortening by regulating [Ca^{2+}]$_i$. Both ghrelin and hexarelin prevented the decrease in the amplitude of [Ca^{2+}]$_i$ transients and SR Ca^{2+} content after I/R by maintaining the ratio of p-PLB to total PLB and therefore the SERCA2a activity. Their positive inotropic effect on the cardiomyocytes and corresponding increase in [Ca^{2+}]$_i$ transients is mainly mediated by the activation of GHS-R1a.

Acknowledgments

We thank the careful editing of Dr Tamara Paravicini at the School of Biomedical Sciences, University of Queensland.

Author Contributions

Conceived and designed the experiments: LZ JNE BSL CC. Performed the experiments: YM. Analyzed the data: YM. Contributed reagents/materials/analysis tools: JNE BSL CC. Wrote the paper: YM LZ JNE BSL CC.

Reference

1. Ostadal B, Kolář F (1999) Cardiac ischemia: from injury to protection: Springer.
2. Murphy E, Steenbergen C (2008) Mechanisms underlying acute protection from cardiac ischemia-reperfusion injury. Physiol Rev 88: 581–609.
3. Headrick JP, Peart J, Hack B, Flood A, Matherne GP (2001) Functional properties and responses to ischaemia-reperfusion in Langendorff perfused mouse heart. Exp Physiol 86: 703–716.
4. Furman E, Acad BA, Sonn J, Raul A, Kedem J (1985) Effect of global vs regional ischaemia upon myocardial contractility and oxygen balance. Cardiovasc Res 19: 606–612.
5. Chambers DJ, Fallouh HB (2010) Cardioplegia and cardiac surgery: pharmacological arrest and cardioprotection during global ischemia and reperfusion. Pharmacol Ther 127: 41–52.

6. del Monte F, Lebeche D, Guerrero JL, Tsuji T, Doye AA, et al. (2004) Abrogation of ventricular arrhythmias in a model of ischemia and reperfusion by targeting myocardial calcium cycling. Proc Natl Acad Sci U S A 101: 5622–5627.
7. Xu XL, Chen XJ, Ji H, Li P, Bian YY, et al. (2008) Astragaloside IV improved intracellular calcium handling in hypoxia-reoxygenated cardiomyocytes via the sarcoplasmic reticulum Ca-ATPase. Pharmacology 81: 325–332.
8. Kojima M, Hosoda H, Date Y, Nakazato M, Matsuo H, et al. (1999) Ghrelin is a growth-hormone-releasing acylated peptide from stomach. Nature 402: 656–660.
9. Bulgarelli I, Tamiazzo L, Bresciani E, Rapetti D, Caporali S, et al. (2009) Desacyl-ghrelin and synthetic GH-secretagogues modulate the production of

inflammatory cytokines in mouse microglia cells stimulated by beta-amyloid fibrils. J Neurosci Res 87: 2718–2727.

10. Torsello A, Bresciani E, Rossoni G, Avallone R, Tulipano G, et al. (2003) Ghrelin plays a minor role in the physiological control of cardiac function in the rat. Endocrinology 144: 1787–1792.

11. Bodart V, Febbraio M, Demers A, McNicoll N, Pohankova P, et al. (2002) CD36 mediates the cardiovascular action of growth hormone-releasing peptides in the heart. Circ Res 90: 844–849.

12. Gnanapavan S, Kola B, Bustin SA, Morris DG, McGee P, et al. (2002) The tissue distribution of the mRNA of ghrelin and subtypes of its receptor, GHS-R, in humans. J Clin Endocrinol Metab 87: 2988.

13. Sun Y, Garcia JM, Smith RG (2007) Ghrelin and growth hormone secretagogue receptor expression in mice during aging. Endocrinology 148: 1323–1329.

14. Sax B, Nadasy GL, Turi K, Hirschberg K, Furjesz D, et al. (2011) Coronary vasoconstrictor effect of ghrelin is not mediated by growth hormone secretagogue receptor 1a type in dogs. Peptides 32: 362–367.

15. Baldanzi G, Filigheddu N, Cutrupi S, Catapano F, Bonissoni S, et al. (2002) Ghrelin and des-acyl ghrelin inhibit cell death in cardiomyocytes and endothelial cells through ERK1/2 and PI 3-kinase/AKT. J Cell Biol 159: 1029–1037.

16. Cassoni P, Papotti M, Ghe C, Catapano F, Sapino A, et al. (2001) Identification, characterization, and biological activity of specific receptors for natural (ghrelin) and synthetic growth hormone secretagogues and analogs in human breast carcinomas and cell lines. J Clin Endocrinol Metab 86: 1738–1745.

17. Frascarelli S, Ghelardoni S, Ronca-Testoni S, Zucchi R (2003) Effect of ghrelin and synthetic growth hormone secretagogues in normal and ischemic rat heart. Basic Res Cardiol 98: 401–405.

18. Chang L, Ren Y, Liu X, Li WG, Yang J, et al. (2004) Protective effects of ghrelin on ischemia/reperfusion injury in the isolated rat heart. J Cardiovasc Pharmacol 43: 165–170.

19. Zhang GG, Teng X, Liu Y, Cai Y, Zhou YB, et al. (2009) Inhibition of endoplasm reticulum stress by ghrelin protects against ischemia/reperfusion injury in rat heart. Peptides 30: 1109–1116.

20. Berti F, Muller E, De Gennaro Colonna V, Rossoni G (1998) Hexarelin exhibits protective activity against cardiac ischaemia in hearts from growth hormone-deficient rats. Growth Horm IGF Res 8 Suppl B. pp 149–152.

21. Sun Q, Ma Y, Zhang L, Zhao YF, Zang WJ, et al. (2010) Effects of GH secretagogues on contractility and Ca2+ homeostasis of isolated adult rat ventricular myocytes. Endocrinology 151: 4446–4454.

22. Santiago DJ, Curran JW, Bers DM, Lederer WJ, Stern MD, et al. (2010) Ca sparks do not explain all ryanodine receptor-mediated SR Ca leak in mouse ventricular myocytes. Biophys J 98: 2111–2120.

23. Kawamura K, Sato N, Fukuda J, Kodama H, Kumagai J, et al. (2003) Ghrelin inhibits the development of mouse preimplantation embryos in vitro. Endocrinology 144: 2623–2633.

24. Fung JN, Seim I, Wang D, Obermair A, Chopin LK, et al. (2010) Expression and in vitro functions of the ghrelin axis in endometrial cancer. Horm Cancer 1: 245–255.

25. Ceylan-Isik AF, Sreejayan N, Ren J (2011) Endoplasmic reticulum chaperon tauroursodeoxycholic acid alleviates obesity-induced myocardial contractile dysfunction. J Mol Cell Cardiol 50: 107–116.

26. Kuster GM, Lancel S, Zhang J, Communal C, Trucillo MP, et al. (2010) Redox-mediated reciprocal regulation of SERCA and Na+-Ca2+ exchanger contributes to sarcoplasmic reticulum Ca2+ depletion in cardiac myocytes. Free Radic Biol Med 48: 1182–1187.

27. Launikonis BS, Stephenson DG (1997) Effect of saponin treatment on the sarcoplasmic reticulum of rat, cane toad and crustacean (yabby) skeletal muscle. J Physiol 504 (Pt 2): 425–437.

28. Bers DM (2002) Cardiac excitation-contraction coupling. Nature 415: 198–205.

29. Halem HA, Taylor JE, Dong JZ, Shen Y, Datta R, et al. (2004) Novel analogs of ghrelin: physiological and clinical implications. Eur J Endocrinol 151 Suppl 1: S71–75.

30. Asakawa A, Inui A, Kaga T, Katsuura G, Fujimiya M, et al. (2003) Antagonism of ghrelin receptor reduces food intake and body weight gain in mice. Gut 52: 947–952.

31. McDonough JL, Arrell DK, Van Eyk JE (1999) Troponin I degradation and covalent complex formation accompanies myocardial ischemia/reperfusion injury. Circ Res 84: 9–20.

32. Yu W, Wang JJ, Gan WY, Lin GS, Huang CX (2010) [Effects of verapamil preconditioning on cardiac function in vitro and intracellular free Ca2+ and L-type calcium current in rat cardiomyocytes post ischemia-reperfusion injury]. Zhonghua Xin Xue Guan Bing Za Zhi 38: 225–229.

33. Zima AV, Bovo E, Bers DM, Blatter LA (2010) Ca(2)+ spark-dependent and -independent sarcoplasmic reticulum Ca(2)+ leak in normal and failing rabbit ventricular myocytes. J Physiol 588: 4743–4757.

34. Xu XB, Cao JM, Pang JJ, Xu RK, Ni C, et al. (2003) The positive inotropic and calcium-mobilizing effects of growth hormone-releasing peptides on rat heart. Endocrinology 144: 5050–5057.

35. Seehase M, Quentin T, Wiludda E, Hellige G, Paul T, et al. (2006) Gene expression of the Na-Ca2+ exchanger, SERCA2a and calsequestrin after myocardial ischemia in the neonatal rabbit heart. Biol Neonate 90: 174–184.

36. Feng DD, Yang SK, Loudes C, Simon A, Al-Sarraf T, et al. (2011) Ghrelin and obestatin modulate growth hormone-releasing hormone release and synaptic inputs onto growth hormone-releasing hormone neurons. Eur J Neurosci 34: 732–744.

37. Ogawa A, Mochiki E, Yanai M, Morita H, Toyomasu Y, et al. (2011) Interdigestive migrating contractions are coregulated by ghrelin and motilin in conscious dogs. Am J Physiol Regul Integr Comp Physiol.

38. Iwasaki E, Suzuki H, Masaoka T, Nishizawa T, Hosoda H, et al. (2011) Enhanced Gastric Ghrelin Production and Secretion in Rats with Gastric Outlet Obstruction. Dig Dis Sci.

39. Yang CG, Qiu WC, Wang ZG, Yu S, Yan J, et al. (2011) Down-regulation of ghrelin receptors in the small intestine delays small intestinal transit in vagotomized rats. Mol Med Report 4: 1061–1065.

19

A Device for Performing Automated Balloon Catheter Inflation Ischemia Studies

Silas J. Leavesley[1,2,3]*, **Whitley Ledkins**[1], **Petra Rocic**[4]

1 Chemical and Biomolecular Engineering, University of South Alabama, Mobile, Alabama, United States of America, 2 Pharmacology, University of South Alabama, Mobile, Alabama, United States of America, 3 Center for Lung Biology, University of South Alabama, Mobile, Alabama, United States of America, 4 Pharmacology, New York Medical College, Valhalla, New York, United States of America

Abstract

Coronary collateral growth (arteriogenesis) is a physiological adaptive response to transient and repetitive occlusion of major coronary arteries in which small arterioles (native collaterals) with minimal to no blood flow remodel into larger conduit arteries capable of supplying adequate perfusion to tissue distal to the site of occlusion. The ability to reliably and reproducibly mimic transient, repetitive coronary artery occlusion (ischemia) in animal models is critical to the development of therapies to restore coronary collateral development in type II diabetes and the metabolic syndrome. Current animal models for repetitive coronary artery occlusion implement a pneumatic occluder (balloon) that is secured onto the surface of the heart with the suture, which is inflated manually, via a catheter connected to syringe, to effect occlusion of the left anterior descending coronary artery (LAD). This method, although effective, presents complications in terms of reproducibility and practicality. To address these limitations, we have designed a device for automated, transient inflation of balloon catheters in coronary artery occlusion models. This device allows repeated, consistent inflation (to either specified pressure or volume) and the capability for implementing very complex, month-long protocols. This system has significantly increased the reproducibility of coronary collateral growth studies in our laboratory, resulting in a significant decrease in the numbers of animals needed to complete each study while relieving laboratory personnel from the burden of extra working hours and enabling us to continue studies over periods when we previously could not. In this paper, we present all details necessary for construction and operation of the inflator. In addition, all of the components for this device are commercially available and economical (Table S1). It is our hope that the adoption of automated balloon catheter inflation protocols will improve the experimental reliability of transient ischemia studies at many research institutions.

Editor: Rajesh Gopalrao Katare, University of Otago, New Zealand

Funding: The authors would like to acknowledge support from NIH grant R01 HL093052 and the ISAC Scholar's Program (http://isac-net.org/ISAC-Cytometry/ISAC-Scholars.aspx). The funders had no role in study design, data collection and analysis, decision to publish, or preparation of the manuscript.

Competing Interests: The authors have declared that no competing interests exist.

* E-mail: leavesley@southalabama.edu

Introduction

Type II diabetes and the metabolic syndrome – a cluster of risk factors including abdominal obesity, insulin resistance, hyperglycemia, dyslipidemia and hypertension – affect ~30% of the U.S. population with increasing prevalence [1]. These pathologies are also associated with increased severity of ischemic coronary artery disease (CAD). For example, higher numbers of metabolic syndrome components have been correlated with more severe CAD [1,2] and increased CAD-associated mortality. Patients with type II diabetes are ~2 times more likely to die of CAD, whereas patients with all component pathologies of the metabolic syndrome are ~3.6–4.4 times more likely to die of CAD [3,4]. Moreover, current revascularization therapies, coronary artery bypass grafting (CABG), and percutaneous transluminal coronary angioplasty (PTCA) in type II diabetics and metabolic syndrome patients are associated with higher procedural risk and poorer long-term outcomes then in patients without type II diabetes or the metabolic syndrome [5–7].

Coronary collateral growth (arteriogenesis) is a physiological adaptive response to transient and repetitive occlusion of major coronary arteries in which small arterioles (native collaterals) with minimal to no blood flow remodel into larger conduit arteries capable of supplying adequate perfusion to tissue distal to the site of occlusion. Transient repetitive coronary artery occlusion and resultant myocardial ischemia stimulate coronary collateral growth in healthy humans and normal animals [8–11]. Clinically, patients with stable angina have decreased incidence of fatal myocardial infarction, which is associated with better developed collateral networks [8]. In addition, well-developed collateral networks seem to promote long term patency of coronary bypass grafts. However, this normal physiological response is impaired in patients with type II diabetes and the metabolic syndrome [12–15]. Graft closure, and consequent need for revascularization, is a significant problem in type II diabetic and metabolic syndrome patients [6]. Therefore, the ability to reliably and reproducibly mimic transient, repetitive coronary artery ischemia in animal models is critical to the development of therapies to restore coronary collateral development in type II diabetes and the metabolic syndrome.

Like in human metabolic syndrome, coronary collateral growth has been shown to be impaired in most animal models of the metabolic syndrome [10,16–18]. However, normal collateral development has been reported in a swine model of the metabolic syndrome [19]. The most obvious difference in the swine model is that this was a model of progressive chronic ischemia whereas the other animal models used transient, repetitive coronary artery occlusion to stimulate collateral development, which mimics the pathophysiology of the human. Since the exact timing and duration of coronary occlusions has been associated with the extent of collateral growth [20,21], the difference between these two methods of inducing coronary occlusion is a likely explanation for the different outcomes between the models and emphasizes the necessity of using transient and repetitive coronary occlusion models vs. progressive occlusion (ameroid constrictors) when studying coronary collateral development.

We and others have recently successfully used both normal and metabolic syndrome rat models of transient, repetitive left anterior descending coronary artery (LAD) occlusion to study coronary collateral development [10,16,18,22–25]. A pneumatic occluder (balloon) is secured onto the surface of the heart with the suture, which is also passed under the LAD so that when the balloon is inflated, the LAD is occluded [23]. The occluder has a catheter, which is externalized for easy access for manual inflation, using an air-filled syringe, post-surgically. This method, although effective, presents complications in terms of reproducibility and practicality. Most significantly, manual inflation allows for regulation of the volume of air injected into the occluder but provides no indication of consistent pressure from animal to animal. Since occluders are manufactured individually and manually, some variation in their size is inevitable. Therefore, despite identical volumes being injected, the varying inflation pressure and consequent varying extent of LAD occlusion introduces a small, yet unnecessary confounding variable into the experimental design. Secondly, it can be difficult to maintain a stringent schedule demanded by manual occlusion inflation protocols for periods of several weeks or months, especially in smaller laboratories. Because the timing and duration of transient coronary occlusions has been associated with the extent of collateral growth (as mentioned above), these small variations in LAD occlusion or frequency may also effect variations in the extent of collateral growth.

To overcome these obstacles, we have developed an automated inflation system. This system allows reproducible pressurized inflation of up to four pneumatic occluders simultaneously. In addition, complex and varied experimental protocols can be defined including inflation times, repetition rates, resting times, and the number of cycles for each occlusion protocol (of up to indefinite duration). This system has significantly increased the reproducibility of coronary collateral growth studies in our laboratory, resulting in a significant decrease in the numbers of animals needed to complete each study while relieving laboratory personnel from the burden of extra working hours and enabling us to continue studies over periods when we previously could not.

In this paper, we describe the construction and operation of a device for automated inflation of pneumatic occluders in transient LAD ischemia studies. The device consists of electronics and pneumatics hardware, and corresponding control software. Each element of the device is described in detail, so as to allow construction of similar devices at other research institutions. In addition, a detailed list of all components, with supplier, and description of the operating software are included in the supplemental information. All of the components for this device are commercially available, with a total cost of under $1300 (U.S., not including computer). It is our hope that the adoption of automated balloon catheter inflation protocols will improve the experimental reliability of transient ischemia studies at many research institutions.

Materials and Methods

The automated balloon catheter inflation device consisted of an electronic subsystem, an pneumatic subsystem, and control software with corresponding user interface. The control software communicated with the electronic subsystem via an USB interface board. The electronic subsystem supplied power to solenoid pressure valves, which controlled the pressurizing and depressurizing of the balloon catheters. A list of the parts required for the automated catheter inflation device is given in Table S1.

Electronic Subsystem

The electronic subsystem consisted of an USB interface (USB-6009, National Instruments, Inc.), 24V DC power supply (VOF-25-24, CUI, Inc.), and TTL-controlled 24V relay board (RLY102-24V, Winford Engineering), along with supporting electrical components (Figure 1). Digital input/output lines from the USB interface were used to switch the relays, controlling 24 V power to the solenoid valves. A snubber circuit was used for each solenoid, consisting of a diode connected in reverse polarity from the negative terminal of the solenoid to the positive DC voltage supply. This circuit protects against high reverse potentials generated from solenoid closing. AC Power to the 24 V supply (and hence, the relay board) was controlled by a manual switch.

An air flow meter (D6F-01A1-110, Omron) was used to measure the volume of air delivered. The flow meter output signal was read via an analog input (0–5 V, 14 bit) and integrated using a Labview script (see Control Software section).

All components for the electronic subsystem were placed in a water-tight enclosure. Water-resistant electrical fittings were used for the solenoid valve and flow meter connections.

Pneumatic Subsystem

The pneumatic subsystem consisted of a master pressure control valve, two solenoid valves, the flow meter, and the pressure manifold (Figure 2). Using the dual relay, the two solenoid valves could be operated independently. Three valve combinations were used for catheter inflation: 1) the first solenoid valve (component (7) in Figure 2) was opened and the second solenoid valve (component (8) in Figure 2) was closed, allowing pressurized air to flow into the catheters; 2) the first and second solenoid valves were both closed, maintaining a fixed pressure within the catheters balloons, 3) the first solenoid valve was closed and the second solenoid valve was opened, allowing pressurized air to vent to the atmosphere. Valves were kept in the third configuration between inflation cycles, allowing balloon catheters to remain deflated.

Control Software

Control software was written using Labview software (National Instruments, Inc.). The control software consisted of a series of timed loops, implementing a series of balloon inflation and deflation cycles (see Figure S1 for a detailed description). A user interface was also generated using Labview software, in order to facilitate changing the inflation protocol for different experiments.

The factory calibration for the flowmeter was also applied using the control software, using a signal scaling function. The calibrated signal was then integrated to yield a measure of the total air volume delivered. The exact Labview functions for performing these steps are shown in Figure S1.

Comparison of Manual and Automated Balloon Catheter Inflation

Variation in collateral dependent blood flow in rat repetitive myocardial ischemia (RI) studies was used as an indicator of

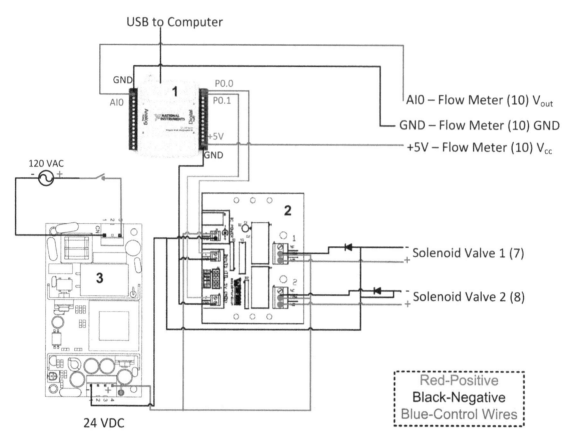

Figure 1. Electronic subsystem schematic. Red lines indicate positive voltage supply (+), black lines indicate negative (−), and blue lines indicate control (digital TTL or analog 0–5 V). Component images for the USB interface (1), relay board (2), and 24 VDC power supply (3), are taken from National Instruments [28], CUI [29], and Winford Engineering [30], respectively.

balloon catheter inflation reproducibility. Data was tabulated from both unpublished and published [23–26] results from our group. Inclusion criteria for the retrospective comparison included: matching the mouse line (different breeds may introduce inherit physiological variance), matching the study protocol, and matching (as closely as possible) the sample size for the study. Two of the more recent automated inflation experiments performed by our

group [24,27] were excluded, as these studies involved much smaller sample sizes than the manual inflation studies (n = 5 vs. n = 12, respectively). Blood flow measurements were performed using either radioactive microspheres or gold-labeled and samarium-labeled microspheres, as described previously [23,25] (for unpublished results, the methodology is described in detail in the following sub-sections). Data from two rat lines was used for comparison: Wistar Kyoto (WKY) rats and Sprague-Dawley (SD) rats. For both rat lines, collateral dependent blood flow measurements were made either before and after RI or in RI-affected collateral zone (CZ) and normal zone (NZ) tissues. All measurements were made using both manual inflation and the automated balloon catheter inflation device described in these studies.

Rat model of coronary collateral growth (CCG)/repetitive ischemia (RI). Male, 10–12 week old Sprague-Dawley (SD; Charles Rivers, Wilmington, MA) (300–350 g) were used for chronic (9 days) implantation of a pneumatic occluder over the left anterior descending coronary artery (LAD). A suture was passed under the proximal portion of the LAD and the occluder was sown onto the surface of the heart. The occluder catheter was externalized between the scapulae. When the occluder is inflated, the suture is pulled towards the surface of the heart and the LAD is occluded. The LAD perfusion territory is termed the collateral-dependent zone (CZ) because perfusion in this area, while the LAD is occluded, depends on the development of coronary collaterals. The animals underwent a RI protocol consisting of eight 40 sec occlusions, once every 20 min (2 h, 20 min total)

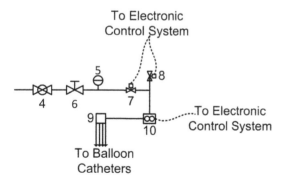

Figure 2. Pneumatic subsystem schematic: main pressure valve (4), pressure dial (5), pressure regulator (6), pressurizing solenoid valve (7), venting solenoid valve (8), pressure manifold (9), and air flow meter (10). Solid lines indicate pneumatic connections. Dashed lines indicate electrical connections (see Figure 1).

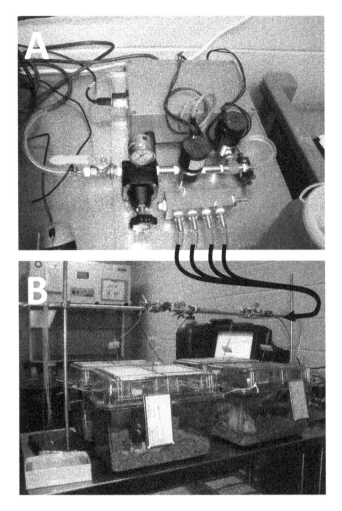

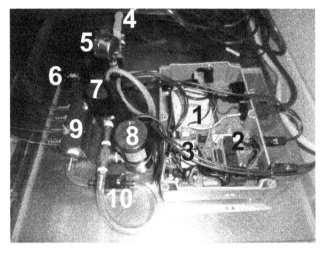

Figure 4. The completed balloon catheter inflation device consists of: the USB interface (1), relay board (2), 24 VDC power supply (3), main pressure valve (4), pressure dial (5), pressure regulator (6), pressurizing solenoid valve (7), venting solenoid valve (8), pressure manifold (9), and air flow meter (10). Components 1–3 comprise the electronic system while components 4–10 comprise the pneumatic subsystem.

Figure 3. The automated catheter inflation device (A) and example of cardiac ischemia study using the device (B). The curved arrows indicate the pressure lines which exit from the manifold in (A) and are connected to the implanted balloon catheters in (B) via rotating couplers.

followed by a rest period of 5 h, 40 min. This 8-hour cycle was repeated 3 times/day for 0–9 days. Surgical procedures were performed in accordance with the Animal Welfare Act and are approved by the IACUC of the University of South Alabama.

Myocardial and collateral-dependent blood flow measurements. Color microspheres (5×10^5, 15 µM diameter) labeled with samarium (day 0 RI (initial surgery) or gold (day 10 RI) or radioactive microspheres (5×10^5, 15 µM diameter) labeled with ^{57}Co (day 0 RI (initial surgery) or ^{103}Ru (day 10 RI) were injected into the LV during LAD occlusion. There are no differences in blood flows measured by colored or radioactive microspheres. Arterial reference blood samples (carotid) and heart tissue from the NZ and the CZ were collected, weighed and sent to BioPal (Worcester, MA) for analysis. Blood flows to the NZ and the CZ (ml/min/g) were calculated from the formula: Blood Flow = [(radioactive counts in myocardial tissue)X(blood reference withdrawal rate)/(radioactive count in blood reference)]/(weight of myocardial tissue). Results were analyzed by calculating the standard error of the mean (SEM):

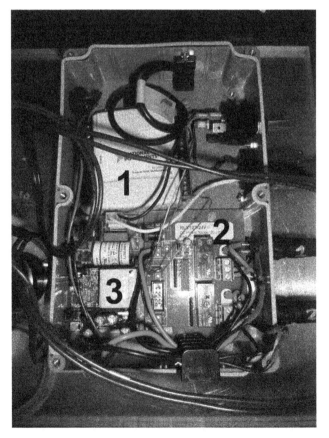

Figure 5. Detailed photograph of the electronics control system: the USB interface (1), relay board (2), and 24 VDC power supply (3).

$$SEM = \frac{SD}{\sqrt{n}} \qquad (1)$$

where SD is the standard deviation and n is the number of samples. The coefficient of variation (CV) was then calculated:

$$CV = \frac{SD}{\mu} \qquad (2)$$

where μ is the mean value. The CV was used as a metric to characterize the reproducibility of each study evaluated.

Results

System Description

The automated catheter inflation device provided consistent inflation volumes and balloon pressures. The manifold allowed up to four catheters to be inflated and deflated simultaneously (Figure 3). All components were integrated on a 2 ft×2 ft piece of Plexiglas for easy transport (Figure 4). 120 VAC and 24 VDC wire connections were enclosed in appropriate connectors or solder connections were enclosed in heat-shrink tubing to minimize the risk for short circuits. The electronic subsystem was placed in a water-tight enclosure (Figure 5).

The user interface allowed relatively complex or lengthy experimental protocols to be performed automatically – up to several weeks in duration (Figure 6). The user interface also allowed for monitoring of the protocol progress through a series of counters and timers. The software was compiled into an executable file (with a corresponding installer) that could be run on any windows-based computer.

Comparison of Manual and Automated Balloon Catheter Inflation

One of the central outcomes of automated balloon catheter inflation is to ensure reproducible occlusion during repetitive myocardial ischemia (RI) studies. A key outcome of these studies is the development of coronary collateral growth, which can be assessed through the measurement of collateral dependent blood flow. Hence, variation in collateral dependent flow among animals in the same study group is one of the most important indicators of the reproducibility of balloon catheter inflation experiments. We have previously performed manual inflation protocols in WKY rats that resulted in collateral dependent blood flows of 0.26 ± 0.09 mL/min/g ($\pm$ indicates standard error of the mean (SEM); coefficient of variation (CV) = 1.038) and 1.63 ± 0.3 (CV = 0.552) for pre- and post-RI, respectively (n = 9 animals) [23]. We have more recently performed these same protocols using the automated inflation device described in this paper, resulting in collateral dependent blood flows of 0.15 ± 0.03 (CV = 0.470) and 2.04 ± 0.05 (CV = 0.064) for pre- and post-RI, respectively (n = 6, see Figure 7, A–C for graphical representation) [25]. Similar studies were attempted using Sprague-Dawley rats, where manual studies resulted in highly variant blood flows (CV = 0.523 and 0.463) that were not publishable, even with a

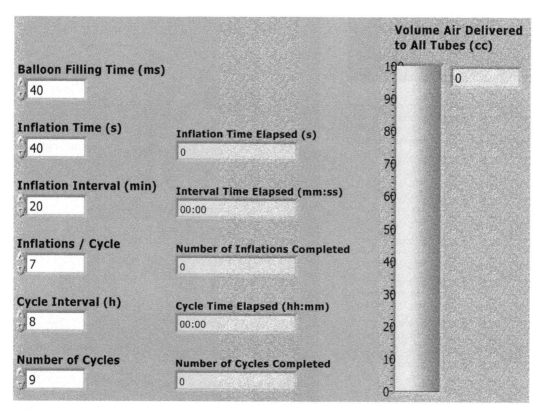

Figure 6. The software user interface (Labview front panel) allows the user to adjust parameters for automated inflation: the catheter pressurization (balloon filling time); the duration that the catheter remains inflated (inflation time); the interval between subsequent, shortly-spaced inflations in a cycle (inflation interval); the number of inflations per cycle (inflations/cycle); the interval between cycles (cycle interval); and the total number of cycles. For each of these sequences, a timer or counter displays the progress of the automated inflation. A bar plot displays the inflation volume, as measured by the flow meter.

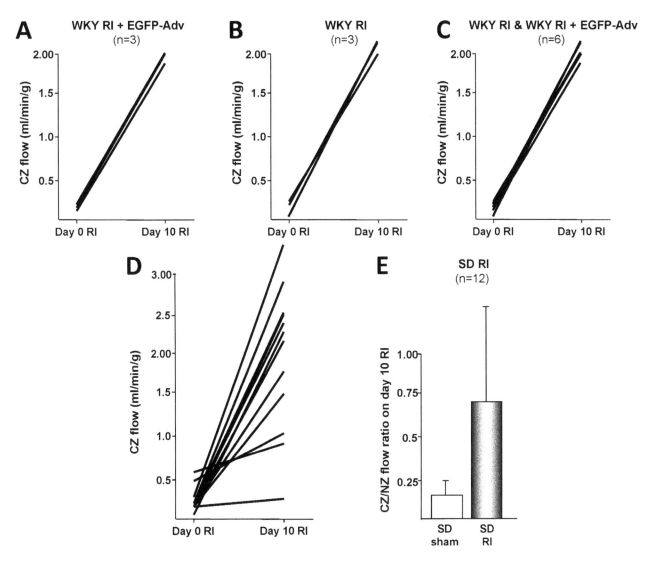

Figure 7. Collateral dependent blood flow measurements made after transient repetitive myocardia ischemia (RI) studies using the automated balloon catheter inflation device described in this manuscript displayed greatly reduced variance compared to blood flow measurements made after transient ischemia using manual inflation. Blood flow measurements made in WKY rats after using the automated inflation device (A–C) not only displayed greatly reduced variance than our previous manual inflation studies (compare to Figure 2 in Toyota, et al., 2005) [23], but also required fewer animals to complete a similar study (n = 3 or n = 6, compared to n = 9, for a study group). Note that panel C represents data from panels A and B combined. Similarly, blood flow measurements made in SD rats after manual inflation (D, E) had such high variance that they were not statistically significant (even with an n = 12), while measurements made after automated inflation (compare to Figure 7 in Dodd, et al., 2011 and Figure 4C in Hutcheson, et al., 2013) [24] achieved a high level of significance (p<0.05) with fewer animals (n = 5 and n = 7, respectively). A summary of results with coefficients of variation is given in Table 1.

large sample size (n = 12, Figure 7, D). By comparison, automated inflation studies provided blood flows with reduced variation (CV = 0.039 and 0.067) and statistically-significant results, while requiring fewer animals (n = 7) [26]. A summary of the multi-study comparison is presented in Table 1.

Discussion

Balloon catheter inflation experiments have been vital for simulating myocardial ischemia in animal models [16,18,23]. In these approaches, a catheter balloon is inflated to reduce or eliminate blood flow to a desired region. Manual approaches for balloon catheter inflation have been successfully used in previous studies. However, we have found that manual balloon inflation requires intermittent-to-constant supervision, depending on the

type of inflation protocol used. As shown (Table 1), the common method for supplying pressurized air – through a hand-held syringe – introduces a non-negligible amount of human error into the inflation protocol, resulting in higher variance in subsequent collateral dependent blood flow measurements, with coefficients of variation (CV) of 1 or greater. Also, some aspects of manual balloon catheter inflation (such as the rate of inflation and deflation) are operator dependent, and hence, difficult to reproduce in varied settings. Because of all of these reasons, we have designed the automated balloon catheter inflation device reported here, which reduces the need for operator supervision, increases the reproducibility of balloon inflation, and allows multi-week experimental protocols to be performed. We have controlled the balloon catheter inflation device with a software package that allows for easy set-up and alteration of the inflation protocol, as

Table 1. Summary of collateral dependent blood flow measurements made using manual and automated inflation protocols for before and after transient repetitive myocardia ischemia (RI).

Study Group	Manual Inflation				Automated Inflation			
	Collateral Dependent Blood Flow (mL/min/g)	SEM	CV	n	Collateral Dependent Blood Flow (mL/min/g)	SEM	CV	n
WKY	0.26	0.09	1.038	9	0.15	0.03	0.470	6
WKY RI	1.63	0.3	0.552	9	2.04	0.05	0.064	6
SD	0.25	0.04	0.523	12	2.33*	0.03	0.039	7
SD RI	1.97	0.26	0.463	12	1.95	0.05	0.067	7

Automated inflation produced a marked decrease in the standard error of the mean (SEM) and coefficient of variation (CV), even with reduced sample numbers (n). Data were tabulated from several studies for this comparison: WKY manual inflation studies [23], WKY automated inflation studies [25], SD manual inflation studies (unpublished), SD automated inflation studies [26].
*Indicates normal-zone blood flow (not collateral dependent flow) measured at 0 days RI.

well as monitoring of the progress of the inflation protocol and an estimate of the volume of pressurized air delivered to the balloons. This device has resulted in reduced variation in collateral dependent blood flow measurements. The highest CV reported with automated inflation was 0.470, which was measured at conditions of very low blood flow rate (likely close to the instrumentation error of the flow measurement technique). All other CVs for automated inflation were <0.1. By contrast, CVs for manual inflation ranged from 0.436–1.038. It should also be noted that, in both WKY and SD rats, fewer animals were required for each study using automated inflation, while still yielding blood flow measurements with decreased CVs.

The automated balloon catheter inflation device that we have developed provides several significant advantages over previous manual inflation studies. First, collateral dependent blood flow measurements made after using automated inflation have greatly reduced variance when compared to those made after manual inflation (Figure 7 and Table 1). Second, this reduced variance has allowed us to reduce the number of animals needed to achieve statistically-significant results, and hence has allowed a decreased morbidity (mortality) rate associated with transient ischemia studies. Third, automated inflation has significantly reduced the number of man-hours required to complete an animal study – both due to the need for less monitoring and interaction with animals and due to a fewer number of animals needed. Finally, we anticipate that automated balloon catheter inflation greatly reduces the potential for over-inflation of the balloon, which may serve to better preserve the mechanical integrity of the balloon. Consistent mechanical integrity may, in turn, be one of the factors leading to reduced variance among animals with automated balloon catheter inflation. While beyond the scope of this study, the integrity of the balloon catheter could be assessed using stress-strain testing and a load failure analysis.

The automated balloon catheter inflation device costs roughly $1,200–$2,000 (US) to build, depending on the availability of parts (listed in Table S1) and technical support. Hence, this represents a very economical investment, when compared to the number of man-hours required for a single, multi-week catheter inflation protocol (which is usually repeated multiple times for statistical significance). Although routine monitoring of any animal protocol is necessary, using an automated inflation device reduced the need for human supervision from hourly to daily. In addition, the dependence of the accuracy of the protocol on operator interaction was largely eliminated.

The volumetric flowrate that was measured (by integrating the flowmeter signal) represents an estimate of the total volume delivered to all four balloon catheters. However, because of changes in pressure, and because of the compliance of catheter lines and connecting tubing, this measured volume was not interpreted as an absolute volume of air delivered, but was rather used to verify the reproducibility of the device. Because the balloon catheters are pressurized in parallel, it should also be noted that the volume expansion of each balloon catheter may vary, depending on manufacturing differences in the balloon. In our previous work, we have seen significant manufacturing variation in balloon volume. Hence, prior to beginning an animal protocol, it is important to test each of the balloon catheters used. The automated inflation device we have developed also aids in this pre-experimental testing, a multiple balloons can be simultaneously inflated and their volumes compared. In addition, a series of rapid inflation/deflation cycles can be run to check for defects in the balloons or catheter lines. It should also be noted that this device can easily be modified to allow connection to more than four catheter lines by replacing the pressure manifold with a manifold having more ports.

The automated inflation device was controlled through a custom Labview program with user interface. This program was compiled as an executable, to allow easy access by users and to allow the program to be installed on multiple PCs. However, it should be noted that the executable still requires a deployable version of Labview with associated virtual instrument libraries. Because of this, there is some amount of computational overhead required to run the automated inflation device software. If very high speed inflation/deflation cycles were required (on the order of μs-ms), it would be advisable to develop a stand-alone version of the software, that did not require the overhead of the deployable version of Labview. However, for the time scales of most studies (inflation times of seconds), the Labview-based software we have developed provides more-than-adequate response speed and reproducibility.

Conclusion

The ability to repetitively occlude the coronary artery is critical to the use of animal models for transient coronary ischemia. In our previous work, we have found that repeated occlusion of the coronary artery through manual inflation of balloon catheters can achieve reproducible changes in collateral dependent blood flow. However, relatively large numbers of animals and man-hours were often required to achieve statistical significance, and a high level of variance was often noted among study animals. In this work, we have developed a device for repetitive automated inflation of balloon catheters. We have also compared manual and automated inflation studies and shown that studies using this automated inflation device have demonstrated greatly reduced variance, reduced need for animals, and reduced man-hours to complete a given study. We have fully documented the parts, equipment, procedures, and software needed, enabling the automated inflation device to be constructed by technical or engineering staff at most institutions. Finally, in addition to the reduced variance, reduced need for animals, and reduced man-hours required to complete a study, adoption of automated inflation protocols using this (or similar) device should result in enhanced data quality in the field of transient ischemia studies and a better ability to compare results amongst research groups.

Supporting Information

Figure S1 Labview back panel. The main portion of the software consists of a series of "filmstrip" timing loops, indicated by the thick lines with squares.

Table S1 Table of parts required to build the automated balloon catheter inflator.

Author Contributions

Conceived and designed the experiments: SJL PR. Performed the experiments: SJL WEL PR. Analyzed the data: SJL WEL PR. Contributed reagents/materials/analysis tools: SJL PR. Wrote the paper: SJL PR.

References

1. Roger VL, Go AS, Lloyd-Jones DM, Adams RJ, Berry JD, et al. (2011) Heart disease and stroke statistics—2011 update: a report from the american heart association. Circulation 123: e18–e209.
2. Kim JY, Mun HS, Lee BK, Yoon SB, Choi EY, et al. (2010) Impact of metabolic syndrome and its individual components on the presence and severity of angiographic coronary artery disease. Yonsei medical journal 51: 676–682.
3. Schernthaner G (1996) Cardiovascular mortality and morbidity in type-2 diabetes mellitus. Diabetes Research and Clinical Practice 31, Supplement: S3–S13.
4. Lakka H, Laaksonen DE, Lakka TA, Niskanen LK, Kumpusalo E, et al. (2002). The metabolic syndrome and total and cardiovascular disease mortality in middle-aged men. JAMA 288: 2709–2716.
5. Kajimoto K, Kasai T, Miyauchi K, Hirose H, Yanagisawa N, et al. (2008). Metabolic syndrome predicts 10-year mortality in non-diabetic patients following coronary artery bypass surgery.
6. Brackbill ML, Sytsma CS, Sykes K (2009). Perioperative outcomes of coronary artery bypass grafting: effects of metabolic syndrome and patient's sex. American Journal of Critical Care 18: 468–473.
7. Hoffmann R, Stellbrink E, Schröder J, Grawe A, Vogel G, et al. (2007). Impact of the metabolic syndrome on angiographic and clinical events after coronary intervention using bare-metal or sirolimus-eluting stents. The American Journal of Cardiology 100: 1347–1352.
8. Seiler C (2003). The human coronary collateral circulation. Heart 89: 1352–1357.
9. Chen W, Gabel S, Steenbergen C, Murphy E (1995). A redox-based mechanism for cardioprotection induced by ischemic preconditioning in perfused rat heart. Circulation Research 77: 424–429.
10. Reed R, Kolz C, Potter B, Rocic P (2008). The mechanistic basis for the disparate effects of angiotensin II on coronary collateral growth. Arterioscler Thromb Vasc Biol 28: 61–67.
11. Matsunaga T, Warltier DC, Weihrauch DW, Moniz M, Tessmer J, et al. (2000). Ischemia-induced coronary collateral growth is dependent on vascular endothelial growth factor and nitric oxide. Circulation 102: 3098–3103.
12. Sasmaz H, Yilmaz MB (2009). Coronary collaterals in obese patients: impact of metabolic syndrome. ANGIOLOGY 60: 164–168.
13. Yilmaz MB, Caldir V, Guray Y, Guray U, Altay H, et al. (2006). Relation of coronary collateral vessel development in patients with a totally occluded right coronary artery to the metabolic syndrome. The American Journal of Cardiology 97: 636–639.
14. Turhan H, Yasar AS, Erbay AR, Yetkin E, Sasmaz H, et al. (2005). Impaired coronary collateral vessel development in patients with metabolic syndrome. Coronary artery disease 16: 281–285.
15. Mouquet F, Cuilleret F, Susen S, Sautière K, Marboeuf P, et al. (2009). Metabolic syndrome and collateral vessel formation in patients with documented occluded coronary arteries: association with hyperglycaemia, insulin-resistance, adiponectin and plasminogen activator inhibitor-1. Eur Heart J 30: 840–849.
16. Hattan N, Chilian WM, Park F, Rocic P (2007). Restoration of coronary collateral growth in the Zucker obese rat. Basic research in cardiology 102: 217–223.
17. Weihrauch D, Lohr NL, Mraovic B, Ludwig LM, Chilian WM, et al. (2004). Chronic hyperglycemia attenuates coronary collateral development and impairs proliferative properties of myocardial interstitial fluid by production of angiostatin. Circulation 109: 2343–2348.
18. Pung YF, Rocic P, Murphy MP, Smith RAJ, Hafemeister J, et al. (2012). Resolution of mitochondrial oxidative stress rescues coronary collateral growth in zucker obese fatty rats. Arteriosclerosis, thrombosis, and vascular biology 32: 325–334.
19. Lassaletta AD, Chu LM, Robich MP, Elmadhun NY, Feng J, et al. (2012). Overfed Ossabaw swine with early stage metabolic syndrome have normal coronary collateral development in response to chronic ischemia. Basic Res Cardiol 107: 1–11.
20. Mohri M, Tomoike H, Noma M, Inoue T, Hisano K, et al. (1989). Duration of ischemia is vital for collateral development: repeated brief coronary artery occlusions in conscious dogs. Circulation Research 64: 287–296.
21. Yamanishi K, Fujita M, Ohno A, Sasayama S (1990). Importance of myocardial ischaemia for recruitment of coronary collateral circulation in dogs. Cardiovasc Res 24: 271–277.
22. Reed R, Potter B, Smith E, Jadhav R, Villalta P, et al. (2009). Redox-sensitive Akt and Src regulate coronary collateral growth in metabolic syndrome. Am J Physiol Heart Circ Physiol 296: H1811–H1821.
23. Toyota E, Warltier DC, Brock T, Ritman E, Kolz C, et al. (2005). Vascular endothelial growth factor is required for coronary collateral growth in the rat. Circulation 112: 2108–2113.
24. Dodd T, Jadhav R, Wiggins L, Stewart J, Smith E, et al. (2011). MMPs 2 and 9 are essential for coronary collateral growth and are prominently regulated by p38 MAPK. Journal of Molecular and Cellular Cardiology 51: 1015–1025.
25. Jadhav R, Dodd T, Smith E, Bailey E, DeLucia AL, et al. (2011). Angiotensin type I receptor blockade in conjunction with enhanced Akt activation restores coronary collateral growth in the metabolic syndrome. Am J Physiol Heart Circ Physiol 300: H1938–H1949.
26. Hutcheson R, Terry R, Chaplin J, Smith E, Musiyenko A, et al. (2013). MicroRNA-145 Restores Contractile Vascular Smooth Muscle Phenotype and Coronary Collateral Growth in the Metabolic SyndromeSignificance. Arteriosclerosis, thrombosis, and vascular biology 33: 727–736.

27. Dodd T, Wiggins L, Hutcheson R, Smith E, Musiyenko A, et al. (2013). Impaired Coronary Collateral Growth in the Metabolic Syndrome Is in Part Mediated by Matrix Metalloproteinase 12–Dependent Production of Endostatin and Angiostatin. Arteriosclerosis, thrombosis, and vascular biology 33: 1339–1349.

28. National Instruments: Test, Measurement, and Embedded Systems. at http://www.ni.com/.

29. CUI Inc | Electromechanical products for an interconnected world. at http://www.cui.com/.

30. Winford Engineering. at http://www.winford.com/.

20

Transient Focal Cerebral Ischemia/Reperfusion Induces Early and Chronic Axonal Changes in Rats: Its Importance for the Risk of Alzheimer's Disease

Qinan Zhang[1,2⑨], Teng Gao[2⑨], Yi Luo[1⑨], Xijuan Chen[2], Ge Gao[3], Xiaoqun Gao[2,3], Yiwu Zhou[4], Jiapei Dai[1]*

1 Wuhan Institute for Neuroscience and Neuroengineering, South-Central University for Nationalities, Wuhan, China, 2 Department of Anatomy, Medical College of Zhengzhou University, Zhengzhou, China, 3 Brain Paralysis Research Center, Medical College of Zhengzhou University, Zhengzhou, China, 4 Department of Forensic Medicine, Tongji Medical College of Huazhong University of Science & Technology, Wuhan, China

Abstract

The dementia of Alzheimer's type and brain ischemia are known to increase at comparable rates with age. Recent advances suggest that cerebral ischemia may contribute to the pathogenesis of Alzheimer's disease (AD), however, the neuropathological relationship between these two disorders is largely unclear. It has been demonstrated that axonopathy, mainly manifesting as impairment of axonal transport and swelling of the axon and varicosity, is a prominent feature in AD and may play an important role in the neuropathological mechanisms in AD. In this study, we investigated the early and chronic changes of the axons of neurons in the different brain areas (cortex, hippocampus and striatum) using in vivo tracing technique and grading analysis method in a rat model of transient focal cerebral ischemia/reperfusion (middle cerebral artery occlusion, MCAO). In addition, the relationship between the changes of axons and the expression of β-amyloid 42 (Aβ42) and hyperphosphorylated Tau, which have been considered as the key neuropathological processes of AD, was analyzed by combining tracing technique with immunohistochemistry or western blotting. Subsequently, we found that transient cerebral ischemia/reperfusion produced obvious swelling of the axons and varicosities, from 6 hours after transient cerebral ischemia/reperfusion even up to 4 weeks. We could not observe Aβ plaques or overexpression of Aβ42 in the ischemic brain areas, however, the site-specific hyperphosphorylated Tau could be detected in the ischemic cortex. These results suggest that transient cerebral ischemia/reperfusion induce early and chronic axonal changes, which may be an important mechanism affecting the clinical outcome and possibly contributing to the development of AD after stroke.

Editor: Stephen D. Ginsberg, Nathan Kline Institute and New York University School of Medicine, United States of America

Funding: This work was supported by a project of the China Ministry of Human Resources for Return Overseas Chinese Scholarship (2007) and the Research Foundation for the Key Laboratory of Neuroscience and Neuroengineering from South-Central University for Nationalities (XJS09001), and partly by a joint research project between China and the Netherlands, Royal Netherlands Academy of Arts and Sciences (05CDP030). The funders had no role in study design, data collection and analysis, decision to publish, or preparation of the manuscript.

Competing Interests: The authors have declared that no competing interests exist.

* E-mail: jdai@mail.scuec.edu.cn

⑨ These authors contributed equally to this work.

Introduction

Alzheimer's disease (AD) and vascular dementia (VaD) are widely accepted as the most common forms of dementia and demonstrate similar increases with age [1,2]. AD is a severe neurodegenerative disorder defined histologically by the presence of senile plaques (SPs) containing β-amyloid (Aβ), and neurofibrillary tangles (NFTs). In previous studies, cerebral ischemia has been generally considered an exclusion criterion for clinical diagnosis of AD [3], however, recent advances in the epidemiology of AD reveal that ischemic disease significantly affects 60% to 90% of patients with AD and increases the risk of developing AD [4–6]. It is estimated that AD is three times more likely to precipitate in old age after a transient ischemia attack (TIA) [2], and it is clear that cerebral ischemia may exacerbate dementia and worsen outcomes in AD patients [4,6,7]. There are several isolated reports suggesting an interaction between AD and cerebral ischemia [2,4,8,9], nevertheless, we have not yet understood the processes and nature of the acute ischemic events triggering the onset and progression of AD.

Various hypotheses regarding the causes of AD have been debated, and there is currently no consensus on this issue [10–13]. An increasing body of evidence has implicated that axonopathy, mainly manifesting as impairment of axonal transport and swelling of the axon and varicosity, may play an important role in the etiology of AD. Such changes have been identified in living AD patients, in postmortem AD brains and in different animal models [14–20], however, so far no study has investigated long-term axonal changes after transient focal cerebral ischemia.

To explore the importance of cerebral ischemia for the risk of AD, we observed the morphological changes of axons of neurons in the different brain areas (cortex, hippocampus and striatum) following transient focal cerebral ischemia/reperfusion in rats. In addition, we determined whether axonal changes after transient focal cerebral ischemia/reperfusion were related to AD-associated neuropathological changes such as SPs and NFTs.

Results

Transient focal cerebral ischemia/reperfusion induced early and chronic axonal changes

Using in vivo tracing, we examined the effects of transient focal cerebral ischemia/reperfusion on axonal changes in the ischemic or perilesional cortex, caudoputamen (striatum) and hippocampus of the MCAO hemisphere. The typical axonal changes presenting swollen axons and varicosities were detected in the different brain areas (Fig. 1A–D). Swollen axons and varicosities appeared in the

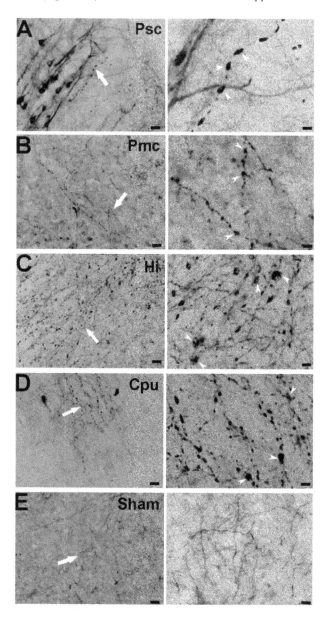

Figure 1. Axonal morphological changes demonstrated by in vivo tracing in the different brain areas after transient cerebral ischemia/reperfusion. Right panels were high magnification views of the areas in left panels in A–E (single arrow), respectively. Typical swollen axons or varicosities (arrowheads) could be seen in the primary sensory cortex (Psc) (A), primary motor cortex (Pmc) (B), hippocampus (Hi) (C) and caudoputamen (Cpu) (D) of the ischemic hemisphere after transient cerebral ischemia/reperfusion. No obvious axonal changes were noticed in the primary sensory cortex from the sham group (E). Scale bars: 20 µm for left panels and 5 µm for right panels in A–E.

ischemic sensory and motor cortex, perilesional cortex, hippocampus and caudoputamen as early as 6 h (Fig. 2A–E) after transient cerebral focal ischemia/reperfusion as compared to the corresponding contralateral regions and the sham-operated group (Fig. 1E). Such axonal changes even extended to 4 w after transient cerebral focal ischemia/reperfusion (Fig. 2A–E).

We determined the degree of axonal changes from axonal tracing evaluation using a grade system and found that the degree of swollen axons and varicosities was particularly obvious (similar to grade 2) at 2 w after transient cerebral ischemia/reperfusion (Table 1, Fig. 3) and extended to 4 w, although such axonal damages appeared to recover gradually after 2 w. Unexpectedly, obvious changes found at 24 h seemed to self-recover temporarily at 1 w after transient cerebral ischemia/reperfusion compared to the corresponding sham-operated group (Table 1, Fig. 3).

Lack of Aβ plaques or overexpression of Aβ42 after transient focal cerebral ischemia/reperfusion

Assemblies of Aβ42 are believed to contribute to the formation of senile plaques, one of the classic neurodegenerative changes in AD. To investigate the relationship between the axonal changes induced by cerebral ischemia and the formation and development of Aβ plaques, we used double immunohistochemical staining for tracer and Aβ42. We did not observe the classic Aβ plaques and overexpression of Aβ42 within and/or close to the swollen axons and varicosities in the ischemic brain regions at each time point after reperfusion (Figure not shown).

Aberrant Tau hyperphosphorylation occurs in the ischemic cortex

To characterize the phosphorylation status of Tau in the ischemic regions, double immunohistochemical staining for tracer and phosphorylated Tau protein (P-tau and AT8) or the total Tau (Tau-5) was performed. It was found that only some Tau protein staining for AT8 and Tau-5 could be detected within the ischemic and perilesional cortex (Fig. 4A and B), whereas the staining for P-tau was very weak (Fig. 4C).

To further explore the detailed effect in the cortex of cerebral ischemia on Tau phosphorylation over time, we used protein immunoblotting for quantitative analysis and found that there was an enhancement of Tau phosphorylation at 6 h after reperfusion (Fig. 5A). The level of AT8 was increased significantly in the ischemic cortex at 1 w as compared to the ipsilateral side of ischemic cortex at 6 h, 24 h, 2 w, 3 w or 4 w, respectively (Fig. 5A and B). Whereas the level of P-tau was significantly increased only 6 h after transient cerebral ischemia/reperfusion (Fig. 5A and C). Similar to AT8, the total amount of Tau detected with Tau-5 reached the peak at 1 w after transient cerebral ischemia/reperfusion (Fig. 5A and D).

Discussion

In the present study, using an in vivo tracing technique, we could observe the development process of the morphological changes of axons after transient cerebral ischemia/reperfusion, mainly manifesting as axonal swellings or spheroids, which were similar to the axonopathy in AD brains and in animal models of AD [14–20]. Even 6 h after the reperfusion, the swellings of axons and varicosities had obviously appeared in the ischemic and perilesional regions, including the sensory and motor cortex, hippocampus and striatum. Axonal damages did not increase gradually after transient cerebral ischemia/reperfusion, however, such axonal changes could exist for up to 4 w after reperfusion. To our surprise, no obvious changes were found at 1 w after transient

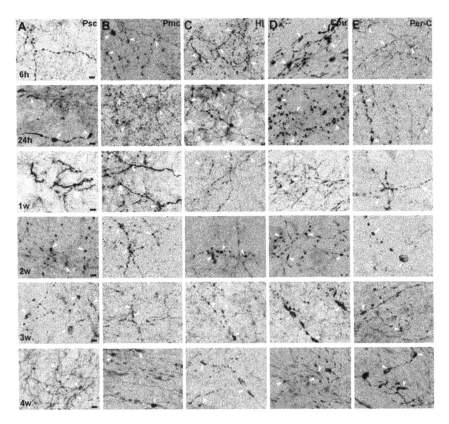

Figure 2. Transient cerebral ischemia/reperfusion induces early and chronic axonal changes. Representative axonal changes (swellings of axons and varicosities) can be seen at 6 h, 24 h, 1 w, 2 w, 3 w and 4 w after transient cerebral ischemia/reperfusion in different brain regions, including the ischemic primary sensory cortex (Psc) (A), primary motor cortex (Pmc) (B), hippocampus (Hi) (C), caudoputamen (Cpu) (D) and peri-lesional cortex (E). Arrowheads in each figure mark the swollen axons or varicosities. Scale bars: 5 μm for A–E.

cerebral ischemia/reperfusion compared to the corresponding sham-operated group, the underlying mechanisms are not clear and need to be further elucidated.

As an acute neurodegenerative and dementia-causing disorder in the elderly, ischemic stroke has been recognized as contributing to the pathogenesis of AD [1,8,21]. Nevertheless, the pathological mechanism of AD induced by cerebral ischemia seems poorly understood. Recent advances suggest that axonopathy may play a key role in the initiation of the neuropathological processes and cognitive defects in AD. For example, axonopathy has been identified in mouse models of AD preceding known disease-related pathology, and it is considered as an early stage of AD [15]. Axonal transport impairment and the swellings of the axons and varicosities have also been observed both in living AD patients and in other animal models [14–20]. In the current study, such axonal changes were detected in several ischemic or perilesional regions, including sensory and motor cortex, hippocampus and striatum, suggesting that axonopathy may be an important neuropathological change linking cerebral ischemia with AD.

The classic pathological hallmarks of AD are SPs and NFTs, which are potentially linked to alterations of the axonal compartment [22]. Although the formation and development of SPs and NFTs are two defining characteristics of neuropathological processes in AD, a debate still persists over whether SPs or NFTs play key and causal roles in the neuropathological mechanisms of AD [10–13], and a proposal has been raised that the formation of Aβ plaques and hyperphosphorylated Tau may be the consequences of axonopathy [9,15,20]. In the present study, we tested the expression of Aβ42 and Tau hyperphosphorylation by using double immunohistochemical staining for tracer and Aβ42 or Tau protein (P-tau, Tau-5, AT8) in order to study the possible relationship between AD and cerebral ischemia. Consequently, we did not observe Aβ plaques or overexpression of Aβ42 in the ischemic and perilesional brain areas, but found weak staining against hyperphosphorylated Tau (AT8 or P-tau) or the total Tau (Tau-5), accompanied by a few tracer-labeled fibers observed in the ischemic cortex. In addition, we performed a quantitative analysis for Tau protein in ischemic cortex over time after transient cerebral ischemia/reperfusion using western blotting and found significant increases in the total Tau and hyperphosphorylated Tau (pS202 and pS199), suggesting that a specific set of kinases were activated during the short period after reperfusion, which may contribute to the formation of intracellular Tau aggregates. Moreover, our study demonstrated no significant increase in Tau protein expression in the ischemic caudoputamen, suggesting that the lesions restricted to the caudoputamen were different from the lesions in the ischemic cortex.

In conclusion, our data have demonstrated that the swellings of axons and varicosities occurred early and could exist for up to 4 w after transient cerebral ischemia/reperfusion accompanied by weak Tau expression, but without the over-expression of β-amyloid and amyloid deposition, which may be important for understanding the role of ischemic stroke in the pathogenesis of AD. It has been found that patients with cerebrovascular disease often show AD pathology at autopsy, even if there is no hint or clinical expression of pre-existing AD [21]. Thus, we propose that cerebral ischemia that induces axonal changes, including the swellings of axons and varicosities and impaired axonal transport,

Table 1. Semi-quantitative analysis of the degree of axonal changes in different brain regions in transient cerebral ischemia/ reperfusion and control rats from axonal tracing evaluation.

MCAO	Case No	Psc	Pmc	Per-C	Hi	Cpu	Sham	Case No	Psc	Pmc	Per-C	Hi	Cpu
6 h	N1	2	3	1	1	1	6 h	N1	1	0	0	0	0
	N2	2	1	2	0	2		N2	0	0	0	0	0
	N3	1	1	1	2	ND		N3	0	0	0	0	ND
	N4	1	2	0	2	ND		N4	0	0	0	1	0
24 h	N1	2	ND	3	2	1	24 h	N1	0	0	0	1	ND
	N2	3	2	1	2	3		N2	0	0	0	ND	1
	N3	1	2	1	2	2		N3	1	0	0	0	ND
								N4	0	0	0	0	0
1 w	N1	1	2	1	1	1	1 w	N1	0	1	0	ND	1
	N2	1	1	0	2	ND		N2	1	1	0	1	1
	N3	1	1	0	ND	1		N3	1	ND	0	0	1
2 w	N1	2	2	2	3	ND	2 w	N1	1	1	1	1	1
	N2	2	3	2	ND	3		N2	1	1	1	1	1
	N3	2	2	2	2	2		N3	1	0	0	0	1
	N4	2	3	2	3	3							
3 w	N1	2	2	0	2	ND	3 w	N1	0	0	0	1	0
	N2	2	1	2	3	1		N2	0	0	0	1	0
	N3	1	2	1	2	3		N3	0	0	0	0	0
	N4	2	2	1	1	3							
4 w	N1	1	2	2	1	1	4 w	N1	0	ND	0	1	0
	N2	ND	2	1	2	2		N2	0	0	0	1	0
	N3	2	2	1	2	1		N3	1	1	0	ND	1

The numbers (1–3) represent the degree of axonal changes (see also in method). MCAO: middle cerebral artery occlusion and reperfusion; Psc: primary sensory cortex; Pmc: primary motor cortex; Hi: hippocampus; Cpu: caudoputamen; Per-C: perilesional cortex; ND: not detected.

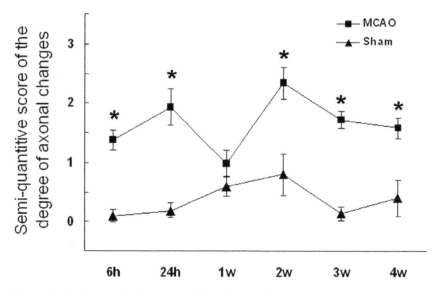

Figure 3. Semi-quantitative score of the degree of axonal changes in ischemic brain regions of transient cerebral ischemia/ reperfusion and control rats from axonal tracing evaluation. The degree of swollen axons and varicosities was particularly obvious at 2 w after transient cerebral ischemia/reperfusion. Such axonal damages could extend to 4 w as compared to the corresponding contra-lateral brain regions in sham groups, although appeared to self-recover temporarily at 1 w. The score at each time point represents 13–19 values (Mean±SD) obtained from 3–4 rats in each subgroup. The asterisk indicates a highly significant difference (P<0.01) between the transient cerebral ischemia/ reperfusion subgroup and the corresponding sham subgroup.

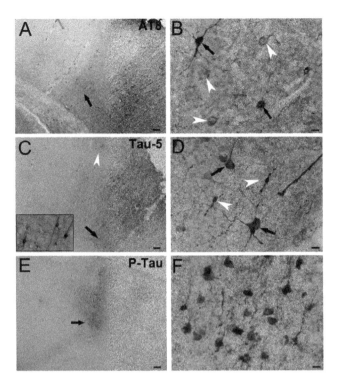

Figure 4. Tracing and immunohistochemical double staining show the tracer-labeled neurons and the expression of hyperphosphorylated Tau induced by transient cerebral ischemia/reperfusion. B, D and F are the magnification of an area in A, C and E, respectively. Some staining for AT8 (brown color) was found in the ischemic cortex (A) and AT8 labeled neuronal bodies could be noticed (B, arrowheads). The arrows in B indicate the tracer-labeled neurons (dark blue color). Strong staining for Tau-5 (brown color) was found in the ischemic cortex (C) and the extensive Tau-5 labeled neurons (D, arrows) and swollen axons (D, arrowheads) were noticed. Inserted figure in C showed the magnification of an area (arrowhead), demonstrating the tracer-labeled neurons (dark blue color). Only very weak staining could be observed for P-tau (E) and tracer-labeled neurons presented the morphological changes as cell shrinkage occurred. Scale bars: 10 μm for B, D, and F, 100 μm for A and C, 200 μm for E.

may be an important mechanism affecting the clinical outcome and possibly contributing to the development of AD after stroke.

Materials and Methods

Rat model of transient focal cerebral ischemia/reperfusion

3-month-old male Wistar rats weighing 280–320 g (from the Experimental Animal Center of Hubei Province, Wuhan, China) were housed in a room with a 12-hour light/dark cycle (lights on at 7:00 AM) with access to food and water ad libitum throughout the experimental period. All animal experiments were conducted with the approval of the Animal Care Committee of South-Center University for Nationalities.

The animals were anesthetized with 10% chloral hydrate (0.3 ml/100 g) and subjected to either middle cerebral artery occlusion (MCAO) or sham operation. The right middle cerebral artery (MCA) was occluded using the intraluminal suture technique described previously [23]. Briefly, the right carotid region was exposed through a midline cervical incision, the external carotid was ligated with a 4-0 suture and the common

carotid artery was blocked with an artery clip. A 4-0 monofilament nylon suture, whose tip had been rounded by heating, was introduced from the carotid bifurcation into the internal carotid artery until a resistance was encountered (18±0.5 mm), thereby occluding the origin of the MCA. After 30 min, recirculation was established by gentle withdrawal of the suture. For the rats in the sham group, the right carotid region was only exposed but not cut. The body temperature of rats was maintained in the normal range during surgery using a heating lamp. The rats in the MCAO group and the sham-operated group were assigned to six subgroups according to the time of sacrifice (6 h, 24 h, 1 w, 2 w, 3 w and 4 w after surgery).

Neurological assessment

Neurological deficit was evaluated after surgery by Zea Longa test on a four-point scale (0 = no deficit, 1 = failure to extend right forepaw fully, 2 = circling to the right, 3 = falling to the right, and 4 = no spontaneous walking with a depressed level of consciousness) [23]. Rats scoring 1–3 points indicated successful model establishment.

In vivo tracing

All rats were subjected to in vivo tracing 3–5 days before sacrifice at the desired time point on 1 w, 2 w, 3 w and 4 w (four subgroups) with exception of other two subgroups, in which the tracing was executed 3 days before MCAO and the animals were killed at 6 h and 24 h after MCAO, respectively. For in vivo tracing, animals were anesthetized with 10% chloral hydrate (0.3 ml/100 g) and mounted with their heads in a standard stereotaxic apparatus (Stoelting, USA) before receiving tracer injection [10% biotinylated dextran amine (BDA) in 0.05 M TBS (0.05 M Tris, 0.9% NaCl, pH 7.6), molecular weight 10,000, Molecular Probes, Invitrogen] under pressure (Microsyringe pump controller, WPI, USA), using a glass pipette with a tip of maximally 40–50 μm in diameter; the glass pipette was filled with an injection volume of 15 nl. All coordinates for the injected regions were adapted from the Rat Brain in Stereotaxic Coordinates (by George Paxinos and Charles Watson). The tracer was injected into the motor cortex (bregma 0 mm, lateral 2 mm, ventral 2 mm), the sensory cortex (bregma −2 mm, lateral 5 mm, ventral 3 mm), the hippocampus (bregma −4 mm, lateral 3 mm, ventral 3 mm) and the striatum (bregma 1 mm, lateral 3.5 mm, ventral 5 mm) of the MCAO hemisphere. The injection sites in the cortex were located at the ischemic area or in part of the perilesional cortex. In addition, the tracer was injected into the contralateral cortex for comparison in one or two animals in each subgroup in order to observe the possible damage effects of glass pipette during the tracer injection.

Tracer detection and immunohistochemistry

After tracer injection, the animals were allowed to survive for 3–5 days in the same housing conditions. Then animals were deeply anesthetized with 10% chloral hydrate and perfused with saline, followed by a solution of 4% paraformaldehyde in 0.1 M PBS (pH 7.4) at 4°C. The brains were removed and kept in the same fixative at 4°C for overnight postfixation, equilibrated 48 h with 30% sucrose in 0.1 M PBS. Brains were coronally cut in a cryostat into 30 μm sections, and then sections were collected in sequential order in six vials and rinsed in 0.05 M TBS. Sections were treated with 3% H_2O_2 for 10 min and rinsed in 0.05 M TBS for 30 min, and then sections were stored for further experiments in 50% glycerol in 0.05 M TBS in refrigeration (4°C). One vial was used to perform tracer staining, four vials for double staining and remaining one vial for reservation.

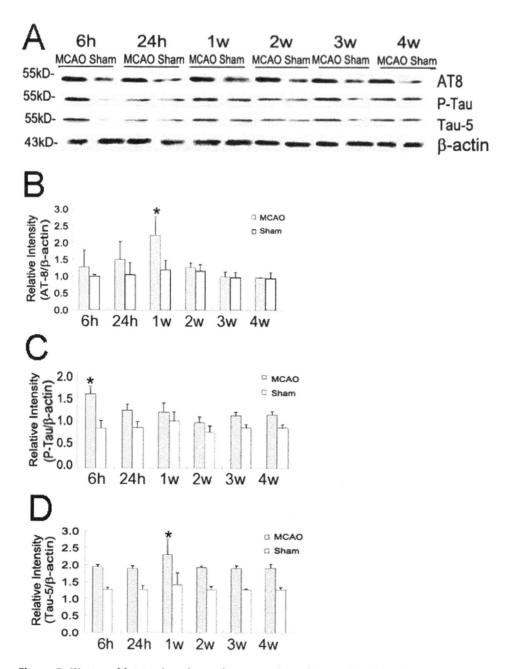

Figure 5. Western blot testing shows the expression of hyperphosphorylated Tau induced by transient cerebral ischemia/ reperfusion. The level of Tau protein increased in the ischemic cortex of the transient cerebral ischemia/reperfusion subgroup compared to the corresponding region in the sham group (A through D). The levels of AT8 and Tau-5 increased obviously at 1 w after transient cerebral ischemia/ reperfusion (B and D), whereas a similar increase was detected in the level of P-tau only at 6 h after transient cerebral ischemia/reperfusion (C). The asterisk indicates a significant difference (P<0.05) between this subgroup and the other five subgroup.

For tracer detection, the sections from in vivo tracing were incubated with the Avidin-Biotin Complex (Vector Laboratories, Burlingame, CA, USA, 1:800) in a mixture of 0.05 M Tris, 0.9% NaCl, 0.25% gelatin, and 0.5% Triton-X 100, pH 7.4 for 2 h at room temperature. After several rinses with TBS, the sections were incubated with 0.05% 3,3′-diaminobenzidine tetrahydrochloride (DAB), 0.2% nickel ammoniumsulphate, and 0.003% H_2O_2 in 0.05 M TBS (pH 7.4), mounted on gelatin-coated slides, and then dehydrated, cleared, and coverslipped.

The double staining combining tracer detection with immuno-cytochemistry was carried out following the procedures described

in detail in a previous article [20]. After visualization of the tracer with DAB + nickel ammoniumsulphate, some sections were processed for immunocytochemical detection of Aβ42 or hyper-phosphorylated Tau (P-tau, Tau-5 and AT8) with the ABC Elite detection method (Vector; Burlingame, CA, USA). Polyclonal antibody against Aβ42 (1:500) was produced in rabbit by immunization with a synthetic peptide corresponding to residues Aβ42 of human (Bioss, Beijing, China; catalog no: Bs-0107R). This antibody was tested to identify the Aβ deposits and plaques in the brain sections from AD brains [20], rat and mouse. Rabbit polyclonal antibody P-tau (1:5000) recognizing Tau when serines

199 and 202 are phosphorylated (Invitrogen, USA; catalog no: 44–768G). Tau-5 (1:5000) monoclonal antibody reacting with non-phosphorylated Tau and the phosphorylated form of Tau (Invitrogen, USA; catalog no: AHB0042). Antihuman PHF-tau monoclonal antibody (AT8) reacting with an epitope including phosphorylated Ser202 and Thr205 residues (1:10, 000; Pierce; Appleton, WI, USA; catalog no: MN1020). AT8 can stain pre-tangles, NFTs and extracellular tangles due to the recognition of hyperphosphorylated tau according to the previous report [24].

Semi-quantitative analysis of axonal changes

Quantitative analysis of the number of axonal changes was hampered because of the variable distribution pattern of the tracer labeled fibers; thus we semi-quantitatively evaluated the degree of axonal changes using a grading system referred to a previous article with a little modification [15]. All sections from a vial containing a tracer labeled injection spot were processed to evaluate the grading of axonal changes using a motorized microscope (ECLIPSE 90i, Nikon, Japan) equipped with a Nikon cooled color CCD camera (DS-5MC-U2) and controlled by a Nikon image analysis software (NIS-Elements BR 3.1). Changes were scored separately in each brain area according to the following metric: 0 = no signs of axonal changes; 1 = sparse/slight axonal changes but less than moderate; 2 = moderate, 3–5 instances of axonal change/0.035 mm^2 (field of view of the 40× objective lens on the microscope) only if they appeared in at least 3 different labeled fibers and were repeated in at least 3 different sections. Each instance of axonal change was scored only when swollen axons (≥1 μm in diameter) and varicosities (≥3 μm in diameter) were identified; 3 = frequent/severe, a greater than moderate amount of axonal changes. Two investigators were blind to case type during the semi-quantitative analysis.

Western blot analysis

At 6 h, 24 h, 1 w, 2 w, 3 w or 4 w after surgery, animals were sacrificed (n = 4 per experimental condition) and then the cortex was immediately removed and stored at −86°C until use. The tissues were homogenized on ice in a Tris-Triton buffer (10 M Tris-HCl, 100 mM NaCl, 1 mM EDTA, 1% TritonX-100, 10% glycerol, 0.1% sodium dodecyl sulfate, 0.5% deoxycholate and 1 mM PMSF, pH 7.4). The total protein was isolated by centrifugation. Sample (30–50 g of protein) were electrophoresed onto a 12% SDS/polyacrylamide gel (SDS/PAGE) and transferred to nitrocellulose membranes, then blocked for 2 h at room temperature in TBS containing 0.05% Tween-20 and 5% (W/V) bovine serum albumin (BSA). Then the blot was incubated overnight at 4°C with the primary antibodies P-tau (1:1000), Tau-5 (1:500), AT8 (1:2500), and β-actin (1:500), respectively. The membranes were washed in TBS containing 0.05% Tween-20 and were incubated for 1 h at room temperature with the appropriate HRP-conjugated secondary antibody (Goat anti-rabbit IgG or Goat anti-mouse IgG, Vector, USA, 1:8000). Blots were developed using SuperSignal West Pico Chemiluminescent substrate (Pierce, USA) in a dark chamber and were imaged by EM-CCD in a dark box. The protein bands were quantitatively analyzed using Nikon image analysis software (NIS-Elements BR 3.1). All data concerning the level of specific proteins were normalized at the level of β-actin.

Statistical analysis

A statistical analysis of significant differences in the degree of axonal changes at the different time points between MCAO and sham group was carried out by means of Rank test. All data for mean values obtained from Western blotting were compared statistically using one-way ANOVA with the S-N-K multiple comparison method and SPSS 13.0 statistical software (SPSS Inc, Chicago, Illinois, USA). Significance level was set at P<0.05.

Author Contributions

Conceived and designed the experiments: JD XG. Performed the experiments: QZ TG YL XC GG. Analyzed the data: QZ TG YL XC GG. Contributed reagents/materials/analysis tools: YZ. Wrote the paper: JD QZ YL.

References

1. Kalaria R (2002) Similarities between Alzheimer's disease and vascular dementia. J Neurol Sci 203–204: 29–34.
2. Zhu X, Smith MA, Honda K, Aliev G, Moreira PI, et al. (2007) Vascular oxidative stress in Alzheimer disease. J Neurol Sci 257: 240–246.
3. McKhann G, Drachman D, Folstein M, Katzman R, Price D, et al. (1984) Clinical diagnosis of Alzheimer's disease: report of the NINCDS-ADRDA Work Group under the auspices of Department of Health and Human Services Task Force on Alzheimer's disease. Neurology 34: 939–944.
4. White L, Petrovitch H, Hardman J, Nelson J, Davis DG, et al. (2002) Cerebrovascular pathology and dementia in autopsied Honolulu-Asia Aging Study participants. Ann N Y Acad Sci 977: 9–23.
5. de la Torre JC (2004) Is Alzheimer's disease a neurodegenerative or a vascular disorder? Data, dogma, and dialectics. Lancet Neurol 3: 184–190.
6. Querfurth HW, LaFerla FM (2010) Alzheimer's disease. N Engl J Med 362: 329–344.
7. Troncoso JC, Zonderman AB, Resnick SM, Crain B, Pletnikova O, et al. (2008) Effect of infarcts on dementia in the Baltimore longitudinal study of aging. Ann Neurol 64: 168–176.
8. Koistinaho M, Koistinaho J (2005) Interactions between Alzheimer's disease and cerebral ischemia–focus on inflammation. Brain Res Rev 48: 240–250.
9. Arvanitakis Z, Leurgans SE, Barnes LL, Bennett DA, Schneider JA (2011) Microinfarct Pathology, Dementia, and Cognitive Systems. Stroke 42: 722–727.
10. Terry RD (1996) The pathogenesis of Alzheimer disease: an alternative to the amyloid hypothesis. J Neuropathol Exp Neurol 55: 1023–1025.
11. Neve RL, Robakis NK (1998) Alzheimer's disease: a re-examination of the amyloid hypothesis. Trends Neurosci 21: 15–19.
12. Hardy J, Selkoe DJ (2002) The amyloid hypothesis of Alzheimer's disease: progress and problems on the road to therapeutics. Science 297: 353–356.
13. Armstrong RA (2011) The pathogenesis of Alzheimer's disease: a reevaluation of the "amyloid cascade hypothesis". Int J Alzheimers Dis 2011: 630865.
14. Dai J, Buijs RM, Kamphorst W, Swaab DF (2002) Impaired axonal transport of cortical neurons in Alzheimer's disease is associated with neuropathological changes. Brain Res 948: 138–144.
15. Stokin GB, Lillo C, Falzone TL, Brusch RG, et al. (2005) Axonopathy and transport deficits early in the pathogenesis of Alzheimer's disease. Science 307: 1282–1288.
16. Wirths O, Weis J, Szczygielski J, Multhaup G, Bayer TA (2006) Axonopathy in an APP/PS1 transgenic mouse model of Alzheimer's disease. Acta Neuropathol 111: 312–319.
17. Lazarov O, Morfini GA, Pigino G, Gadadhar A, Chen X, et al. (2007) Impairments in fast axonal transport and motor neuron deficits in transgenic mice expressing familial Alzheimer's disease-linked mutant presenilin 1. J Neurosci 27: 7011–7020.
18. Smith KD, Kallhoff V, Zheng H, Pautler RG (2007) In vivo axonal transport rates decrease in a mouse model of Alzheimer's disease. Neuroimage 35: 1401–1408.
19. Minoshima S, Cross D (2008) In vivo imaging of axonal transport using MRI: aging and Alzheimer's disease. Eur J Nucl Med Mol Imaging 35(Suppl 1): S89–92.
20. Xiao A, He J, Wang Q, Luo Yi, Sun Y, et al. (2011) The origin and development of plaques and phosphorylated tau are associated with axonopathy in Alzheimer's disease. Neurosci Bull 27(5): 287–299.
21. Kalaria RN (2000) The role of cerebral ischemia in Alzheimer's disease. Neurobiol. Aging 21: 321–330.
22. Goedert M (1993) Tau protein and the neurofibrillary pathology of Alzheimer's disease. Trends Neurosci 16: 460–465.
23. Longa EZ, Weinstein PR, Carison S, Cummins R (1989) Reversible middle cerebral artery occlusion without craniectomy in rats. Stroke 20: 84–91.
24. van de Nes JA, Nafe R, Schlote W (2008) Non-tau based neuronal degeneration in Alzheimer's disease - an immunocytochemical and quantitative study in the supragranular layers of the middle temporal neocortex. Brain Res 1213: 152–165.

21

Impact of Pulmonary Arteriovenous Malformations on Respiratory–Related Quality of Life in Patients with Hereditary Haemorrhagic Telangiectasia

Sandra Blivet[1], Daniel Cobarzan[1], Alain Beauchet[2], Mostafa El Hajjam[1], Pascal Lacombe[1], Thierry Chinet[1]*

1 Aphp, Université De Versailles Saint Quentin En Yvelines, Consultation Pluridisciplinaire Maladie De Rendu-Osler, Hôpital Ambroise Paré, Boulogne, France, 2 Aphp, Université De Versailles Saint Quentin En Yvelines, Département De Santé Publique, Hôpital Ambroise Paré, Boulogne, France

Abstract

Fifteen to fifty percent of patients with hereditary haemorrhagic telangiectasia have pulmonary arteriovenous malformations. The objective of this study was to measure the effect of the presence of pulmonary arteriovenous malformations and of their embolisation on respiratory-related quality of life (QoL). We prospectively recruited patients with a diagnosis of hereditary haemorrhagic telangiectasia based on the Curaçao criteria and/or the identification of a pathogenic mutation. Respiratory-related quality of life was measured using the Saint George's Respiratory Questionnaire (SGRQ). Patients who underwent embolisation of pulmonary arteriovenous malformations completed the questionnaire before and 6–12 mo after the procedure. The 56 participants were divided into three groups: no pulmonary arteriovenous malformation (group A, $n = 10$), small pulmonary arteriovenous malformations not accessible to embolotherapy (group B, $n = 19$), and large pulmonary arteriovenous malformations accessible to embolotherapy (group C, $n = 27$). The SGRQ score was significantly higher in group C compared to the other groups, indicating a worse respiratory-specific QoL. There was no significant difference between groups A and B. Among the 17 patients who underwent an embolisation, the SGRQ score decreased significantly after the procedure, to a value similar to that in patients without pulmonary arteriovenous malformation. Our results indicate that the presence of large but not small pulmonary arteriovenous malformations negatively affects the respiratory-related quality of life and that embolisation of pulmonary arteriovenous malformations normalizes the respiratory-related quality of life.

Editor: Klaus Brusgaard, Odense University Hospital, Denmark

Funding: This work received financial support from the French HHT patient association, AMRO-France HHT (Association Maladie Rendu-Osler). The funders had no role in study design, data collection and analysis, decision to publish or preparation of the manuscript.

Competing Interests: The authors have declared that no competing interests exist.

* E-mail: Thierry.Chinet@Apr.Aphp.Fr

Introduction

Hereditary haemorrhagic telangiectasia (HHT), also known as Rendu-Osler-Weber syndrome, is a genetic vascular disorder with an autosomal dominant inheritance pattern. Its prevalence is estimated at around 1:5,000–1:10,000 [1,2]. The clinical manifestations of HHT include epistaxis; telangiectasia on the skin and mucosal membrane; and visceral arteriovenous malformations (AVMs), predominantly in the lung, brain, gastrointestinal tract, and liver. HHT is associated with mutations in genes involved in the transforming growth factor β (TGF-β) signaling pathway [3]. Mutations in three genes have been found to be responsible for HHT: the endoglin (*ENG*) gene on chromosome 9, the activin-receptor-like kinase 1 (*ACVRL1*) gene on chromosome 12, and the *SMAD4* gene on chromosome 18 (mutations also lead to juvenile polyposis). Other loci have been identified, but the genes have not yet been discovered. The phenotypic expression of the disease depends on the mutated gene: for instance, patients with *ENG* mutations ("HHT1 phenotype") are more likely to have pulmonary arteriovenous malformations (PAVMs) than patients with *ACVRL1* mutations ("HHT2 phenotype"). In addition, clinical expression of the disease usually worsens with age. A diagnosis of HHT is established based on the Curaçao criteria (nose bleeds, mucocutaneous telangiectasia, visceral arteriovenous malformations, and family history) or on the identification of a pathogenic mutation [2,4].

PAVMs are found in approximately 15–50% of HHT patients [1–4]. The presence of PAVMs exposes the patient to significant clinical risks. PAVMs constitute a right-to-left shunt, leading to hypoxaemia that is poorly responsive to supplemental oxygen. Rupture of the thin wall of the PAVM sac in the airways or pleural cavity may cause haemoptysis or haemothorax [5]. In addition, the shunting of the pulmonary capillary bed may allow thrombi, bacteria, and air bubbles to reach the systemic circulation, mainly the cerebral circulation, resulting in paradoxical systemic embolic complications. Cerebral vascular complications (i.e., stroke and transient ischemic attack) and abscesses occur in approximately 30% of patients with PAVMs [5–7]. Management of PAVMs includes prophylactic administration of antibiotics before dental and surgical procedures and embolisation. The treatment of choice for PAVMs is percutaneous transcatheter embolisation of the feeding arteries, which improves blood oxygenation and decreases the risk of paradoxical embolic stroke and cerebral abscess [4,5,6,8]. Embolisation is usually a safe procedure when performed by expert operators. It is recommended to patients with HHT when PAVMs accessible to the procedure are found, even when patients are asymptomatic. Long-term clinical success for embolisation in patients with PAVMs has been extensively reported [4–6,8,9].

Several studies have shown that HHT negatively impacts quality of life (QoL) [10–14]. One of the most significant clinical manifestations associated with poor QoL is severe epistaxis. However, these studies focused on overall, health-related, and symptom-specific aspects of QoL. Since PAVMs have a substantial clinical impact on patients with HHT, we focused on the impact of PAVMs on QoL in patients with HHT and evaluated the effect of embolisation of PAVMs on QoL.

Materials and Methods

Participants

All consecutive patients with HHT who presented to our center between January 2010 and January 2012 for evaluation of their disease were invited to participate in this prospective study. We also recruited patients who were admitted during the same period of time for embolisation of PAVM following evaluation of their disease during the previous year. To be included in the study, patients had to fulfill the following criteria: (1) diagnosis of HHT ascertained by identification of an *ENG*, *ACVRL1*, or *SMAD4* mutation and/or by the presence of at least three Curaçao criteria; (2) age >15 y; and (3) fluency in the French language (4). Patients were not included if they were suffering from chronic respiratory conditions unrelated to HHT. All participants signed an informed consent form. This study was declared to the Commission Nationale Informatique et Liberté (CNIL), was performed in accordance with French regulations and the Helsinki Declaration and was approved by the Société de Pneumologie de Langue Française (SPLF) institutional review board (CEPRO).

Study Protocol

Our routine work-up for the evaluation of the disease included clinical examination by skin, ENT, neurology, pulmonary, and gastroenterology specialists; blood tests; genetic clinical evaluation and testing; chest and abdominal high-resolution CT scans; transthoracic cardiac echocardiography; cerebral magnetic imaging; and pulmonary function tests.

Patients who underwent embolisation of PAVMs were informed about the risks and benefits of the procedure and gave informed consent. The procedure was performed as previously reported [9].

Quality of Life

Respiratory-specific QoL was evaluated with Saint George's Respiratory Questionnaire (SGRQ) (www.healthstatus.sgul.ac.uk/sgrq). This questionnaire was self-administered to participants. The SGRQ measures three components: the "symptoms component" is concerned with the most common respiratory symptoms; the "activity component" is concerned with activities that cause or are limited by breathlessness; and the "impact component" is concerned with the perceived impact of respiratory symptoms on the patient's social life and psychological status (15). The questionnaire has 50 items. The scale is scored from 0 to 100, where the higher score indicates worse health status and a difference or change of four points is considered clinically significant [16].

Patients were instructed to complete the questionnaire during their evaluation in the department or at the time of admission for the embolisation procedure. Patients who underwent embolisation were instructed to answer a second similar questionnaire approximately 6 mo after the procedure. The questionnaire was sent by mail approximately 5 mo after the procedure. If the patient failed to answer by 6 mo after the procedure, a second questionnaire was sent by mail 1–2 mo later. If the patient failed to answer the second mailing, contact was attempted by telephone.

Data Analysis

Participants were divided into three groups: patients with no PAVM at chest CT scan (group A), patients with "small" PAVMs not accessible to embolotherapy because the diameter of the feeding arteries was too small (i.e., <2.5–3 mm; group B), and patients with "large" PAVMs accessible to embolotherapy (group C).

Quantitative data are expressed as mean ± standard deviation (SD) and range; qualitative data are expressed as frequency and percent. Comparisons of quantitative values were performed using the Wilcoxon rank sum test, the Wilcoxon signed-rank test and the Kruskal–Wallis test as appropriate. The Kruskal-Wallis test was completed in case of significance by multiple comparisons tests. Comparisons of frequencies were performed with the Chi-square test and the Fisher's exact test as appropriate. A p value of <0.05 was considered statistically significant. Statistical analysis was performed with SAS software version 9.3 (SAS Institute Inc, Cary, NC, USA).

Results

Characteristics of Patients

Fifty-seven patients with HHT were invited to participate in the study. One female patient declined the invitation. The 56 participants comprised 24 men and 32 women; their mean age was 42.5±17.2 y (range 16–80 y). Mutations in *ENG* were identified in 31 patients (55%), mutations in *ACVRL1* were identified in 17 patients (30%), and one patient had a mutation in *SMAD4* and presented with juvenile polyposis. No mutation was identified in seven patients (13%); these patients fulfilled three or four Curaçao criteria. All but one of the patients reported recurrent nosebleeds. Eight patients reported gastrointestinal bleeding. Hepatic expression of the disease was identified in 29 patients (52%). Four patients had cerebral vascular malformations, which had been treated by embolisation prior to this study in all cases. Five patients with PAVMs reported a history of cerebral complication of PAVMs (one abscess and four transient ischemic attacks). The average haemoglobin level was 13.8±2.1 g/dl (range 7.5–16.7 g/dl). The characteristics of the 56 participants according to their study group are reported in Table 1.

Evaluation of SGRQ

The global score for the SGRQ was significantly different between the three groups (Table 1 and Figure 1). The global score was significantly higher in group C compared to the other groups ($p = 0.04$ compared to group A and $p = 0.02$ compared to group B), indicating worse respiratory-specific QoL. There was no significant difference between groups A and B.

The score for the impact component was significantly higher in group C than in the other groups ($p = 0.02$ compared to group A and $p = 0.007$ compared to group B); there was no significant difference between groups A and B. We also found no difference among the groups in the score for the symptoms or activity components.

Table 1. Characteristics of the study participants.

	GROUP A	GROUP B	GROUP C	p-VALUE
N	10	19	27	
Age (years)	48.9±13.7	40.0±16.9	41.9±18.5	0.34
Female sex, n (%)	4 (40)	12 (63)	16 (59)	0.46
Mutational status				0.008
ENG mutation	1	11	19	
ACVRL1 mutation	8	6	3	
MADH4 mutation	0	1	0	
No mutation	1	1	5	
Hb levels (g/dL)	14.0±2.3	13.9±1.4	13.6±2.5	0.93
O_2 saturation (%)	98±1	98±1	95±4	0.002
Global score	10.5±7.5	11.5±12.9	22.0±17.2	0.03
«Symptoms» score	9.4±10.5	7.2±10.2	9.6±8.1	0.50
«Activity» score	25.8±19.4	24.1±22.0	40.2±28.3	0.07
«Impact» score	2.1±2.7	5.6±11.7	15.4±18.2	0.01

O_2 saturation was measured in sitting position while breathing room air.
Hb: haemoglobin.

Impact of Embolisation of PAVM on QoL

Eighteen patients underwent embolisation of PAVMs in our center at least 6 months prior to the end of the timeframe of the study. One patient declined to answer the second questionnaire. We therefore report the data for 17 patients. As shown in Table 2, there were no significant differences in the characteristics of these patients and the remaining ten patients of group C. Adverse events related to the procedure were documented in two patients: one transient ischemic attack and one thrombosis of a calf vein.

Both the global score and the score for the activity component decreased significantly after embolisation of PAVMs ($p = 0.003$ and $p = 0.0006$, respectively), whereas the score for the impact and symptoms components did not change significantly (Table 3 and Figure 2). We found no statistically significant differences for any

of the four scores between group C after embolisation and groups A and B.

Discussion

Our results demonstrate that the presence of PAVMs significantly impairs the QoL of patients with HHT and that embolisation of PAVMs not only improves their respiratory-specific QoL but raises it to the same level as observed in HHT patients without PAVM (as measured with the SGRQ). In addition, the presence of "small" PAVM(s) (i.e., not accessible to embolisation) does not appear to affect the respiratory-specific QoL.

To our knowledge, this is the first study to examine the respiratory-specific health status of HHT patients. Health-related

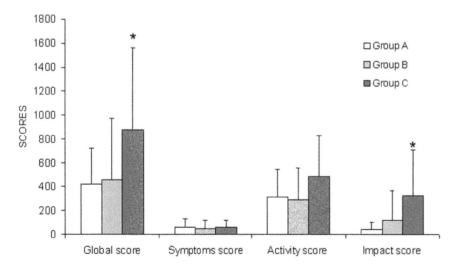

Figure 1. Global score of the Saint George's Respiratory Questionnaire and score of its "symptoms" component, "activity" component and "impact" component in the 3 groups of patients: group A (patients with no PAVM), group B (patients with "small" PAVMs) and group C (patients with "large" PAVMs). Bars indicate standard deviation.

Table 2. Characteristics of the group C patients who participated in the evaluation of the impact of embolisation on the quality of life.

	PARTICIPANTS	NON-PARTICIPANTS	p-VALUE
N	17	10	
Age (years)	42.5±19.4	40.9±17.8	0.82
Female sex, n (%)	10 (59%)	6 (60%)	0.95
Hb levels (g/dL)	13.8±2.0	13.3±3.2	0.86
O₂ saturation (%)	95±5	94±4	0.85
Global score	21.5±16.0	22.8±18.4	1.00
«Symptoms» score	7.6±7.5	13.1±8.3	0.24
«Activity» score	43.4±28.6	34.8±28.4	0.45
«Impact» score	13.4±17.7	19.0±19.3	0.35

O_2 saturation was measured in sitting position while breathing room air.
Hb: haemoglobin.

QoL has been measured before in HHT patients, but the impact of the presence of PAVMs on QoL has not been evaluated to date. Most studies on health-related QoL in HHT patients used a general health questionnaire such as the Short Form-36 (SF-36) questionnaire [10–14]. This questionnaire measures eight dimensions: role limitation due to physical health problems, physical functioning, role limitation due to emotional problems, bodily pain, general health, vitality, social functioning, and mental health. For instance, Geistholl UW et al. found that in 77 HHT patients, impairment of QoL, as measured by the SF-36 questionnaire, was associated with digestive bleeding and the severity of epistaxis [12]. The negative impact of severe epistaxis on QoL has been confirmed in other studies [10,11,13,17,18]. Interestingly, Pfister et al. reported that HHT2 patients have a higher health-related QoL than HHT1 patients and suggested that this might be due to the fact that 30–40% of HHT1 patients have PAVMs compared to 0–14% of HHT2 patients [14]. Our study confirms this hypothesis: in addition to other manifestations of HHT, such as

severe epistaxis and digestive bleeding, the presence of PAVMs significantly impairs health-related QoL.

The presence of PAVMs predisposes patients to severe complications. It is therefore recommended that clinicians screen all HHT patients for the presence of PAVMs (e.g., by contrast echocardiography). In patients with PAVMs, an embolisation procedure should be performed whenever technically possible. Complications related to the procedure include device migration, stroke, gaseous embolism, pulmonary infarction and haemoptysis, and reperfusion of embolised PAVMs [4–6,8]. However, the risks of procedure-related complications are considered to be outweighed by the benefits of embolotherapy when the procedure is performed in centers of excellence [4,8]. Unfortunately, it is sometimes difficult to convince patients to undergo such a procedure when no complications due to PAVMs have yet occurred. Patients are usually more concerned with issues that have an immediate daily impact, such as epistaxis and gastrointestinal blood loss, than with theoretical risks from a PAVM,

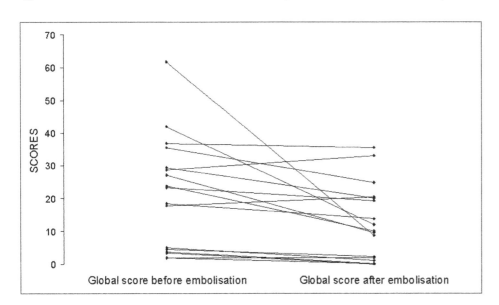

Figure 2. Global score of the Saint George's Respiratory Questionnaire in 17 HHT patients before and 6–12 months after embolisation of PAVMs.

Table 3. Impact of embolisation on quality of life.

	BEFORE EMBOLISATION	AFTER EMBOLISATION	p-VALUE
Global score	21.5±17.0	12.5±11.5	0.003
«Symptoms» score	7.6±7.5	6.4±7.4	0.19
«Activity» score	43.4±28.6	25.9±23.5	0.0006
«Impact» score	13.4±17.7	6.8±8.6	0.11

however potentially debilitating that risk might be. It is therefore crucial to help patients to understand the risks related to the presence of PAVMs [8]. In addition, Gupta et al. conducted a poll of current practice related to embolisation of PAVMs among 21 HHT experts in nine countries [19]; most of these experts indicated that fewer than one-half of physicians practicing outside of HHT centers recommended embolisation for an asymptomatic PAVM with a feeding artery of at least 3 mm, often resulting in major complications. Our results highlight additional reasons to recommend the procedure for all patients with PAVMs when technically feasible.

Interestingly, the presence of "small" PAVMs was not associated in our study with an impairment in respiratory-related QoL. The impact of small PAVMs in terms of risk of systemic complications is subject to debate. A recent study reported that the presence of small PAVMs, as demonstrated by a grade I shunt on contrast echocardiography, is not associated with an increased risk of systemic emboli [20]. The authors suggested that prophylactic antibiotherapy might not be necessary in these patients. Our results also submit that the presence of small PAVMs might not be deleterious in terms of QoL. Another explanation for our results is that the SGRQ is not sensitive enough to detect small impairments in respiratory-specific QoL.

Our study has several limitations. First, we used the SGRQ to measure respiratory-specific QoL. Our objective was to minimize the impact on the SGRQ score of other clinical manifestations of the disease, such as gastrointestinal bleeding or epistaxis. The SGRQ was developed initially for patients with airway diseases, such as asthma and chronic obstructive pulmonary disease [15]. It has also been used in a variety of respiratory disorders, such as pulmonary fibrosis [21], pulmonary hypertension [22], and chronic pulmonary aspergillosis [23]. It has been validated in the French language [24]. Our results suggest that the SGRQ can also be used in patients with HHT and PAVMs, since it is able to differentiate between different levels of lung disease severity and to detect a beneficial effect of embolisation of PAVMs on health status. Second, the SGRQ score itself can be affected by other manifestations of HHT, such as anemia or cardiac insufficiency

secondary to liver disease. However, the level of haemoglobin was similar in the three groups and there was one patient with severe liver disease (i.e., responsible for pulmonary hypertension) in each group. Third, there was no randomization with respect to the decision to perform embolisation, because we felt that it was not ethical not to advise embolisation whenever possible to all patients, as recommended in the international guidelines. However, this was a prospective study and the QoL was evaluated twice in patients who underwent embolisation of PAVMs (immediately prior to the embolisation and approximately 6 mo after); this enabled us to use the subjects as their own controls.

In summary, in patients with HHT, the presence of PAVMs negatively impacts QoL when the size of the feeding artery is large enough to be embolised. Moreover, embolisation of PAVMs normalises respiratory-specific QoL. These results may constitute an additional argument to convince patients to undergo this procedure, not only because it is beneficial in terms of prevention of systemic and cerebral complications, but also because it may increase QoL.

Acknowledgments

The authors would like to thank the the French HHT patient association, AMRO-France (Association Maladie Rendu-Osler) and the patients who agreed to participate in this study. The authors acknowledge the contributions of the staff at our HHT-dedicated centre, and in particular Jean-Hugues Blondel, MD, Marcel Bonay, MD, Isabelle Bourgault, MD, Gilles Lesur, MD, Augustin Ozanne, MD, Joëlle Roume, MD, Bernadette Raffestin, MD, Alexandre Cordier, MD, Carole Fagnou, MD, Bénédicte Chesneau and Lorela Renard (Assistance Publique Hôpitaux de Paris, Consultation Pluridisciplinaire Maladie de Rendu-Osler, Hôpital Ambroise Paré, Boulogne, France).

Author Contributions

Conceived and designed the experiments: SB DC TC PL ME. Performed the experiments: DC SB. Analyzed the data: SB TC AB. Wrote the paper: TC SB AB. Performed embolisations of pulmonary arteriovenous malformations: ME PL.

References

1. Guttmacher AE, Marchuk DA, White RI Jr (1995) Hereditary hemorrhagic telangiectasia. N Engl J Med 333: 918–924.
2. Shovlin Cl, Guttmacher AE, Buscarini E, Faughnan ME, Hyland RH et al. (2000) Diagnostic criteria for hereditary hemorrhagic telangiectasia (Rendu-Osler-Weber syndrome). Am J Med Genet 91: 66–67.
3. Abdalla SA, Le Tarte M (2006) Hereditary haemorrhagic telangiectasia: current views on genetics and mechanisms of disease. J Med Genet 43: 97–110.
4. Faughnan ME, Palda VA, Garcia-Tsao G, Geisthoff UW, McDonald J, et al. (2011) International Guidelines for the diagnosis and management of Hereditary Hemorrhagic Telangiectasia. J Med Genet 48: 73–87.
5. Gossage JR, Kanj G (1998) Pulmonary arteriovenous malformations. Am J Respir Crit Care Med 158: 643–661.
6. Faughnan ME, Granton JT, Young LH (2009) The pulmonary vascular complications of hereditary hemorrhagic telangiectasia. Eur Respir J 33: 1186–1194.

7. Moussouttas M, Fayad P, Rosenblatt M, Hashimoto M, Pollak J, et al. (2000) Cerebral ischemia and neurologic manifestations. Neurology 55: 959–964.
8. Trerotola SO, Pyeritz RE (2010) PAVM embolisation: an update. Am J Roentgenol 195: 837–845.
9. Lacombe P, Lagrange C, Beauchet A, El Hajjam M, Chinet T, et al. (2009) Diffuse Pulmonary Arteriovenous Malformations in Hereditary Hemorrhagic Telangiectasia: Long-term results of Embolization According to the Extent of Lung Involvement. Chest 135: 1031–1037.
10. Pasculli G, Resta F, Guastamacchia E, Di Gennaro L, Suppressa P, et al. (2004) Health-related quality of life in a rare disease: Hereditary hemorrhagic telangiectasia (HHT) or Rendu–Osler–Weber Disease. Qual Life Res 13: 1715–1723.
11. Lennox PA, Hitchings AE, Lund VJ, Howard DJ (2005) The SF-36 health status questionnaire in assessing patients with epistaxis secondary to hereditary hemorrhagic telangiectasia. Am J Rhinol 19: 71–74.

12. Geisthoff UW, Heckmann K, D'Amelio R, Grunewald S, Knobber D, et al. (2007) Health-related quality of life in hereditary hemorrhagic telangiectasia. Otolaryngol Head Neck Surg 136: 726–733.

13. Geirdal AØ, Dheyauldeen S, Bachmann-Harildstad G, Heimdal K (2012) Quality of life in patients with hereditary hemorrhagic telangiectasia in Norway: A population-based study. Am J Med Genet Part A 158A: 1269–1278.

14. Pfister M, Zalaman IM, Blumenstock G, Mauz PS, Baumann I (2009) Impact of genotype and mutation type on health-related quality of life in patients with hereditary hemorrhagic telangiectasia. Acta Otolaryngol 129: 862–866.

15. Jones PW, Quirk FH, Baveystock CM, Littlejohns P (1992) A self-complete measure of health status for chronic airflow limitation. The St. George's Respiratory Questionnaire. Am Rev Respir Dis 145: 1321–1327.

16. Jones PW (2002) Interpreting thresholds for a clinically significant change in health status in asthma and COPD. Eur Respir J 19: 398–404.

17. de Gussem EM, Snijder RJ, Disch FJ, Zanen P, Westermann CJ, et al. (2009) The effect of N-acetylcysteine on epistaxis and quality of life in patients with HHT: A pilot study. Rhinology 47: 85–88.

18. Karapantzos I, Tsimpiris N, Goulis DG, Van Hoecke H, Van Cauwenberge P, et al. (2005) Management of epistaxis in hereditary hemorrhagic telangiectasia by Nd:YAG laser and quality of life assessment using the HR-QoL questionnaire. Eur Arch Otorhinolaryngol 262: 830–833.

19. Gupta S, Faughnan ME, Bayoumi AM (2009) Embolization for pulmonary arteriovenous malformation in hereditary haemorrhagic telangiectasia. A decision analysis. Chest 136: 849–858.

20. Velthuis S, Buscarini E, van Gent MWF, Gazzaniga P, Manfredi G, et al. (2013) Grade of pulmonary right-to-left shunt on contrast echocardiography and cerebral complications. A striking association. Chest 144: 542–548.

21. Nishiyama O, Taniguchi H, Kondoh Y, Kimura T, Ogawa T, et al. (2005) Health-related quality of life in patients with idiopathic pulmonary fibrosis. What is the main contributing factor? Respir Med 99: 408–414.

22. Rubenfire M, Lippo G, Bodini BD, Blasi F, Allegra L, et al. (2009) Evaluating Health-Related Quality of Life, Work Ability, and Disability in Pulmonary Arterial Hypertension: An Unmet Need. Chest 136: 597–603.

23. Al-Shair K, Atherton GTW, Kennedy D, Powell G, Denning DW, et al. (2013) Validity and reliability of the St George's respiratory questionnaire in assessing health status in patients with chronic pulmonary aspergillosis. Chest 144: 623–631.

24. Bouchet Ch, Guillemin F, Hoang Thi TH, Cornette A, Briançon S (1996) Validation du questionnaire St Georges pour mesurer la qualité de vie chez les insuffisants respiratoires chroniques. Rev Mal Resp 13: 43–46.

22

Co-Administration of Resveratrol and Lipoic Acid, or Their Synthetic Combination, Enhances Neuroprotection in a Rat Model of Ischemia/Reperfusion

Monique C. Saleh[1], Barry J. Connell[1], Desikan Rajagopal[3], Bobby V. Khan[1,3], Alaa S. Abd-El-Aziz[2], Inan Kucukkaya[2], Tarek M. Saleh[1]*

1 Department of Biomedical Sciences, Atlantic Veterinary College, University of Prince Edward Island, Charlottetown, P.E.I., Canada, **2** Department of Chemistry, University of Prince Edward Island, Charlottetown, P.E.I., Canada, **3** Carmel BioSciences Inc., Atlanta, Georgia, United States of America

Abstract

The present study demonstrates the benefits of combinatorial antioxidant therapy in the treatment of ischemic stroke. Male Sprague-Dawley rats were anaesthetised and the middle cerebral artery (MCA) was occluded for 30 minutes followed by 5.5 hours of reperfusion. Pretreatment with resveratrol 30 minutes prior to MCA occlusion resulted in a significant, dose-dependent decrease in infarct volume ($p < 0.05$) compared to vehicle-treated animals. Neuroprotection was also observed when resveratrol (2×10^{-3} mg/kg; iv) was administered within 60 minutes following the return of blood flow (reperfusion). Pretreatment with non-neuroprotective doses of resveratrol (2×10^{-6} mg/kg) and lipoic acid (LA; 0.005 mg/kg) in combination produced significant neuroprotection as well. This neuroprotection was also observed when resveratrol and LA were administered 15 minutes following the onset of MCA occlusion. Subsequently, we synthetically combined resveratrol and LA in both a 1:3 (UPEI-200) and 1:1 (UPEI-201) ratio, and screened these new chemical entities in both permanent and transient ischemia models. UPEI-200 was ineffective, while UPEI-201 demonstrated significant, dose-dependent neuroprotection. These results demonstrate that combining subthreshold doses of resveratrol and LA prior to ischemia-reperfusion can provide significant neuroprotection likely resulting from concurrent effects on multiple pathways. The additional protection observed in the novel compound UPEI 201 may present opportunities for addressing ischemia-induced damage in patients presenting with transient ischemic episodes.

Editor: Vardan Karamyan, School of Pharmacy, Texas Tech University HSC, United States of America

Funding: This work was supported by the Atlantic Canada Opportunities Agency Atlantic Innovation fund (AIF; file #1999294). The funders had no role in study design, data collection and analysis, decision to publish, or preparation of the manuscript.

Competing Interests: Dr. Bobby Khan is a cardiologist employed by Carmel BioSciences to conduct phase I clinical trials. Therefore, although Carmel BioSciences is listed in the affiliations for Dr. Khan, none of the authors (including Dr. Khan) received any financial or other resources from this commercial entity. Dr. Khan was involved in his capacity as a research collaborator at UPEI and therefore the authors do not feel that there are any competing interests.

* E-mail: tsaleh@upei.ca

Introduction

Despite ongoing advances in the arena of stroke research, the worldwide consequences of death and disability remain considerable and delivery of successful therapeutics continues to present a challenge. The application of combinatorial drug therapy in treating stroke has become increasingly attractive in recent years. As researchers uncover the complexity of disease progression following stroke which includes both immediate as well as delayed neuronal effects at multiple levels [1], it has become evident that multi-targeted drug therapy may hold more promise in the treatment and/or prevention of stroke than conventional single class drug regimens. In addition, there is evidence that some drug combinations display pharmacological potentiation (ie synergism) which optimistically translates into lower doses, fewer adverse side effects and an extended treatment window. Treatment outcomes for ischemic events involves the reestablishment of blood flow to compromised tissue, with the reintroduction of oxygen transiently adding to the injury due to generation of inflammatory mediators and toxic levels of oxidative free radicals [2] culminating in lipid

peroxidation, protein synthesis arrest, and ultimately cell death [3]. Successful treatment options are therefore required to address several critical mediators of neuronal death simultaneously.

With the increasing popularity of natural products, science has sought to exploit the medicinal potential of common extracts as is evident in the growing literature of natural product drug discovery. In the current study, we test 2 novel compounds combining resveratrol (3, 5, 4′-trihydroxystilbene), a naturally-occurring component of grapes, and α-lipoic acid (LA), a potent anti-oxidant found in common foods, for neuroprotective effects in 2 animal models of ischemic stroke. Separately, resveratrol and LA possess potent anti-oxidant and anti-inflammatory activities and have been shown to produce neuroprotection in several animal models of neurological disease via complementary pathways [4] [5].

Resveratrol possesses multiple biological activities [6] [7], including being a potent antioxidant [8] and anti-inflammatory [9] agent. These therapeutic uses of resveratrol have led researchers to investigate its protective effects in several animal models of neurological disease, particularly those with unknown

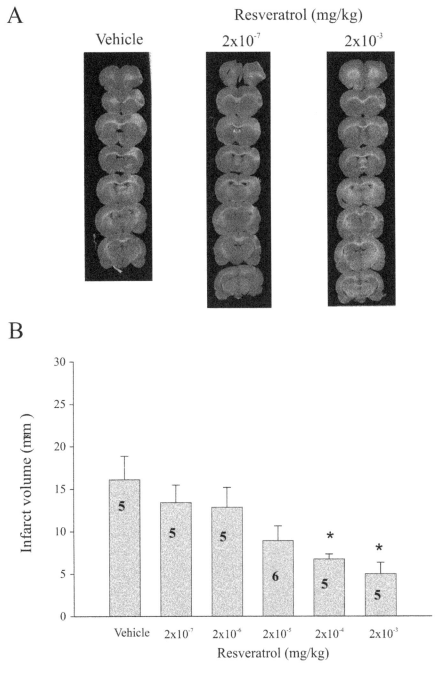

Figure 1. Dose-dependent effect of resveratrol on infarct volume following transient ischemia/reperfusion. (A) Representative photomicrographs of TTC-stained, 1 mm thick coronal slices illustrating the extent of infarct within the prefrontal cortex following pretreatment (30 minutes prior to MCAO; i.v.) with either Vehicle (propylene glycol $4 \times 10^{-3\%}$ (v/v)) or Resveratrol (2×10^{-7} and 2×10^{-3} mg/kg) following ischemia/reperfusion (tMCAO). (B) Bar graph summarizing the dose-response relationship between increasing doses of resveratrol and infarct size (mm^3) calculated from TTC-stained, 1 mm thick coronal sections following tMCAO. Each bar represents the mean ± S.E.M. (n = 5–6/group) and * indicates significance ($p \leq 0.05$) from the vehicle-treated control group.

etiology, or where inflammation and oxidative stress may play a role in the pathogenesis. Consequently, resveratrol has shown promise as a neuroprotectant in animal models of cerebral ischemia through its ability to attenuate ischemia-induced cell death [10].

Also a powerful antioxidant, α-lipoic acid (LA) is characterized by high reactivity towards free radicals [11] and demonstrates potent neuroprotective effects in several animal models of stroke including models of reperfusion injury [12] [13] [14] [15] [16] [17]. Further, the co-administration of LA with other compounds has been shown to enhance the protective effect of the drug in various animal models of pathology [18] [19] [20] [21] [22]. Our own research has shown that co-administration of non-protective (sub-threshold) doses of both LA and apocynin, an NADPH oxidase inhibitor, provided significant neuroprotection against ischemic injury [23].

Thus, the current study investigated the potential for enhanced neuroprotective effects with LA by combining it with resveratrol in a rodent model of acute stroke and reperfusion injury [24]. In addition, the effects of resveratrol and lipoic acid were compared to UPEI-200 and UPEI-201, two novel synthetic compounds linking resveratrol with LA in both a transient occlusion-reperfusion model (tMCAO) as well as in a permanent occlusion model (pMCAO). Lastly, the feasibility of delayed treatment intervention was investigated for all drug combinations.

Methods

Ethics Statement

All experiments were carried out in accordance with the guidelines of the Canadian Council on Animal Care and were approved by the University of Prince Edward Island Animal Care Committee (protocol #11-045 and 13-036).

General Surgical Procedures for in vivo Studies

All experiments were conducted on male Sprague-Dawley rats (250–350 g; Charles Rivers; Montreal, PQ, CAN). For all animals, food and tap water were available *ad libitum*. Rats were anaesthetized with sodium thiobutabarbital (Inactin; Sigma-Aldridge; St.Louis, MO, USA; 100 mg/kg; ip) and supplemented as needed. For intravenous administration of drugs, a polyethylene catheter (PE-10; Clay Adams, Parsippany, NJ, USA) was inserted into the right femoral vein. An endotracheal tube was inserted to facilitate breathing. Body temperature was monitored and maintained at $37 \pm 1°C$ using a feedback system (Physitemp Instruments; Clifton, NJ, USA).

A separate group of animals were instrumented for the recording of blood pressure and heart rate via an indwelling catheter (PE-50; ; Clay Adams, Parsippany, NJ, USA) placed inside the right femoral artery. Arterial blood pressure was measured with a pressure transducer (Gould P23 ID, Cleveland, OH) connected to a Gould model 2200S polygraph. Heart rate was determined from the pulse pressure using a Gould tachograph (Biotach). These parameters were displayed and analyzed using

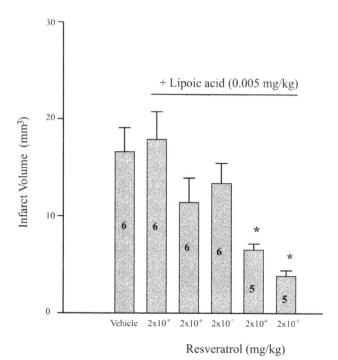

Figure 3. Effect of increasing doses of resveratrol in combination with lipoic acid on infarct volume. Bar graph summarizing the effect of co-administration of a sub-threshold dose of lipoic acid (0.005 mg/kg) with increasing doses of resveratrol on infarct volume following ischemia/reperfusion. Each bar represents the mean ± S.E.M. (n = 5–6/group) and * indicates significance ($p \le 0.05$) from the vehicle-treated (propylene glycol $4 \times 10^{-3\%}$ (v/v)) control group.

PolyviewPro/32 data acquisition and analysis software (Grass Technologies, Warwick, RI).

Transient and Permanent Middle Cerebral Artery Occlusions (tMCAO and pMCAO)

We have previously published the detailed methodology for transient occlusion of the middle cerebral artery [24]. Briefly, animals were placed in a David Kopf stereotaxic frame (Tujunga, CA, USA) and the right middle cerebral artery (MCA) approached through a rostra-caudal incision of the skin and frontalis muscle at the approximate level of bregma. Blood flow through the MCA was impeded by the placement of surgical suture behind the MCA at 3 designated positions along the exposed vessel for 30 minutes in the transient model (tMCAO), or left in place for a total of 6 hours in the permanent model (pMCAO). The sutures were positioned such that the middle of each suture applied pressure to the underside of the MCA and impeded blood flow (ischemia) as previously confirmed using laser Doppler flowmetry (OxyFlo, Oxford-Optronix, Oxford, UK) (Connell and Saleh 2010). This 3-point placement of surgical sutures produced a highly reproducible and consistent focal ischemic lesion restricted to the prefrontal cerebral cortex. Blood flow in the tMCAO model was re-established (reperfusion) for an additional 5.5 hours following removal of the sutures.

Drug Preparation

Resveratrol (trans-3,5,4′-trihydroxy stilbene; Sigma Aldrich, St. Louis, MO, USA) stock solutions were prepared in 40% propylene glycol and diluted 10,000X in 0.9% saline The concentration of propylene glycol in each solution was $4 \times 10^{-3\%}$ (v/v). Lipoic acid

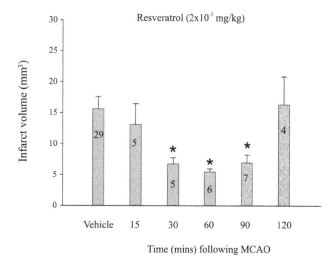

Figure 2. Time course of resveratrol-induced neuroprotection. Bar graph summarizing the effect of resveratrol injected 15 minutes into middle cerebral artery occlusion (15), or at 30 min intervals post-reperfusion. Each bar represents the mean ± S.E.M. (n = 5–6/group) and * indicates significance ($p \le 0.05$) from the pooled vehicle-treated (propylene glycol $4 \times 10^{-3\%}$ (v/v)) control group.

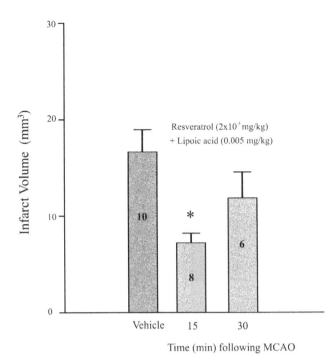

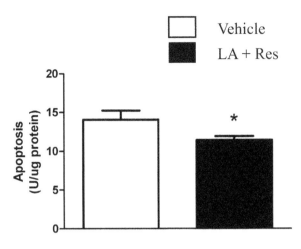

Figure 5. Effect of lipoic acid and resveratrol combination on a marker of apoptotic cell death. Bar graph of the quantified cytoplasmic histone-associated-DNA fragmentation (an indicator of apoptotic cell death) as obtained from a tissue sample (see methods for detailed description). Each bar represents the mean ± S.E.M. and * indicates significance ($p \leq 0.05$) from the vehicle-treated (propylene glycol $4 \times 10^{-3\%}$ (v/v)) control group.

Figure 4. Time course of effect of combining lipoic acid and resveratrol on infarct volume. Bar graph summarizing the effect on infarct volume of administering a non-protective dose of lipoic acid in combination with a protective dose of resveratrol 15 minutes during the occlusion (15 min), or immediately after reperfusion (30 min). Each bar represents the mean ± S.E.M. (n = 5–8/group) and * indicates significance ($p \leq 0.05$) from the vehicle-treated (propylene glycol $4 \times 10^{-3\%}$ (v/v)) control group.

(LA; Sigma-Aldridge; St. Louis, MO, USA; 0.005 mg/ml) was prepared in physiological saline (0.9% sodium chloride) and the pH was adjusted to 7.0–7.4 with sodium hydroxide. The concentration of LA used was previously determined to be non-neuroprotective in our tMCAO model [12]. Appropriate vehicle solutions were prepared for each drug and dose.

Synthesis of UPEI-200

The chemical synthesis of UPEI-200 was performed as follows; resveratrol (0.01 M) was combined with 0.05 M LA and 0.04 M of dimethylaminopyridine (DMAP) in 80 ml of anhydrous dichloromethane (CH_2Cl_2). 1-Ethyl-3-(3-dimethylaminopropyl) carbodimide hydrochloride (EDCI; 0.05 M) was added in small quantities over a period of 2 hours. The entire reaction was performed under nitrogen atmosphere at room temperature. After stirring overnight, the crude mixture of compounds was quickly purified by passing through a silica column following an aqueous work up. The product was again purified on a Chromatotran silica plate using 2 mm pre-coated UV active plate. Appropriate fractions were mixed and concentrated in a rotary evaporator keeping the water bath temperature at 45°C. The final pure compound was obtained as a pale yellow viscous solid in very low yield and was characterized by proton nuclear magnetic resonance spectroscopy and mass spectrometry.

Synthesis of UPEI-201

Resveratrol (1 mmol) in 20 ml dimethylformamide (DMF) was combined with DMAP (10 mmol) and LA (1 mmol). Dicyclohexylcarbodiimide (DCC; 1 mmol) was added to the reaction mixture

at 0°C under nitrogen atmosphere, which is then stirred for 5 min at 0°C and 3 h at 20°C. Precipitated urea is then filtered off and the filtrate evaporated down *in vacuo*. The residue was taken up in dichloromethane (CH_2Cl_2) and, if necessary, filtered free of any further precipitated urea. The solvent was removed by evaporation and the crude compound was purified by silica column chromatography (Eluent, Hexanes:Ethylacetate (1:1; yellow oil), Yield; 57%.^{1}H NMR (300 MHz, Acetone) δ 7.40 (2H, d, $J = 8.6$ Hz), 7.05–6.79 (4H,m), 6.52 (2H, d, $J = 2.1$ Hz), 6.25 (1H, t, $J = 2.1$ Hz), 3.58 (1H, tt, $J = 12.7$, 6.4 Hz), 3.24–3.04 (2H, m), 2.45 (1H, tt, $J = 12.3$, 6.2 Hz), 2.28 (1H, t, $J = 7.2$ Hz), 1.95–1.80 (1H, m), 1.79–1.52 (4H, m), 1.45 (2H, dtd, $J = 11.1$, 7.1, 4.1 Hz).

Effect of Resveratrol on tMCAO Model

In the first experiment, resveratrol (2×10^{-3} (n = 5), 2×10^{-4} (n = 5), 2×10^{-5} (n = 6), 2×10^{-6} (n = 5), 2×10^{-7} (n = 5) mg/kg; 1 ml/kg; i.v.) or vehicle (propylene glycol; $4 \times 10^{-3\%}$ (v/v); 1 ml/kg; i.v.; n = 5) was administered 30 minutes prior to the onset of MCAO. The sutures were left in place for 30 minutes, followed by 5.5 hours of reperfusion.

The feasibility of extended treatment options was investigated by administering the highest dose of resveratrol (2×10^{-3} mg/kg; i.v.) or vehicle (propylene glycol; $4 \times 10^{-3\%}$ (v/v); 1 ml/kg; i.v.) at the following intervals during the I/R protocol; 15 minutes (n = 5/group) following the onset of MCAO, and 0, 30, 60, 90 minutes (n = 5,6,7,4 respectively) following the onset of reperfusion.

Co-administration of Resveratrol and Lipoic Acid (tMCAO)

To examine neuroprotection following co-administration of various doses of resveratrol (2×10^{-5} (n = 5), 2×10^{-6} (n = 5), 2×10^{-7} (n = 6), 2×10^{-8} (n = 6), or 2×10^{-9} (n = 6) mg/kg) with LA (0.005 mg/kg) on ischemia-reperfusion injury in our tMCAO model, resveratrol and LA were combined into a single solution and administered (1.0 ml/kg; iv) 30 minutes prior to MCAO. The MCA was occluded for 30 minutes followed by 5.5 hours of reperfusion.

Delayed treatment effects were also studied by co-injecting resveratrol (2×10^{-5} mg/kg) and LA (0.005 mg/kg; i.v) at the

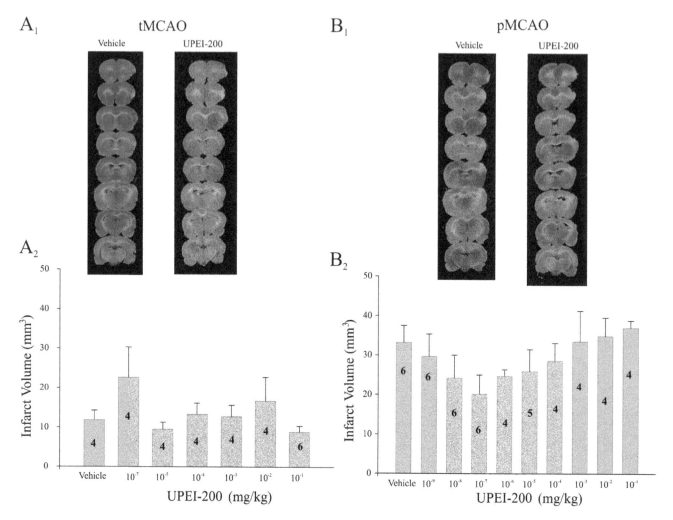

Figure 6. Lack of an effect of UPEI-200 on ischemic or reperfusion injury-induced cell death. (A_1) Representative photomicrographs of TTC-stained sections from vehicle and UPEI-200-treated animals prior to either ischemia/reperfusion (tMCAO; A_1) or permanent middle cerebral artery occlusion (6 hr pMCAO; B_1). Bar graphs illustrating the lack of effect on infarct volume of UPEI-200 (3:1 ratio of lipoic acid to resveratrol) at increasing doses or a vehicle (propylene glycol $4 \times 10^{-3\%}$ (v/v)) injected 30 minutes prior to either tMCAO (A_2) or pMCAO (B_2). Each bar represents the mean ± S.E.M. (n = 4–6/group).

following intervals during the I/R protocol; 15 minutes (n = 8) following the onset of MCAO, and 0, 30, 60, 90 minutes (n = 6,6,7,4 respectively) following the onset of reperfusion.

Co-administration of Resveratrol and Lipoic Acid and Permanent Occlusion (pMCAO)

To determine if the co-administration of resveratrol and LA was neuroprotective on ischemia-induced cell death only, co-injection of resveratrol and LA (2×10^{-5} mg/kg and LA, 0.005 mg/kg; i.v.; n = 4) or vehicle (propylene glycol; $4 \times 10^{-3\%}$ (v/v); 1 ml/kg; i.v.; n = 4) were made 30 minutes prior to pMCAO. The experiments were terminated at the end of 6 hours of occlusion with no reperfusion period.

UPEI-200 or 201 Effects in tMCAO or pMCAO

The effects of UPEI-200 and UPEI-201 on infarct volume in both transient and permanent MCAO models were investigated. Dose-response curves were generated for both entities (n = 4–7/ group). UPEI-201 was further studied for its effectiveness in delayed intervention by administering a neuroprotective dose

(1×10^{-6} mg/kg) 15 minutes post-occlusion as well as 0, 30 and 60 minutes into the 5.5 hr reperfusion period (n = 4–7/group).

Histological Procedures

At the end of each experiment, in which infarct volume was measured, animals were transcardially perfused with phosphate buffered saline (PBS; 0.1 M; 200 mL). The brains were removed and sliced into 1 mm coronal sections with the aid of a rat brain matrix (Harvard Apparatus; Holliston, MA, USA). Sections were incubated in a 2% solution of 2,3,5-triphenol tetrazolium chloride (TTC; Sigma-Aldrich; St. Louis; MO, USA) for 5 minutes. Infarct volumes were calculated with measurements taken from scanned digital images of each brain section. The infarct area for opposing views of each brain section was calculated using a computer-assisted imaging system (Scion Corporation; Frederick, MD, USA), averaged and multiplied by section thickness (1 mm) to give a measure of infarct volume for each section. The sum total of the individual infarct volumes provided the infarct volume for each rat.

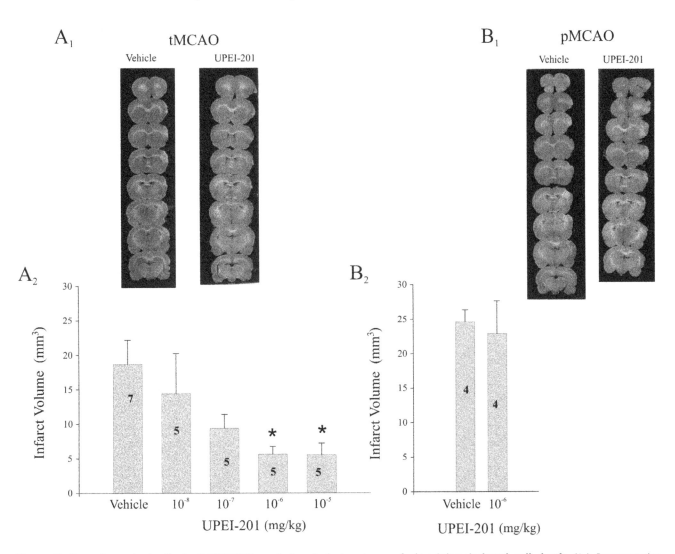

Figure 7. Dose-dependent effect of UPEI-201 on ischemic but not reperfusion injury-induced cell death. (A₁) Representative photomicrographs of TTC-stained sections from vehicle and UPEI-201-treated animals prior to either ischemia/reperfusion (tMCAO; A₁) or permanent middle cerebral artery occlusion (6 hr pMCAO; B₁). Bar graph illustrating the effect on infarct volume of UPEI-201 (1:1 ratio of lipoic acid to resveratrol) at increasing doses or a vehicle (propylene glycol $4\times10^{-3\%}$ (v/v)) injected 30 minutes prior to either ischemia/reperfusion (tMCAO; A₂) or permanent middle cerebral artery occlusion (6 hr pMCAO; B₂). Each bar represents the mean ± S.E.M. (n = 5–7/group) and * indicates significance ($p\leq0.05$) from the vehicle-treated control group.

Co-administration of Resveratrol - Lipoic Acid and Apoptosis

In a separate set of experiments, the co-administration of resveratrol (2×10^{-5} mg/kg) and LA (0.005 mg/kg; i.v.; n = 4) or vehicle (propylene glycol; $4\times10^{-3\%}$ (v/v); 1 ml/kg; i.v.; n = 4) were made 30 minutes prior to tMCAO. The sutures were left in place for 30 minutes followed by 5.5 hours of reperfusion. Animals were transcardially perfused with 200 mL of 0.1 M phosphate buffered saline (pH 7.4), the brains removed and the ipsilateral cerebral cortex isolated by careful dissection. A biopsy needle having an internal diameter of 8 mm was used to collect tissue from the region of infarct. The region of infarct was visually identified as that area which displayed a grayish hue and was slightly swollen compared to the surrounding healthy tissue. The biopsy needle was centered on this area and the tissue sample removed.

The tissue was weighed and homogenized (20% w/v) in ice cold PBS. The homogenate was centrifuged 12 000×g for 15 min at 4°

C. Aliquots of the supernatant were stored at −80°C until assayed for protein. Apoptotic cell death was quantified using an ELISA based assay for determination of cytoplasmic histone-associated DNA fragments (Roche Diagnostics, Montreal, QC, CAN).

Statistical Analysis

Data were analyzed using a statistical software package (SigmaStat and SigmaPlot; Jandel Scientific, Tujunga, CA). All data are presented as a mean ± standard error of the mean (S.E.M). Differences were considered statistically significant if $p\leq0.05$ by an analysis of variance (ANOVA) followed by a Bonferroni post-hoc analysis. When only two groups were being compared the Student's t-test was used.

Results

Resveratrol and tMCAO

Pre-administration of resveratrol provided dose-dependent neuroprotection in our model of ischemia-reperfusion. This was

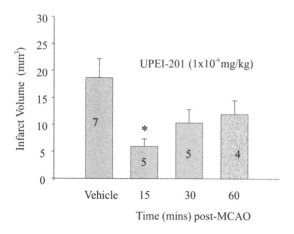

Figure 8. Time course of the effect of UPEI-201 on infarct volume. (A) Bar graph illustrating the effect on infarct volume of UPEI-201 (1:1 ratio of lipoic acid to resveratrol) at a dose of 1×10^{-6} mg/kg or a vehicle (propylene glycol $4 \times 10^{-3\%}$ (v/v)) injected during the occlusion (15) or at 30 minute intervals immediately following reperfusion. Each bar represents the mean $\pm$ S.E.M. (n = 5–7/group) and * indicates significance ($p \leq 0.05$) from the vehicle-treated control group.

evident by a reduction in mean infarct volume with increasing doses of resveratrol (Figs. 1A and B). A significant difference in infarct volume between resveratrol treated animals and vehicle treated controls was observed at the 2 highest doses tested (2×10^{-3} and 2×10^{-4} mg/kg; $p \leq 0.05$).

Resveratrol or vehicle was injected during MCAO or during the period of reperfusion (Figure 2). There were no significant differences in the mean infarct volumes when vehicle was injected during MCAO or at any time point during reperfusion ($p \geq 0.05$), therefore, the vehicle data for all time points was pooled (n = 29). However, all statistical comparisons were made between the infarct volumes measured following resveratrol and vehicle administration for each time point. When resveratrol treatment (2×10^{-3} mg/kg; i.v.) was delayed until 15 minutes into the ischemic period or 90 minutes into the reperfusion period (120 min post occlusion) there was no effect on infarct volume when compared to vehicle injected controls ($p \geq 0.05$; Fig. 2). However, significant neuroprotection was observed when resveratrol (2×10^{-3} mg/kg) was administered at the start of the reperfusion period (30 minutes post-occlusion), or at 30 and 60 minutes into the reperfusion period (60 and 90 minutes post-occlusion; $p \leq 0.05$ at each time point; Fig. 2).

Co-administration of Resveratrol and Lipoic Acid

The combined pre-administration of resveratrol and LA 30 minutes prior to tMCAO produced a dose-dependent reduction in infarct volume compared to vehicle injected controls when measured following 5.5 hrs of reperfusion (Fig. 3). This effect was significant at the 2 highest doses of resveratrol (2×10^{-6} and 2×10^{-5} mg/kg; $p \leq 0.05$; Fig. 3). Delaying treatment of resveratrol (2×10^{-5} mg/kg) and LA (0.005 mg/kg) until 15 minutes following the onset of tMCAO was neuroprotective however no significant effect was observed when the same combination of resveratrol and LA was injected immediately prior to suture removal and the onset of reperfusion (30 minutes post occlusion; Fig. 4).

Tissue sampled from the infarct region of rats injected with resveratrol (2×10^{-5} mg/kg) and LA (0.005 mg/kg) 30 minutes prior to tMCAO displayed lower levels of cytoplasmic histone-

associated-DNA fragmentation. This biomarker suggests decreased apoptotic cell death ($p \leq 0.05$; Fig. 5).

Co-injection of resveratrol (2×10^{-5} mg/kg) and LA (0.005 mg/kg) 30 minutes prior to 6 hours of permanent MCAO did not produce significant neuroprotection ($p \geq 0.05$; data not shown). The average infarct volumes following 6 hrs of permanent MCAO in the vehicle and resveratrol - LA treated groups were 25.3 ± 6 and 19.9 ± 5 mm^3 respectively.

UPEI-200 and UPEI-201 in tMCAO and pMCAO

UPEI-200 is a chemical construct composed of 3 LA moieties bonded to a single resveratrol molecule (3:1). When administered 30 minutes prior to MCA occlusion in either tMCAO or pMCAO models, there was no significant neuroprotection observed at any of the doses tested ($p \geq 0.05$; Fig. 6A, 6B).

Conversely, UPEI-201, which is composed of a single LA moiety bound to resveratrol (1:1), displayed potent neuroprotection when administered 30 minutes prior to MCA in tMCAO (Fig. 7A; $p \leq 0.05$). Delayed intervention with UPEI-201 (1×10^{-6} mg/kg) was successful in reducing infarct volume when administered 15 minutes into the occlusion period (15 min; $p \leq 0.05$, Fig. 8), but not when administered at the start or reperfusion or 30 minutes into the 5.5 hr reperfusion period (30, 60 min; Fig. 8).

Effects of UPEI-201 on Blood Pressure and Heart Rate

Since UPEI-201 was observed to provide neuroprotection in the tMCAO model, the following experiment was designed to determine the effect of UPEI-201 on arterial pressure and heart rate for a period of 2 hrs following administration. Baseline MAP and mean HR prior to drug administration were 109 ± 9 mm/Hg and 378 ± 27 bpm, respectively. Intravenous administration of UPEI-201 (1×10^{-6} mg/kg; n = 4) did not significantly alter mean arterial blood pressure or mean HR at any time point during the 2 hrs of continuous recording compared with vehicle (n = 4; $P \geq 0.05$; data not shown).

Discussion

Dietary plant phenolics such as resveratrol are being widely used in supplement form to prevent and treat common health concerns. Potential safety issues exist as high doses of resveratrol have been shown to cause renal toxicity [25] and contribute to hepatic oxidative stress [26]. In the presence of peroxidase and/or transition metals, resveratrol may function as a pro-oxidant ultimately contributing to DNA damage and mitochondrial dysfunction [27] [28]. As well, resveratrol has been shown to inhibit cytochrome P450 enzyme CYP1A1 [29], an interference which may render other drugs in a patient's treatment plan ineffective at therapeutic doses. Clearly, the health benefits of resveratrol are extensive and hence, finding ways to harness the potency of resveratrol in the absence of adverse side effects is desirable.

To this end, we show in this study that resveratrol on its own produced dose-dependent neuroprotection against neuronal cell death in a rodent model of transient ischemia-reperfusion injury [24]. Combined injection of resveratrol with a non-neuroprotective dose of α-lipoic acid [12] prior to tMCAO produced neuroprotection at doses of resveratrol 100 fold less than when injected alone. By chemically bonding resveratrol to lipoic acid in a 1:1 ratio (UPEI-201), we were able to show a further dose reduction (ten-fold lower) coincident with significant neuroprotection which supports the advantage of combination therapy in stroke treatment.

Numerous studies have proven the efficacy of treatment with lipoic acid in disease states reflective of pro- and antioxidant imbalance such as diabetes, Alzheimer's disease, cancer and cerebrovascular disease [30] [31] [32]. The chemical characteristics of LA, as well as its reduced form dihydrolipoic acid, qualify it as an effective scavenger of hydroxyl radicals, nitric oxide, peroxyl radicals and peroxynitrites, singlet oxygen species and hypochlorous acid [33]. Previously in our laboratory, we showed that LA pretreatment was effective as a neuroprotectant in both reperfusion injury following tMCAO [12] as well as in permanent ischemia (pMCAO) [13]. In the present study, combination of LA with resveratrol did not protect against neuronal death in a model of pMCAO. Prolonged ischemia is characterized by glutamate-induced neuronal toxicity ultimately leading to necrosis [3]. Generation of oxidative radicals is minimal owing to the lack of blood flow and dampening of mitochondrial activity, thereby rendering anti-oxidant therapy ineffectual. In contrast, anti-oxidants are highly effective in combating the oxidative stress generated during reperfusion injury which is demonstrated in the current study in our model of tMCAO. The reduction in infarct volume associated with resveratrol-LA treatment correlates with fewer necrotic cells at the ischemic core as evidenced with TTC staining, as well as reduced apoptotic cell death in the area of the penumbra as demonstrated by reduced oxidative DNA damage.

Other potential implications of combining resveratrol treatment with LA include their complementary participation in cell preserving pathways. For example, resveratrol and LA have both been shown to enhance aldehyde dehydrogenase-2-mediated detoxification of aldehydes in models of ethanol toxicity and ischemia-reperfusion injury respectively [4] [5]. Both compounds influence antioxidant status, in part through direct reduction of reactive oxygen species, but also as modulators of endogenous anti-oxidant systems. Resveratrol was shown to induce MnSOD activity in isolated rat liver mitochondria while LA inhibited glutathione peroxidase activity and induced mitochondrial uncoupling in the same model [34]. It is also noteworthy, that the LA/dihyrolipoate system is highly efficient in the reduction of the oxidized forms of antioxidants essentially aiding in their recycling allowing them to work more effectively without saturation [35]. Its dual solubility in water and lipid allows LA to interact with antioxidants in extracellular (blood) as well intracellular (both cytoplasmic and mitochondrial) compartments and to effectively cross the blood-brain barrier [36].

To utilize the strategy of combinatorial therapy, we created 2 new chemical entities, UPEI-200 and 201 and determined that a 1:1 ratio of resveratrol-LA moieties (UPEI-201) was preferred in providing neuroprotection following ischemia-reperfusion (tMCAO). UPEI-201 effectively provided neuroprotection when injected 15 minutes into the period of occlusion but not when injected during reperfusion. With dosing in the nanomolar range providing significant neuroprotection in our model of transient ischemia, UPEI-201 is clearly a potent neuroprotectant against oxidative damage. Future studies will be necessary to address mechanism of action, bioactivation, plasma stability, and preconditioning applications. Recent figures estimate medication non-compliance at around 50% at a cost of $300 hundred billion a year [37]. Novel compounds such as UPEI-201 which aim to provide multi-level care in a single dose, may improve compliance and could make a significant contribution to global health initiatives in treating and/or preventing cerebrovascular disease. In contrast, the ineffectiveness of UPEI-200 to provide neuroprotection in either tMCAO or pMCAO paradigms clearly demonstrates the utility of bioassay-guided optimization to achieve the ideal ratio of newly synthesized bioactive molecules.

In conclusion, the results presented above support the notion that combining antioxidants at subthreshold doses can produce equal or enhanced neuroprotective effects. In addition, creation of novel chemical entities via the synthetic bonding of these antioxidants can produce comparable effects to those observed by the co-administration of the 2 compounds, but at lower doses. The clear advantage to lowering the dose required to gain therapeutic effect is to minimize off-target effects on other organ systems which may lead to side effects as is seen in so many of the prescription drugs on the market today.

Author Contributions

Conceived and designed the experiments: TS MS BC AA BK DR IK. Performed the experiments: BC MS DR IK. Analyzed the data: BC TS MS IK DR. Contributed reagents/materials/analysis tools: DR IK AA BK. Wrote the paper: MS TS AA IK.

References

1. Wang M, Iliff J, Liao Y, Chen MJ, Shinseki MS, et al. (2012) Cognitive deficits and delayed neuronal loss in a mouse model of multiple microinfarcts. J Neuroscience 32(50): 17948–17960.
2. Ginsberg MD (2008) Current status of neuroprotection for cerebral ischemia: Synoptic overview. Stroke 40: S111–S114.
3. Lipton P (1999) Ischemic cell death in brain neurons. Physiological Reviews 79: 1431–1568.
4. He L, Liu B, Dai Z, Zhang HF, Zhang YS, et al. (2012) Alpha lipoic acid protects heart against myocardial ischemia-reperfusion injurt through a mechanism involving aldehyde dehydrogenase 2 activation. Eur J Pharmacology 678: 32–38.
5. Yan Y, Yang J, Chen G, Mou Y, Zhao Y, et al. (2011) Protection of resveratrol and its analogues against ethanol-induced oxidative DNA damage in human peripheral lymphocytes. Mutation Research 721: 171–177.
6. de la Lastra CA, Villegas I (2005) Resveratrol as an anti-inflammatory and anti-aging agent: mechanisms and clinical implications. Molecular Nutrition and Food Research 49: 405–430.
7. Delmas D, Jannin B, Latruffe N (2005) Resveratrol: preventing properties against vascular alterations and ageing. Molecular Nutrition and Food Research 49: 377–395.
8. Candelario-Jalil E, de Oliveira AC, Graf S, Bhatia HS, Hull M, et al. (2007) Resveratrol potently reduces prostaglandin E2 production and free radical formation in lipopolysaccharide-activated primary rat microglia. J Neuroinflammation 4: 25.
9. Kang OH, Jang HJ, Chae HS, Oh YC, Choi JG, et al. (2009) Anti-inflammatory mechanisms of resveratrol in activated HMC-1 cells: pivotal roles of NF-kappaB and MAPK. Pharmacol Res. 59: 330–7.
10. Saleh MC, Connell BJ, Saleh TM (2013) Resveratrol induced neuroprotection is mediated via both estrogen receptor subtypes, ER alpha and ER beta. Neurosci. Lett., 548: 217–221.
11. Biewenga GP, Haenen GRM, Bast A (1997) The pharmacology of the antioxidant lipoic acid. Gen Pharm 29: 315–331.
12. Connell BJ, Saleh M, Khan BV, Saleh TM (2011) Lipoic acid protects against reperfusion injury in the early stages of cerebral ischemia. Brain Res. 1375: 128–136.
13. Richard MJP, Connell BJ, Khan BV, Saleh TM (2011) Cellular mechanisms by which lipoic acid confers protection during the early stages of cerebral ischemia: a possible role for calcium. Neurosci. Res. 69: 299–307.
14. Clark WM, Rinker LG, Lessov NS, Lowery SL, Cipolla MJ (2001) Efficacy of antioxidant therapies in transient focal ischemia in mice. Stroke 32: 1000–1004.
15. Panigrahi M, Sadguna Y, Shivakumar BR, Kolluri SVR, Roy S, et al. (1996) α-Lipoic acid protects against reperfusion injury following cerebral ischemia. Brain Res. 717: 184–188.
16. Wolz P, Krieglstein J (1996) Neuroprotective effects of α-Lipoic acid and its enantiomers demonstrated in rodent models of focal cerebral ischemia. Neuropharmacol. 35: 369–375.
17. Cao XH, Phillis JW (1995) The free radical scavenger α-lipoic acid protects against cerebral ischemia-reperfusion injury in gerbils. Free Radical Res 23: 365–370.
18. Mukherjee R, Banerjee S, Joshi N, Singh PK, Baxi D, et al. (2011) A combination of melatonin and alpha lipoic acid has greater cardioprotective effect than either of them singly against cadmium-induced oxidative damage. Cardiovasc. Toxicol. 11: 78–88.

19. Garcia-Estrada J, Gonzalez-Perez O, Gonzalez-Castaneda RE, Martinez-Contreras A, Luquin S, et al. (2003) An alpha-lipoic acid-vitamin E mixture reduces post-embolism lipid peroxidation, cerebral infarction, and neurological deficit in rats. Neurosci. Res. 47: 219–224.

20. Sola S, Mir MQS, Cheema FA, Khan-Merchant N, Menon RG, et al. (2005) Irbesartan and lipoic acid improve endothelial function and reduce markers of inflammation in the metabolic syndrome. Results of the Irbesartan and lipoic acid in endothelial dysfunction (ISLAND) study. Circ. 111: 242–248.

21. Shotton HR, Broadbent S, Lincoln J (2004) Prevention and partial reversal of diabetes-induced changes in enteric nerves of the rat ileum by combined treatment with α-lipoic acid and evening primrose oil. Autonomic Neurosci.: Basic and Clinical 111: 57–65.

22. Gonzalez-Perez O, Gonzalez-Castaneda RE, Heurta M, Luquin S, Gomez-Pinedo U, et al. (2002) Beneficial effects of α-lipoic acid plus vitamin E on neurological deficit, reactive gliosis and neuronal remodeling in the penumbra of the ischemic rat brain. Neurosci. Lett. 321: 100–104.

23. Connell BJ, Saleh TM (2012) Co-administration of apocynin with lipoic acid enhances neuroprotection in a rat model of ischemia/reperfusion. Neurosci. Lett. 507(1): 43–46.

24. Connell BJ, Saleh TM (2010) A novel rodent model of reperfusion injury following occlusion of the middle cerebral artery. J. Neurosci. Methods 190: 28–33.

25. Crowell JA, Korytko PJ, Morrissey RL, Booth TD, Levine BS (2004) Resveratrol-associated renal toxicity. Toxicol. Sci. 82(2): 614–619.

26. Rocha KKR, Souza GA, Ebaid GX, Seiva FRF, Cataneo AC, et al. (2009) Resveratrol toxicity: effects on risk factors for atherosclerosis and hepatic oxidative stress in standard and high-fat diets. Food and Chemical Toxicology 47(6): 1362–1367.

27. Galati G, Sabzevari O, Wilson JX, O'Brien PJ (2002) Prooxidant activity and cellular effects of the phenoxyl radicals of dietary flavonoids and other polyphenolics. Toxicology 177: 91–104.

28. Ahmed A, Asad SF, Singh S, Hadi SM (2000) DNA breakage by resveratrol and Cu(II): reaction mechanism and bacteriophage inactivation. Cancer Lett. 154: 29–37.

29. Chun YJ, Kim MY, Guengerich FP (1999) Resveratrol is a selective human cytochrome P450 1A1 inhibitor. Biochem. Biophys. Res. Commun. 262: 20–24.

30. Ibrahimpasic K (2013) Alpha lipoic acid and glycaemic control in diabetic neurophathies at type 2 diabetes treatment. Med. Arh. 67(1): 7–9.

31. Fava A, Pirritano D, Plastino M, Cristiano D, Puccio G, et al. (2013) The effect of lipoic acid therapy on cognitive functioning in patients with alzheimer's disease. J. Neurodegen. Diseases 2013: ID 454254, 7 pages.

32. Michikoshi H, Nakamura T, Sakai K, Suzuki Y, Adachi E, et al. (2013) α-Lipoic acid-induced inhibition of proliferation and met phosphorylation in human non-small cell lung cancer cells. Cancer Lett. 335(2): 472–478.

33. Gulcin I (2010) Antioxidant properties of resveratrol: a structure-activity insight. Innov. Food Sci. Emerg. Tech. 11: 210–218.

34. Valdecantos MP, Perez-Matute P, Quintero P, Martinez JA (2010) Vitamin C, resveratrol and lipoic acid actions on isolated rat liver mitochondria: all antioxidants but different. Redox Rep. 15(5): 207–216.

35. Smith AR, Shenvi SV, Widlansky M, Suh JH, Hagen TM (2004) Lipoic acid as a potential therapy for chronic disease associated with oxidative stress. Curr. Med. Chem. 11: 1135–1146.

36. Bilska A, Wlodek L (2005) Lipoic acid – the drug of the future? Pharmacol. Reports 57: 570–577.

37. Jin J, Sklar GE, Oh VMS, Li SC (2008) Factors affecting therapeutic compliance: a review from the patient's perspective. Therapeutics and Clinical Risk Management 4(1): 269–286.

Permissions

All chapters in this book were first published in PLOS ONE, by The Public Library of Science; hereby published with permission under the Creative Commons Attribution License or equivalent. Every chapter published in this book has been scrutinized by our experts. Their significance has been extensively debated. The topics covered herein carry significant findings which will fuel the growth of the discipline. They may even be implemented as practical applications or may be referred to as a beginning point for another development.

The contributors of this book come from diverse backgrounds, making this book a truly international effort. This book will bring forth new frontiers with its revolutionizing research information and detailed analysis of the nascent developments around the world.

We would like to thank all the contributing authors for lending their expertise to make the book truly unique. They have played a crucial role in the development of this book. Without their invaluable contributions this book wouldn't have been possible. They have made vital efforts to compile up to date information on the varied aspects of this subject to make this book a valuable addition to the collection of many professionals and students.

This book was conceptualized with the vision of imparting up-to-date information and advanced data in this field. To ensure the same, a matchless editorial board was set up. Every individual on the board went through rigorous rounds of assessment to prove their worth. After which they invested a large part of their time researching and compiling the most relevant data for our readers.

The editorial board has been involved in producing this book since its inception. They have spent rigorous hours researching and exploring the diverse topics which have resulted in the successful publishing of this book. They have passed on their knowledge of decades through this book. To expedite this challenging task, the publisher supported the team at every step. A small team of assistant editors was also appointed to further simplify the editing procedure and attain best results for the readers.

Apart from the editorial board, the designing team has also invested a significant amount of their time in understanding the subject and creating the most relevant covers. They scrutinized every image to scout for the most suitable representation of the subject and create an appropriate cover for the book.

The publishing team has been an ardent support to the editorial, designing and production team. Their endless efforts to recruit the best for this project, has resulted in the accomplishment of this book. They are a veteran in the field of academics and their pool of knowledge is as vast as their experience in printing. Their expertise and guidance has proved useful at every step. Their uncompromising quality standards have made this book an exceptional effort. Their encouragement from time to time has been an inspiration for everyone.

The publisher and the editorial board hope that this book will prove to be a valuable piece of knowledge for researchers, students, practitioners and scholars across the globe.

List of Contributors

Laura Rota Nodari, Daniela Ferrari, Fabrizio Giani and Lidia De Filippis
Department of Biotechnologies and Biosciences, University Milano Bicocca, Milan, Italy

Mario Bossi, Giovanni Tredici and Virginia Rodriguez-Menendez
Department of Neurosciences and Biomedical Technologies, University Milano Bicocca, Milan, Italy

Domenico Delia
Department of Experimental Oncology, Fondazione IRCSS Istituto Nazionale Tumori, Milan, Italy

Angelo Luigi Vescovi
Department of Biotechnologies and Biosciences, University Milano Bicocca, Milan, Italy
IRCCS Casa Sollievo della Sofferenza, Opera di San Pio da Pietralcina, San Giovanni Rotondo, Italy

Xiaogang Guo, Xiuren Gao, Yesong Wang and Longyun Peng
Department of Cardiology, The First Affiliated Hospital of Sun Yat-sen University, Guangzhou, China

Yingying Zhu
Intensive Care Unit, Central Hospital, Tai'an, China

Shenming Wang
Department of Vascular Surgery, The First Affiliated Hospital of Sun Yat-sen University, Guangzhou, China

Jenna L. Ross
Department of Pharmacology, Dalhousie University, Halifax, Nova Scotia, Canada

Susan E. Howlett
Department of Pharmacology, Dalhousie University, Halifax, Nova Scotia, Canada
Division of Geriatric Medicine, Dalhousie University, Halifax, Nova Scotia, Canada

Simon S. F. Cheung, Justin W. C. Leung and Amy K. M. Lam
Department of Anatomy, The University of Hong Kong, Hong Kong, China

Karen S. L. Lam
Department of Medicine, The University of Hong Kong, Hong Kong, China
Research Centre of Heart, Brain, Hormone and Healthy Aging, Li Ka Shing Faculty of Medicine, The University of Hong Kong, Hong Kong, China

Amy C. Y. Lo and Sookja K. Chung
Department of Anatomy, The University of Hong Kong, Hong Kong, China
Research Centre of Heart, Brain, Hormone and Healthy Aging, Li Ka Shing Faculty of Medicine, The University of Hong Kong, Hong Kong, China

Stephen S. M. Chung
Department of Physiology, The University of Hong Kong, Hong Kong, China
Research Centre of Heart, Brain, Hormone and Healthy Aging, Li Ka Shing Faculty of Medicine, The University of Hong Kong, Hong Kong, China

Yong-Hui Xiang, Xin-Jia Han, Ying Xu and Kwok-Fai So
Department of Central Nervous System Regeneration, Guangdong – Hongkong - Macau Institute of CNS Regeneration (GHMICR), Jinan University, Guangzhou, Guangdong, China

An-Ding Xu and Ying Zhao
Department of Neurology, the First Affiliated Hospital, Jinan University, Guangzhou, Guangdong, China

Yi-Wen Ruan
Department of Central Nervous System Regeneration, Guangdong – Hongkong - Macau Institute of CNS Regeneration (GHMICR), Jinan University, Guangzhou, Guangdong, China
Department of Human Anatomy, Jinan University School of Medicine, Guangzhou, Guangdong, China

Bo Yu
Department of Human Anatomy, Medical College, Shanghai University of Traditional Chinese Medicine, Shanghai, China

Michele Hepponstall
Haematology Research, Murdoch Childrens Research Institute; Melbourne, Victoria, Australia
Cardiac Surgery Unit and Cardiology, Royal Children's Hospital; Melbourne, Victoria, Australia
Department of Paediatrics, The University of Melbourne; Melbourne, Victoria, Australia
Bioscience Research Division, Department of Primary Industries, Melbourne, Victoria, Australia

Michael H. H. Cheung and Igor E. Konstantinov
Haematology Research, Murdoch Childrens Research Institute; Melbourne, Victoria, Australia
Cardiac Surgery Unit and Cardiology, Royal Children's Hospital; Melbourne, Victoria, Australia
Department of Paediatrics, The University of Melbourne; Melbourne, Victoria, Australia

Bryn Jones and Yves d'Udekem
Haematology Research, Murdoch Childrens Research Institute; Melbourne, Victoria, Australia
Cardiac Surgery Unit and Cardiology, Royal Children's Hospital; Melbourne, Victoria, Australia

Vera Ignjatovic and Paul Monagle
Haematology Research, Murdoch Childrens Research Institute; Melbourne, Victoria, Australia
Department of Paediatrics, The University of Melbourne; Melbourne, Victoria, Australia

Steve Binos
Bioscience Research Division, Department of Primary Industries, Melbourne, Victoria, Australia

Youshi Fujita, Yoshiki Hase and Ryosuke Takahashi
Department of Neurology, Graduate School of Medicine, Kyoto University, Sakyo-ku, Kyoto, Japan

Masafumi Ihara
Department of Neurology, Graduate School of Medicine, Kyoto University, Sakyo-ku, Kyoto, Japan
Department of Regenerative Medicine and Research, Institute of Biomedical Research and Innovation, Minatojima, Chuo-ku, Kobe, Hyogo, Japan

Shinae Kizaka-Kondoh, Takahiro Kuchimaru and Tetsuya Kadonosono
Department of Biomolecular Engineering, Tokyo Institute of Technology Graduate School of Bioscience and Biotechnology, Nagatsuta-cho, Midori-ku, Yokohama, Japan

Shotaro Tanaka
Department of Biochemistry, School of Medicine, Tokyo Women's Medical University, Tokyo, Japan

Hidekazu Tomimoto
Department of Neurology, Mie University Graduate School of Medicine, Mie, Japan

Masahiro Hiraoka
Department of Radiation Oncology and Image-applied Therapy, Kyoto University Graduate School of Medicine, Shogoin, Sakyo-ku, Kyoto, Japan

Anthony S. Kim, Sharon N. Poisson and J. Donald Easton
Department of Neurology, University of California San Francisco, San Francisco, California, United States of America

S. Claiborne Johnston
Department of Neurology, University of California San Francisco, San Francisco, California, United States of America
Department of Epidemiology and Biostatistics, University of California San Francisco, San Francisco, California, United States of America

Susan Kirkpatrick and Louise Locock
Health Experiences Research Group, Department of Primary Care Health Sciences, University of Oxford, Oxford, United Kingdom

Matthew F. Giles
Stroke Prevention Unit, Nuffield Department of Clinical Neuroscience, University of Oxford, Oxford, United Kingdom

Daniel S. Lasserson
Department of Primary Care Health Sciences, University of Oxford, Oxford, United Kingdom

Frank Bode, Christof Burgdorf, Heribert Schunkert and Volkhard Kurowski
Medical Department II, University of Luebeck, Luebeck, Germany

Pengwei Zhuang, Yanjun Zhang, Guangzhi Cui, Mixia Zhang, Jinbao Zhang,
Yang Liu, Xinpeng Yang, Adejobi Oluwaniyi Isaiah, Yingxue Lin and Yongbo Jiang
Tianjin State Key Laboratory of Modern Chinese Medicine, Key Laboratory of Traditional Chinese

Medicine Pharmacology, Chinese Materia Medica College, Tianjin University of Traditional Chinese Medicine, Tianjin, China

Yuhong Bian
Chinese Medical College, Tianjin University of Traditional Chinese Medicine, Tianjin, China

Sagar Rohailla., Nadia Clarizia., Michel Sourour, Wesam Sourour, Nitai Gelber, Can Wei, Jing Li and Andrew N. Redington
Division of Cardiology, Labatt Family Heart Center, Hospital for Sick Children, University of Toronto, Ontario, Canada

Hongbo Zhang
Department of Pediatrics, First hospital of Jilin University, Changchun, China

Yongxin Luan and Bin Lu
Department of Neurosurgery, First hospital of Jilin University, Changchun, China

Jianmin Liang
Department of Pediatrics, First hospital of Jilin University, Changchun, China
Neuroscience Research Center, First hospital of Jilin University, Changchun, China

Yi-nan Luo and Pengfei Ge
Department of Pediatrics, First hospital of Jilin University, Changchun, China
Department of Neurosurgery, First hospital of Jilin University, Changchun, China
Neuroscience Research Center, First hospital of Jilin University, Changchun, China

Nienke van Rein
Department of Thrombosis and Hemostasis, Leiden University Medical Center, Leiden, The Netherlands
Einthoven Laboratory of Experimental Vascular Medicine, Leiden University Medical Center, Leiden, The Netherlands

Frederikus A. Klok, Menno V. Huisman, Bas Spaans, Koen A. J. van Beers, Judith Kooiman, Jonna R. Bank and Wilke R. van de Peppel
Department of Thrombosis and Hemostasis, Leiden University Medical Center, Leiden, The Netherlands

Antonio Iglesias del Sol
Department of Internal Medicine, Rijnland Hospital, Leiderdorp, The Netherlands

Suzanne C. Cannegieter
Department of Clinical Epidemiology, Leiden University Medical Center, Leiden, The Netherlands

Ton J. Rabelink
Department of Nephrology, Leiden University Medical Center, Leiden, The Netherlands

Gregory Y. H. Lip
Haemostasis, Thrombosis, and Vascular Biology Unit, University of Birmingham Centre for Cardiovascular Sciences, City Hospital, Birmingham, United Kingdom

Michael A. McDonald, Juarez R. Braga and Heather J. Ross
Division of Cardiology, Peter Munk Cardiac Centre, University of Toronto, Toronto, Canada

Andrew N. Redington, Jing Li and Cedric Manlhiot
Division of Cardiology, Hospital for Sick Children, University of Toronto, Toronto, Canada

Agnes Dechartres and Philippe Ravaud
UMR-S 738, INSERM, Paris, France
UMR-S 738, Université Paris Diderot, Paris, France
Université Paris Descartes, Paris, France
Centre d'Epidémiologie Clinique, Hôpital Hôtel-Dieu, APHP, Paris, France

Florence Tubach
UMR-S 738, INSERM, Paris, France
UMR-S 738, Université Paris Diderot, Paris, France
Université Paris Diderot, Paris, France
CIE 801, INSERM, Paris, France
Département d'Epidémiologie, Biostatistique et Recherche Clinique, Hôpital Bichat-Claude Bernard, APHP, Paris, France

Pierre Albaladejo
Pôe d'Anesthésie et de Réanimation, Centre Hospitalier Universitaire, Grenoble, France
Université Joseph Fourier, Grenoble, France

Jean Mantz
Service d'anesthésie réanimation et SMUR, Hôpital Beaujon, APHP, Clichy, France
Université Paris Diderot, Paris, France

Charles Marc Samama
Université Paris Descartes, Paris, France
Service d'anesthésie réanimation, Hôpital Hôtel-Dieu, APHP, Paris, France

Jean-Philippe Collet
Service de cardiologie, Hôpital Pitié-Salpé triére, APHP, Paris, France
Université Pierre et Marie Curie, France

Philippe Gabriel Steg
Université Paris Diderot, Paris, France
INSERM U-698, Paris, France
Service de cardiologie, Hôpital Bichat-Claude Bernard, APHP, Paris, France

Bryan Haines
The Buck Institute for Research on Aging, Novato, California, United States of America

P. Andy Li
Department of Pharmaceutical Sciences, Biomanufacturing Research Institute and Technological Enterprise (BRITE), North Carolina Central University, Durham, North Carolina, United States of America

Yi Ma, Joshua N. Edwards, Bradley S. Launikonis and Chen Chen
School of Biomedical Sciences, University of Queensland, Brisbane, Queensland, Australia

Lin Zhang
School of Biological Sciences, University of Auckland, Auckland, New Zealand

Whitley Ledkins
Chemical and Biomolecular Engineering, University of South Alabama, Mobile, Alabama, United States of America

Silas J. Leavesley
Chemical and Biomolecular Engineering, University of South Alabama, Mobile, Alabama, United States of America
Pharmacology, University of South Alabama, Mobile, Alabama, United States of America
Center for Lung Biology, University of South Alabama, Mobile, Alabama, United States of America

Petra Rocic
Pharmacology, New York Medical College, Valhalla, New York, United States of America

Yi Luo and Jiapei Dai
Wuhan Institute for Neuroscience and Neuroengineering, South-Central University for Nationalities, Wuhan, China

Qinan Zhang
Wuhan Institute for Neuroscience and Neuroengineering, South-Central University for Nationalities, Wuhan, China
Department of Anatomy, Medical College of Zhengzhou University, Zhengzhou, China

Teng Gao and Xijuan Chen
Department of Anatomy, Medical College of Zhengzhou University, Zhengzhou, China

Xiaoqun Gao
Department of Anatomy, Medical College of Zhengzhou University, Zhengzhou, China
Brain Paralysis Research Center, Medical College of Zhengzhou University, Zhengzhou, China

Ge Gao
Brain Paralysis Research Center, Medical College of Zhengzhou University, Zhengzhou, China

Yiwu Zhou
Department of Forensic Medicine, Tongji Medical College of Huazhong University of Science & Technology, Wuhan, China

Sandra Blivet, Daniel Cobarzan, Mostafa El Hajjam, Pascal Lacombe and Thierry Chinet
Aphp, Université De Versailles Saint Quentin En Yvelines, Consultation Pluridisciplinaire Maladie De Rendu-Osler, Hôpital Ambroise Paré, Boulogne, France

Alain Beauchet
Aphp, Université De Versailles Saint Quentin En Yvelines, Département De Santé Publique, Hôpital Ambroise Paré, Boulogne, France

Monique C. Saleh, Barry J. Connell and Tarek M. Saleh
Department of Biomedical Sciences, Atlantic Veterinary College, University of Prince Edward Island, Charlottetown, P.E.I., Canada

Alaa S. Abd-El-Aziz and Inan Kucukkaya
Department of Chemistry, University of Prince Edward Island, Charlottetown, P.E.I., Canada

Bobby V. Khan
Department of Biomedical Sciences, Atlantic Veterinary College, University of Prince Edward Island, Charlottetown, P.E.I., Canada
Carmel BioSciences Inc., Atlanta, Georgia, United States of America

Desikan Rajagopal
Carmel BioSciences Inc., Atlanta, Georgia, United States of America

Index

CPSIA information can be obtained
at www.ICGtesting.com
Printed in the USA
BVHW02*0448020218
506942BV00003B/30/P